Handbook of
Human Genetic Linkage

Umadevi Tundonvahi
June 1994
W & I Hospital
Brown University

Handbook of
Human Genetic Linkage

JOSEPH DOUGLAS TERWILLIGER
Department of Genetics and Development

and

JURG OTT
Department of Genetics and Development and Department of Psychiatry

Columbia University
New York, New York

The Johns Hopkins University Press
Baltimore and London

The authors would like to acknowledge the assistance of Dr. Marcy Speer, Patrick J. Gambino, Yin Yao Shugart, and Dr. Pentti Tienari for their critical comments and assistance in the preparation of this document.

The Johns Hopkins University Press
2715 North Charles Street
Baltimore, Maryland 21218-4319
The Johns Hopkins Press Ltd., London

Library of Congress Cataloging-in-Publication Data

Terwilliger, Joseph Douglas.
   Handbook of human genetic linkage / Joseph Douglas Terwilliger and Jurg Ott.
      p. cm.
   Companion vol. to: Analysis of human genetic linkage / Jurg Ott.
   Includes bibliographical references and index.
   ISBN 0-8018-4803-2 (pbk. : acid-free paper)
   1. Linkage (Genetics)—Data processing. 2. Linkage (Genetics)—Computer programs. 3. Human genetics—Data processing.
   4. Human genetics—Computer programs. I. Ott, Jurg. II. Title.
QH445.2.T47 1994
573.2'13—dc20   93-6460
                                            CIP

A catalog record for this book is available from the British Library

Contents

1. □

Background Material

1.1 The Purpose of This Book

This is a practical guide to human linkage analysis, with emphasis on the use of various computer programs. Little theoretical background will be provided. For theoretical and methodological background and references, we refer the reader to Ott (1991), with which this book may be used as a companion. Because this is predominantly a technical how-to book, we do not want to cite sources already referenced in the companion book except for those on major issues and new sources.

Much of this book consists of detailed instructions on how to carry out linkage analyses presented in such a way that novices will be able to complete them successfully. The book is intended to be used for self-instruction or as a manual in linkage courses. Most exercises employ the LINKAGE programs version 5.1, though brief discussions of other programs are given (version 5.2 is very similar to version 5.1). All exercises in this book are written for execution on a personal computer (IBM PC–compatible computers) under the MS-DOS (Microsoft) operating system (or in a DOS window under IBM's OS/2). Some ILINK results may differ slightly from one machine to another. For example, in this book, ILINK analyses were done on a VAX to illustrate some minor differences between implementations.

To carry out the exercises described in the subsequent chapters on a PC, you need to enter data into a computer file with the aid of a text editor or word-processing program. You may use Microsoft Word or WordPerfect by WordPerfect Corporation for that purpose, but make sure that the files you create are in ASCII or "text" file format. To test whether a file is in ASCII or in a word processor's own format, type it out on the screen, that is, issue the DOS command *TYPE FNAME,* where FNAME is the name of your data file. If it looks like normal text on the screen, then it is in ASCII format; otherwise you will see strange symbols or the lines will not start at the left margin. Useful text editors are the MS-DOS editor, which comes with MS-DOS version 5.0, or PC-WRITE, which is a shareware product.

1.2 Notation and Definitions

We sometimes use mathematical notation, which may not be familiar to all readers.

Intervals are indicated with parentheses or brackets, depending on whether the endpoints do or do not belong to the interval. $[a,b]$ defines an interval between the values a and b, both values inclusive (closed interval), whereas (a,b) denotes an interval excluding the endpoints a and b (open interval).

That x belongs to a certain set of values or to an interval is indicated by $\in$, which stands for "member of" or "element of." For example, $x \in [a,b)$ is equivalent to $a \leq x < b$.

Binomial coefficients are written in the usual manner as

$$\binom{n}{k}$$

(pronounced n choose k), where

$$\binom{n}{k} = \frac{n!}{[k!(n-k)!]}$$

with $n!$ (n factorial) being defined as

$$n \times (n-1) \times (n-2) \times \cdots \times 2 \times 1$$

A vertical bar, $|$, can have more than one meaning. In probability statements, it indicates a condition. For example, $P(X|Y)$ is short for "the conditional probability that X occurs given that Y occurs or is true." For sets of parameter values, the same symbol indicates a restriction on the range of values considered. For example, $\{\theta \mid 0.02 < \theta < 0.15\}$ reads "values of θ such that theta is between 0.02 and 0.15."

1.3 A Review of the Principles of Linkage Analysis

In this section, we give a brief summary of human genetic linkage analysis: what it is, and how it works. There are two different aspects a linkage analysis: testing and estimation. These two ideas are compared and contrasted, and we delineate when and how to use each of these aspects.

1.3.1 A Basic Introduction to Human Genetics

Human beings, like all other mammals, reproduce sexually. A man's sperm cell infiltrates and fertilizes a woman's egg cell, with the resulting zygote containing a complete and unique set of genetic information defining many of the biological characteristics of the newly developing human being. This genetic information is stored in coded form within molecules of deoxyribonucleic acid (DNA). DNA is composed of a linear arrangement of smaller molecules, known as nucleotides, whose sequence forms a code that contains information defining the structure of various protein molecules to be synthesized by the cell, the regulation of the production of these molecules, and a great many other functions, the entirety of which define much of what a person will become. Although the major function of DNA is the encoding of the structure of various protein molecules, only a small fraction of the total DNA in any cell is actually involved in this process. Those sections of the DNA that are responsible for coding protein structures are called *genes*. They are inherited according to the mendelian laws. In general, any piece of DNA (or of a chromosome, such as a secondary restriction) inherited in a mendelian manner is called a *locus*; thus genes are a particular type of loci.

In humans, this linear string of DNA, containing both genes and noncoding sequences, is divided into 23 segments called *chromosomes*. Further, each child receives one copy of each chromosome from its mother and one from its father, for a total of 46 chromosomes, comprising 22 pairs of *autosomes* and one pair of *sex chromosomes*. The sex chromosomes come in variants X and Y and are involved in the determination of the sex of an individual: all men have one X chromosome and one Y chromosome (XY), and all women have two X chromosomes (XX).

As stated above, each offspring has two copies of each chromosome (except that the sex chromosomes in males are X and Y), one derived from each of the parents, and transmits one copy of each chromosome to his or her offspring. Each chromosome segregates independently, meaning, for example, if a mother transmits her maternally derived copy of chromosome 1 to an offspring, she still has an equal chance of transmitting her paternally or maternally derived copy of chromosome 2, etc. This division of the DNA into independently segregating chromosomes allows for an increase in diversity of the population, as opposed to forcing each individual to receive half of his DNA from each of two of his four grandparents (i.e., one entire genome as opposed to 23 separate chromosomal entities). However, nature has a way of increasing the diversity of the species even further through a process known as recombination.

1.3.2 Recombination

Every human produces germ cells (sperm or egg), containing one copy of each chromosome (*haploid* chromosome set). When a sperm fertilizes an egg, the two haploid chromosome sets are combined, making a new zygote containing two copies of each chromosome (*diploid* chromosome set). This diploid cell then develops into a new human, whose every cell contains an identical full diploid set of chromosomes. However, because each cell contains two identical copies of each chromosome, these obvious questions arise: Where do these haploid germ cells come from? and How is it determined which copy they will receive of each chromosome? The answers are found in the complicated process called *meiosis*. Refer to a genetics textbook, such as Ayala and Kiger (1984) for a detailed description of meiosis. In summary, when a germ cell is formed, the two *homologous* copies of each chromosome pair up, each member of which goes into one or the other daughter cell (which may eventually become gametes). In this distribution of homologous chromosomes, the selection of either the paternally or maternally derived chromosome of each pair in a specific daughter cell is random. Consequently, a gamete contains some chromosomes from the father and some chromosomes from the mother of the individual producing the gamete.

There is, however, one additional source of variation, which is the main focus of our study. When the pairs of homologous chromosomes line up side by side, they undergo a process called *crossing over*, which results in what is referred to as *recombination*. In recombination, portions of the maternal homolog recombine with the paternal homolog to form a hybrid chromosome in the place of the original ones. Let us assume we have chromosomes MMMMMMMMM and PPPPPPPPP lined up beside each other, in which

M stands for a maternally derived gene and P for a paternal gene. They could recombine in such a way that a crossover takes place between genes 2 and 3 and another one occurs between genes 6 and 7. The two resulting chromosomes would then be represented by MMPPPPPMMM and PPMMMMMPPP. For a more detailed description of recombination involving four chromosome strands, see Ott (1991).

Recombination occurs frequently, and it appears that at least one chiasma must occur on each chromosomal arm (or chromosome) in each meiosis (Sturt, 1976). Small acrocentric chromosomes typically show few crossovers, with larger chromosomes experiencing multiple crossover events. The entire basis of linkage analysis is that recombination events occur between two genetic loci (genes, DNA markers, chromosomal aberrations, etc.) at a rate related to the distance between them on the same chromosome. In other words, loci that are physically very close to each other tend to be inherited together more often than not. The goal of linkage analysis is to determine whether two loci tend to cosegregate more often than they should if they were not physically close together on the same chromosome.

1.3.3 Linkage Analysis

We discussed how each individual carries two copies of each chromosome, one derived from each parent. Each of the two chromosomes may carry different variations of the DNA sequence at a given locus. These variations are then referred to as *alleles* (some people use the term *gene* instead of *allele*). Traditionally, the term *allele* has referred to the variant forms of a protein-encoding gene that typically had different phenotypic expressions, such as the *A, B,* and *O* alleles of the ABO blood group locus. However, with the advent of DNA polymorphisms that are inherited in a mendelian form, the term *allele* has been expanded to include any mendelianly inherited variation in the DNA sequence at a given locus.

The two homologous chromosomes segregate independently; an allele at one locus on one chromosome, therefore, segregates together with a given allele at another locus on another chromosome with 50% probability. Alleles at loci on the same chromosome should cosegregate at a rate that is somehow related to the distance between them on the chromosome. This rate is the probability, or *recombination fraction* (hereafter denoted by θ), of a recombination event occurring between the two loci. Multiple recombination events can occur on the same chromosome. If in a gamete two loci have experienced two crossovers between them, then the final result shows a *nonrecombination* between the two loci (for example, the first and last loci on chromosome MMPPPPPMMM considered above).

The recombination fraction ranges from $\theta = 0$ for loci right next to each other through $\theta = \frac{1}{2}$ for loci far apart (or on different chromosomes), so that it can be taken as a measure of the *genetic distance,* or *map distance,* between gene loci. This measure works well for small distances. The unit of measurement is 1 map unit = 1 centimorgan (cM), corresponding approximately to a recombination fraction of 1%. However, because of the occurrence of multiple crossovers, the recombination fraction is not an additive distance measure and must therefore be transformed by a *map function* into the map distance. For example, the Haldane map function turns $\theta = 0.27$ (27%) into 39 cM, and the Kosambi map function translates $\theta = 0.27$ into 0.30 Morgans (30 cM, see Ott (1991), or Liberman and Karlin (1984), for more information).

Two loci are said to be genetically *linked* when $\theta < \frac{1}{2}$, and the phenomenon describing this occurrence is *genetic linkage*. The object of *linkage analysis* is to estimate θ and to test if θ is less than $\frac{1}{2}$; that is, whether an observed deviation from 50% recombination is statistically significant. The estimate of the recombination fraction, usually denoted by $\hat{\theta}$, is in simple cases the proportion of recombinants (proportion of children carrying a recombinant gamete) out of all opportunities for recombination and ranges in principle between 0 and 1. Because maximum likelihood estimates are defined on the set of admissible parameter values and the recombination fraction cannot exceed $\frac{1}{2}$ (unless there is chromatid interference), its estimate is usually also restricted to $[0, \frac{1}{2}]$.

Notice that the term *linkage* refers to *loci,* not to specific alleles at these loci. For example, it is wrong to say that, in a given pedigree, the disease gene is linked with the *A* allele at the marker locus. In a child, alleles at different loci are said to be *in coupling* (as opposed to being *in repulsion*) when they originated from the same parent. Furthermore, two loci residing on the same chromosome are said to be *syntenic*; they may or may not be linked.

A rudimentary test of linkage between two loci could be set up by comparing, in a chi-square test, an observed number *k* of recombinations and $n - k$ of nonrecombinations with their expected numbers of $n/2$ each under no linkage. The main problem with this, however, is that in most human pedigree data, it is not possible to count recombinants and nonrecombinants. For this reason, researchers usually use likelihood-based methods in linkage analysis. Using sophisticated analysis programs, such as LINKAGE, it is possible to evaluate the likelihood of a given pedigree under different assumptions about the recombination fraction between two loci. Furthermore, the Neymann-Pearson lemma tells us that if there is a best test of a given hypothesis, it takes the form of a likelihood ratio test. This lemma provides a good theoretical basis for using the likelihood ratio test as our test of choice. In linkage analysis, our likelihood ratio is formed as $L(\theta)/L(\theta = 0.5)$, with the denominator corresponding to the likelihood of our data under the assumption of no linkage. Likelihoods will be discussed in more detail in the exercises to follow.

In linkage analysis, the test is typically formulated in terms of the common (base 10) logarithm of this ratio, or *lod score*. The formula for the lod score is

$$Z(\theta) = \log_{10}\frac{L(\theta)}{L(0.5)}$$

or equivalently

$$Z(\theta) = \log_{10}[L(\theta)] - \log_{10}[L(\theta = 0.5)]$$

These log likelihoods are then calculated via one of the many available linkage analysis programs. The emphasis of this book is using the LINKAGE program package to compute these lod scores in practical situations. In some simple cases, the likelihoods can be evaluated by hand, as you will see later, but in the majority of family data, hand evaluation is either impractical or impossible. This is true especially when a disease with a complicated mode of inheritance is one of our loci.

The most common application of linkage analysis is to try and find the location, in the genome, of a gene responsible for a certain mendelianly inherited disease. In these situations, we often have complicated modes of inheritance, in which we are not certain which individual has which alleles at the disease locus. Consider, for example, the occurrence of a dominant disease. Assuming that *D* represents the dominant disease-causing allele, and + represents the normal or "wild type" allele, we must define the genotype–phenotype relationships or *penetrances*. In this case, we know that unaffected individuals have genotype +/+ and that affected individuals have either genotype D/+ or D/D; however, we cannot discern one from the other phenotypically. The computer programs calculate accurate likelihoods, allowing for both possibilities for each affected individual. As you will see in the course of this book, likelihoods can be computed for these, as well as much more complicated penetrance models. The important thing for our purposes now, is to understand how these likelihoods can then be converted to lod scores and what these lod scores tell us.

1.3.4 Testing

Two basic aspects of linkage analysis can be performed using lod scores. The first is a test of linkage. In other words, do our data provide us with sufficient information to say that we have found linkage between our two genes? Because we usually have marker loci with known genetic location and a disease for which we want to find the genetic cause, we can rephrase this test as "Is there evidence for linkage between our disease gene and our marker locus?" We have already defined a test statistic, the lod score (typically denoted as $Z(\theta)$), but we have not yet decided how to apply this test. In other words, for which critical region does our test statistic provide sufficient evidence to conclude that there is linkage with our disease gene? By convention, a critical value of 3 is accepted as significant evidence of linkage. A theoretical examination of this cutoff point (see Ott, 1991) ensures that in only 1 in 20 times is a lod score of 3 spurious for mendelian disorders. This is therefore taken as the minimum acceptable level for a significant test with a simple autosomal disease. Similarly, for diseases known from segregation analysis to be on the X chromosome, a lod score of 2 is considered to represent a significant linkage finding because the prior probability of linkage is much higher than for an autosomal disease. For complex diseases, however, this lod score threshold of 3 may be too low, but we defer further discussion of this until Chapter 25.

The lod score test is usually performed by maximizing the lod score over all values of θ on the interval [0, 0.5]. If the maximum of this lod score curve exceeds 3, the test of linkage is significant, and the location of our disease has likely been found. If we are doing a genomic screen, however, what should we do when we find a lod score that is not significant yet is still quite large, since typically not all potentially available families are analyzed in the early stages of a linkage analysis? In general, if a lod score of around 2 is found, it may be advisable to type additional families for that marker or to look for other markers in the vicinity of that one. If on typing more individuals, the lod score drops, it was most likely spurious. The lod score may also rise, however, exceeding the threshold of 3, in which case you may have found a significant linkage.

1.3.5 Estimation

After significant evidence for linkage of the disease to a given marker has been found, the next step is to determine the exact location of this gene, to make it easier to isolate, and eventually, easier to study the gene itself. We have already explained that a monotonic relationship exists between the recombination fraction and physical distance on the chromosome, so if we can determine the recombination fraction between the disease and marker, we will have some idea where to look for the gene itself. If you remember, the lod score test was based on the maximum of the lod score, maximized over θ. We know that the maximum of the likelihood function occurs at the same point as the maximum of the log of the likelihood function, so the value of θ at which our lod score is maximized is an estimate of the recombination fraction between disease and marker. This is referred to as the *maximum likelihood estimate* (MLE) of θ, and is denoted by $\hat{\theta}$.

Standard likelihood theory tells us that we can obtain a consistent estimate of any parameter given a set of data (*and* the correct model), by maximizing the likelihood of the data with respect to that parameter; that is, in the limit of a large number of observations, the MLE is unbiased with a variance tending toward zero. For finite data sets, however, MLEs in human genetics are generally biased. In the presence of modelling or diagnostic or marker-typing errors, MLEs may be inconsistent (asymptotically biased).

In addition to point estimates discussed above, we can also obtain interval estimates. Two types of intervals are discussed below: confidence intervals and support intervals.

Confidence intervals for a parameter, such as the recombination fraction or a gene frequency, are intimately connected with statistical tests about the parameter in question. On the basis of a set of observations, we can test the null hypothesis, $H_0 : p = p_0$, that is, whether the parameter estimate is significantly different from an assumed parameter value p_0. The test may be carried out for a multitude of parameter values p_0. The set of all those parameter values p_0 for which the test is not significant constitutes the confidence interval for p. Therefore, a significant test result for some value p_t implies that p_t is outside the confidence interval for p, and vice versa.

A *support interval* is, in principle, quite a different construct. It is based on the *support* (a synonym for $\log_e$ likelihood) for a parameter provided by a set of observations. The m-unit support interval (Edwards, 1992) consists of all those parameter points with associated $\log_e$ likelihood within m units of the maximum $\log_e$ likelihood; the parameter values inside a support interval are considered "plausible" because their support is only m units lower than that of the best supported parameter value. Examples of how to compute confidence and support intervals are given in Appendix A (BINOM program). In human genetics, support is also used to mean $\log_{10}$ likelihood. For example, we speak of 1-lod-unit or 3-lod-unit support intervals.

There is a connection between confidence and support intervals. Consider a regular test situation in which you want to test the null hypothesis that a parameter p has a certain value p_0. You do this by obtaining a maximum likelihood estimate $\hat{p}$ and want to contrast $\hat{p}$ versus p_0. Under the null hypothesis, the test statistic $\chi^2 = 2 \ln[L(\hat{p})/L(p_0)]$, follows an asymptotic chi-square distribution with 1 degree of freedom (df), where $L(p)$ denotes the likelihood at the value p. In this situation, a 2-unit support interval may be interpreted as an approximate 95% confidence interval for p, and a 3.32-unit support interval as an approximate 99% confidence interval.

The previous discussion is relevant to the test of the null hypothesis of no linkage ($H_0 : \theta = 0.5$) versus linkage ($H_1 : \theta < 0.5$). As is well-known, the test is declared significant when $Z_{max} \geq 3$. True to the intimate relation between statistical tests and confidence intervals, a confidence interval should contain those values θ_0 for which the test of $H_0 : \theta = \theta_0$ is not significant. In linkage analysis, we construct support intervals rather than confidence intervals but also expect a meaningful relationship between support interval and test result. Consequently, the support interval associated with the test criterion $Z_{max} \geq 3$ must be a 3-lod-unit support interval. The earlier recommendation (Conneally et al., 1985) of testing with $Z_{max} \geq 3$ but constructing 1-lod-unit support intervals leads to an inconsistency between the statistical test and the support interval when $1 < Z_{max} < 3$. Therefore, that recommendation also states that no support interval should be constructed when $Z_{max} < 3$. We feel that this solution to the problem is unsatisfactory and that the test for linkage and its associated support interval should be consistent. We therefore recommend the use of 3-lod-unit support intervals. The exercises in this book adhere to this rule.

We realize that support interval and confidence interval are constructs belonging to different schools of thought (a likelihood approach versus a statistical testing approach); each has its own merits. We hope that our way of intertwining these two constructs is not offensive to representatives of either school.

1.4 Installing the LINKAGE Programs

We assume here that you obtained the PC version of the LINKAGE programs on diskette from us at Columbia University. If this is not the case you may skip this section. For the installation described below we assume that you are using diskette drive A. If you are planning to install from drive B replace all references to A: with B: in the description given below.

Installation is to a hard disk. Please prepare an appropriate directory (e.g., \LINKAGE) on the hard disk and make that your default directory. For example, if you want to install to the C drive, type

```
C:
MD  \LINKAGE
CD  \LINKAGE
```

You are now in the \LINKAGE directory of the C disk drive. Proceed by copying the contents of each disk to your current directory. For example, assume that you received disk GEN. Then, type the commands

```
COPY  A:*.*
COPY  A:GEN
```

(depending on the size of your diskettes, you may have to change disks between the two commands). After the files from all disks have been transferred, simply type Pk unzip *.zip, which decompresses the program files.

Before you can use the programs, note that the CONFIG.SYS file (in the root directory of the boot drive) must contain the following two lines:

```
FILES = 20
DEVICE = ANSI.SYS
```

The second line above assumes that the ANSI.SYS file is in the root directory. Alternatively, it may reside in the DOS directory in which case that line should read

```
DEVICE =  \DOS\ANSI.SYS
```

The ANSI.SYS driver is necessary only when you want to use the LCP and LRP programs. Be sure to reboot the computer after modifying the CONFIG.SYS file, or else the changes will not take effect. The number given after

FILES = is a minimum; you may specify, for example, FILES = 25 if that is required by another of your programs.

It is generally best to have your input data in different directories from the one containing the LINKAGE programs. For example, the data files for a particular problem may be in the \DISEASEX directory and the LINKAGE programs are in the \LINKAGE directory on the C drive. Make sure that the LINKAGE directory is accessed by DOS, for example, by inserting the following line in your AUTOEXEC.BAT file in the root directory:

```
SET PATH = C:\LINKAGE;%PATH%
```

If, in the use of the LINKAGE programs, you find what appears to be a program error, please let us know so we can alert other users and eliminate the bug.

PART I

Two-point Linkage Analysis

2. □

The File System Used by LINKAGE

In this introductory chapter, we examine the basic file structure of the LINKAGE programs (version 5.1). Topics covered include the basics of how to enter pedigree data in preparation for doing a linkage analysis. A schematic view of how files and programs interact is shown in Figure 2–1.

2.1 Pedigree Drawings

First, we assume the pedigree structure and data shown in Figure 2–2. For those of you not familiar with this type of diagram, circles refer to females, and squares refer to males, circles and squares filled in represent individuals affected with the disease in question, and those who are open represent unaffected persons. In addition, marker data are given under each individual. In this example, one marker locus is indicated.

2.2 Pedigree Files

The first thing you must do is to create a pedigree file with your word processor, in which you describe the pedigree to be analyzed. In such a file, you must enter one line per individual, containing the following information:

Column 1 : Pedigree identifier   ⎰ The identifier can be a number
Column 2 : Individual's ID   ⎱ or a character string.

Column 3 : The individual's father ⎰ If the person is a founder, just put a
Column 4 : The individual's mother ⎱ 0 in each column.

Column 5 : Sex   ⎰ *1* = Male, *2* = Female
Column 6+ : Genetic data   ⎱ Disease and marker phenotypes

In this case, our first genetic locus is the disease, which is coded as an *affection status* type of locus. (In the LINKAGE programs, there are four different ways of entering the phenotypic data, called *locus types*. Their usage

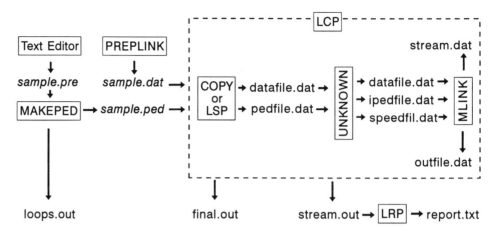

Figure 2–1. Schematic view of how files and programs interact

will be explained in more detail later.) You should then enter the phenotypic data by entering a *2* if the individual is affected, a *1* if unaffected, and a *0* if the person's affection status is unknown. In this case, the second genetic locus is our marker, which we code as an *allele numbers* type of locus. This is the most straightforward way of entering codominant marker information. To do this, you must enter the allele number corresponding to each of the two alleles, separated by at least one space. The most important thing to remember about this type of locus is that you must number your alleles with integers starting from *1*. For example, if you have a two-allele locus with alleles *3.6,* and *5.2,* you must renumber them as *1* and *2* to enter them in your pedigree file as an allele numbers type of locus. If an individual has not been typed, and the marker phenotype is unknown, you must enter *0* for each allele (e.g., phenotype = *0 0*). Note that an individual cannot have one allele known and the other unknown in this type of locus. They must be either both known or both unknown! A clever way of avoiding this problem in simple situations will be dealt with in Chapter 10.

For example, let us enter the pedigree data for the pedigree shown in Figure 2–2, in a file called EX1.PRE. We assign the pedigree the name *ex1,* and give the pedigree members the names *father, mother, dau1, dau2, son1, dau3,* and *son2,* where *dau* represents daughter. If you use PC-WRITE as your text editor, you type *ED EX1.PRE* to which the editor responds by displaying on

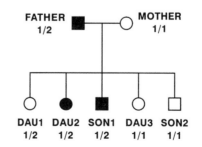

Figure 2–2. Pedigree drawing for EX1.PRE

the top line, *File not found. . . .* Press the ⟨F9⟩ key to create the EX1.PRE file and to prepare the editor for data entry. If you use the MS-DOS editor, simply type *EDIT EX1.PRE* and you are ready for data entry.

To enter the father, we first input the pedigree name *ex1,* followed by a space, and in the next column, type *father,* the individual's name (or ID number). Because he is a founder (i.e. his parents are unknown), we enter zeroes in the next two columns. (*Note:* Either both parents must be unknown, or both known. If one parent is known, but the other is unknown, you must add a "dummy" parent with unknown phenotypes corresponding to the unknown parent). Next, you enter a *1* for his sex (*1* = male, *2* = female). The father is affected, so you type a *2* in the affection status column, and then at the marker he has alleles 1 and 2, so you enter *1* and *2* in the next two columns, followed by ⟨Enter⟩. The line in your pedigree file for this individual should look like the following:

ex1 father 0 0 1 2 1 2

The number of spaces between fields doesn't matter, but making the spacings of different lengths will help you recognize alleles belonging to the same locus. Now, enter the rest of the pedigree on your own. *Caution:* Be certain that your word-processing program produces an ASCII file, with the file ending immediately after the last line. *NO blank lines are permitted at the end nor blank spaces on the line following the last individual.* It is prudent to always insert an end of file mark ([EOF], ASCII no. 26) at the beginning of the line immediately following the last individual.

```
ex1    father  0       0       1  2  1  2
ex1    mother  0       0       2  1  1  1
ex1    dau1    father  mother  2  1  1  2
ex1    dau2    father  mother  2  2  1  2
ex1    son1    father  mother  1  2  1  2
ex1    dau3    father  mother  2  1  1  1
ex1    son2    father  mother  1  1  1  1
[EOF]
```

2.3 MAKEPED

Save this pedigree file as *EX1.PRE* (if you are using PC-WRITE, the file name was specified at the beginning). Next, you need to process this pedigree file with the MAKEPED program, which adds several pointers required by the LINKAGE programs. To do this, type the following at the DOS prompt.

MAKEPED infile outfile n

where *infile* is the name of the pedigree file without pointers (*EX1.PRE* in this case) and *outfile* is the name of the file to be created by MAKEPED (*EX1.PED* in this case). A good general convention is to use the extension .PRE to refer to a pedigree file before it is processed by MAKEPED and to use the extension .PED afterwards. The letter *n* on the command line is optional and tells the program that no loops are present and all probands are to be selected automatically (see below); with *n* as the third parameter on the command line, MAKEPED runs without querying the user as outlined below.

If no *n* is given, the program then asks

```
Does your pedigree file contain any loops? (y/n) ->
```

to which you respond *n*, because there were neither consanguinity nor marriage loops in this simple pedigree. We will discuss how to handle loops in a subsequent exercise. Next, the program asks

```
Do you want probands selected automatically? (y/n) ->
```

In this case, you would enter "*y*," because we are not calculating genetic risks. The MAKEPED program now runs for a few seconds (Actually, the program runs an additional separate program called LOOPS, which checks for undeclared loops, which we will discuss later.) and produces a pedigree file EX1.PED that is readable by the LINKAGE programs. Look at the file in your word processor and notice that all ID numbers are now integers, and not characters any more, and that there are several extra columns. The meanings of each column are as follows:

Column 1: Pedigree number
Column 2: Individual ID number
Column 3: ID of father
Column 4: ID of mother
Column 5: First offspring ID
Column 6: Next paternal sibling ID
Column 7: Next maternal sibling ID
Column 8: Sex (*1* = male, *2* = female. Unknown sex not permitted)
Column 9: Proband status (*1* = proband, higher numbers indicate doubled individuals formed in breaking loops. All other individuals have a *0* in this field.)
Cols 10+: Disease and marker phenotypes (as in the original pedigree file.)

Also, at the end of each line, the program gives the original pedigree names and individual names from your pedigree file, so you can still identify which individual in the processed file corresponds to which person in the *.PRE file. However, to be safe, it is always better to make any future modifications to the pedigree data in the *.PRE file and then rerun MAKEPED.

2.4 Parameter Files (PREPLINK)

You've specified the pedigree to be analyzed; now it is necessary to generate a parameter file, in which you define the model parameters for each locus in the pedigree file, and other parameters required for the analysis. To create this file, use the PREPLINK program. Just type *PREPLINK* at the DOS prompt to begin running this program. The screen should appear similar to the following:

```
******************PRESENT STATUS******************
(a) Number of Loci              : 2
(b) Sex-Linked                  : N
(c) Calculate Risk              : N
(d) Mutation                    : N
(e) Haplotype Frequencies       : N
(f) Locus Order                 : 1 2
(g) Interference                : N
```

```
(h) Recombination Sex Difference    : N
(i) Program Used                     : MLINK
(j) Recombination Values             :
                 0.100


*********************OTHER OPTIONS*********************
(k) See or Modify Loci Description
(l) See or Modify Recombination to Vary
(m) Read Datafile
(n) Write Datafile
(o) Exit
*************************************************************
enter letter to see or modify values
```

Now, we need to make the specifications in this program match our desired analysis. To begin with, we should check the first line *(a) Number of Loci,* which is currently given a value of 2 by default. Because this value is correct for our analysis, we needn't change it. The second line, *(b) Sex-Linked,* is used to tell the program whether we are using autosomal markers or X-linked ones. Currently, the default value is *N,* meaning the disease and markers are autosomal, so we needn't alter this. Next, we come to the option *(c) Calculate Risk.* If we want to compute genetic risks, we select this option to specify the risk locus and allele. Similarly, option *(d) Mutation* allows us to specify one locus at which mutations can occur. There is, however, the additional restriction that mutation can only occur to one specific allele. Hence, it is primarily useful for disease loci, with normal alleles being mutated into disease alleles with a specific frequency. For our purposes, however, we assume the absence of mutation, so we can ignore this option, which by default is set to *No.* Option *(e) Haplotype Frequencies* is also set to *No* by default, because by default, the programs assume linkage equilibrium and compute haplotype frequencies from gene frequencies at each locus. If we want to incorporate linkage disequilibrium data into the analysis, it is imperative to specify haplotype frequencies for all possible haplotypes with this option. We assume linkage equilibrium, so we can leave this set at the default as well. The locus order can be input here as well, but because we have only two loci, the order is immaterial, so we should leave it at the default setting, *1 2. (g) Interference* has only been incorporated in a very rudimentary fashion, as you will see in later chapters. For now, just ignore this option, and leave it set to *no,* because it is unavailable for general use. Option *(h) Recombination Sex Difference* can be very important, because in general there are different rates of recombination in male and female meioses. This option is discussed in detail in Part II; for now we assume there is *None.* Option *(i) Program Used* allows you to choose the program with which to perform the analysis. We stick with the default program MLINK and defer further discussion of this until later. Similarly, the *(j) Recombination Values* option allows you to set the recombination fraction at which to compute lod scores. In general, it is not necessary to specify the program used, recombination values, recombination sex difference, or locus order in PREPLINK, because you can override these choices interactively when running the LCP program, as you will see in upcoming chapters.

Next, we must specify the genetic parameters that define the loci to be analyzed. To do this, you must now choose option *(k) See or Modify Loci*

Description. When you input *k,* followed by pressing the ⟨Enter⟩ key, a screen like the following appears:

```
*********************************************************
(1) Allele Numbers    GENE FREQS : 0.500000 0.500000
(2) Allele Numbers    GENE FREQS : 0.500000 0.500000
*********************************************************
(a) SEE OR MODIFY A LOCUS
(b) DELETE LOCUS
(c) ADD LOCUS
(d) CHANGE ORDER TO CORRESPOND TO PEDIGREE FILE
(NOT CHROMOSOME ORDER)
(e) CHANGE LOCUS TYPE
(f) RETURN TO MAIN MENU
*********************************************************
enter letter to modify values
```

We now make locus 1 correspond to the first locus in our pedigree file, which was the disease locus. To change locus 1 from allele numbers to affection status, choose option *(e),* which prompts you as follows:

```
ENTER LOCUS TO CHANGE
```

to which you should respond 1. Next you are given a menu of options as follows:

```
ENTER NEW LOCUS TYPE:
(a) BINARY FACTORS
(b) QUANTITATIVE TRAIT
(c) AFFECTION STATUS
(d) ALLELE NUMBERS
```

You should choose *(c) AFFECTION STATUS,* after which you see a menu like the one above, with the allele numbers changed to affection status in the description of locus 1. We still must modify the other parameters (gene frequency and penetrances) at locus 1, so choose option *(a) SEE OR MODIFY A LOCUS,* and specify locus 1. You then see a current default description of locus 1, as follows:

```
*************************************************************
LOCUS NUMBER:                      1
*************************************************************
(a) Number of Alleles              : 2
(b) Number of Liability Classes    : 1
(c) Penetrances:
GENOTYPE  1 1  0.000000
GENOTYPE  1 2  0.000000
GENOTYPE  2 2  1.000000
(d) Gene Frequencies :
  0.500000  0.500000
(e) EXIT
*************************************************************
enter letter to modify values
```

Because we assumed two alleles (one normal, one disease), the *(a) Number of Alleles* is correct. Likewise, line *(b) Number of Liability Classes : 1* is correct. We'll get into the meaning and application of liability classes later on. Let us assume for the moment that we have a fully penetrant dominant disease (for more information about penetrance, see Chapter 5) and that allele *2* is the disease allele. If this is the case, our line *(c) Penetrances* must be modified to reflect this. The penetrances given as the default correspond to a recessive disease with full penetrance. Now enter line *(c)* to modify the penetrances to correspond to a fully penetrant dominant disease as follows (the program presents the old penetrance value and prompts you with a question mark (?), at which point you must enter the new value, which may or may not coincide with the old value.)

```
ENTER NEW PENETRANCES
GENOTYPE  1 1  OLD PEN  0.000000
?
0
GENOTYPE  1 2  OLD PEN  0.000000
?
1
GENOTYPE  2 2  OLD PEN  0.000000
?
1
```

Once you respond as above, your locus description is again shown with these modified values. Note that you must enter a new penetrance, followed by ⟨Enter⟩ whenever you are prompted, even if it remains the same as the default value. Next, you must modify the gene frequencies, because the disease allele is certainly not at such a high frequency in the population. Let us assume the disease allele has a population frequency of 0.00001, giving the normal allele a frequency of 0.99999. So, choose option *(d)* and respond as follows:

```
ENTER 2 NEW GENE FREQUENCIES
0.99999 0.00001
```

The order in which you enter the frequencies is important. Because you defined the penetrances above in such a way that allele *2* is the disease-causing allele you must be certain that allele *2* receives the correct gene frequency of 0.00001. Now, this locus is properly specified, so we can choose option *(e)* *Exit* to take us back to the menu screen where each locus is specified. The top should now look like this:

```
************************************************
(1) affection status    GENE FREQS : 0.999990 0.000010
(2) allele numbers       GENE FREQS : 0.500000 0.500000
************************************************
```

Now, we should look at locus 2, by choosing *(a)* *SEE OR MODIFY A LOCUS,* and specifying locus 2. We will then see a screen like this:

```
*********************
Locus Number : 2
*********************
(a) Number of Alleles: 2
(b) Gene Frequencies:
    0.500000 0.500000
(c) EXIT
*********************
enter letter to modify values
```

Because there are only two alleles at this codominant marker locus, and we are assuming equal gene frequencies, we needn't change anything here. In general, the estimates of the gene frequencies *must* be reliable for all alleles at each locus. It has been repeatedly demonstrated (Ott, 1992, for example) that assuming equal gene frequencies for a given marker locus can lead to increased false-positive evidence for linkage when the true gene frequencies deviate from equality (almost always, this is the case). At this time, you should choose option *(c) EXIT,* followed by *(f) RETURN TO MAIN MENU,* and *(n) WRITE DATAFILE.* You are then asked to supply the name of the file to be saved, which should be *EX1.DAT.* The extension **.DAT* is used by convention to refer to the parameter file for the analysis. You may next choose option *(o) EXIT,* when you finish specifying the parameters for the analysis. If you wish, you may now look at this parameter file in your word processor. It should look like the following:

```
2 0 0 5  << NO. OF LOCI, RISK LOCUS, RISK ALLELE, SEXLINKED (IF 1) PROGRAM
0 0.0 0.0 0 << MUT LOCUS, MUT RATE, HAP FREQUENCIES (IF 1)
    1  2
1  2  << AFFECTION, NO. OF ALLELES
 0.999990 0.000010  << GENE FREQUENCIES
 1  << NO. OF LIABILITY CLASSES
 0.0000 1.0000 1.0000  << PENETRANCES
3  2  << ALLELE NUMBERS, NO. OF ALLELES
 0.500000 0.500000  << GENE FREQUENCIES
 0  0  << SEX DIFFERENCE, INTERFERENCE (IF 1 OR 2)
 0.1000  << RECOMBINATION VALUES
 1  0.10000 0.45000  << REC VARIED, INCREMENT, FINISHING VALUE
```

These are just the parameters you selected in PREPLINK, presented in a format readable by the LINKAGE programs. The bottom three lines are specific for the program to be used for the analysis, but for our purposes at this time, we ignore this section of the file.

So far, we have learned how to enter pedigree data in a form readable by the LINKAGE programs. We have also learned how to use the MAKEPED and PREPLINK programs to help in making these files. Throughout your career in linkage analysis, you will keep coming back to these programs, so it is important to understand them and become fluent in their usage. Before going on to the next chapter, where we'll actually begin to do our own linkage analyses, we present an exercise for practicing entering another set of data in the required formats.

□ **Exercise 2**

For the pedigree shown in Figure 2–3, create pedigree and parameter files (USEREX2.*), in the way presented in this chapter. In this drawing, the num-

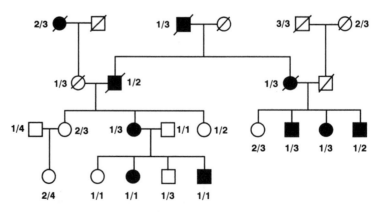

Figure 2–3. Pedigree drawing for USEREX2.*

bers by each individual describe the marker phenotype, if known. Use PREP-LINK to generate a parameter file, specifying the first locus as a fully penetrant dominant disease (affection status locus type) with disease allele frequency of 0.00001, and the second locus to be a codominant locus (allele numbers locus type) with three equally frequent alleles (gene frequencies = 0.33333). Remember that unknown individuals are coded as *0* at an affection status locus, and *0 0* at an allele numbers locus.

3 □

Running the LINKAGE Programs MLINK and ILINK

In this chapter, you will perform your first real two-point linkage analyses, using the pedigree files you created in the previous chapter. We use the MLINK and ILINK programs to perform these analyses. After this chapter, you will be able to do your own basic analyses. In practice, the analysis programs are not typically used directly but analyses are set up using the LCP program, which will be discussed in Chapter 4. For some types of application, however, it is important to know how to handle the analysis programs directly.

3.1 Theoretical Analysis

Let us begin this first linkage analysis with a theoretical examination of the pedigree from Figure 2–2 in the previous chapter, for which you have already made the pedigree file (EX1.PED) and parameter file (EX1.DAT). Let us examine this family more closely. The only way a meiosis can provide information about linkage is when the parent in which the meiosis occurred is heterozygous at both loci. Otherwise, no information can be obtained about linkage from this parent (i.e., if a parent is *1/1* at a marker locus, there is no way to tell which *1* allele was transmitted to any given offspring, so no linkage information is available). Because *mother* is homozygous at the marker locus and also at the disease locus (since it is a fully penetrant dominant disease, she must be homozygous normal to be unaffected), she is uninformative for linkage. So, we need only look at the fate of the paternally derived alleles in this family. We know that *father* is heterozygous at the marker locus (*1/2*) and also at the disease locus (since he is affected, yet to have unaffected children he must carry one disease allele, and one normal allele). Hence, he is informative for linkage. However, we do not know in what *phase* these alleles exist in *father,* but we know there are only two choices, either he has phase <u>D 1</u>/<u>N 2</u> or he has phase <u>N 1</u>/<u>D 2.</u> This type of nuclear family is called a *phase-unknown* pedigree, because only genotype information is available and not haplotype information on the doubly heterozygous parent. Each of these phases then has an equal 50% chance of being correct a priori (since we assumed absence of linkage disequilibrium). So, we can then examine the offspring to count recombinants and nonrecombinants under each phase. We can disregard what each child got from the *mother* and consider the pedigree to be reduced to what is shown in Figure 3–1, containing only the alleles derived from *father.*

Note that there are three different haplotypes observed in the children, (a) D 2, (b) N 1, and (c) N 2. If phase 1 is correct, haplotypes (a) and (b) are both recombinants (i.e., nonparental types), and haplotype (c) is a nonrecombinant (i.e., parental type). Similarly, under phase 2, the opposite situation pertains, and haplotypes (a) and (b) are nonrecombinant, and haplotype (c) is recombinant. Thus, under phase 1, we have four recombinants and one nonrecombinant in this family, and under phase 2, we have four nonrecombinants and one recombinant. Because the probability of a recombination is equal to θ (the *recombination fraction*), and the probability of a nonrecombination is therefore equal to $(1 - \theta)$, we can calculate the likelihood of this pedigree as a function of θ. Under phase 1, the probability of observing the data is equal to $P(\text{data}) = K\theta^4(1 - \theta)$, and under phase 2, the probability of the data is $K\theta(1 - \theta)^4$, where K is a constant coefficient in each case. Because each phase has a prior probability of 0.5, we can compute the probability of the phase-unknown family observed as follows by the law of total probability:

$$P(\text{data}) = P(\text{Phase 1})P(\text{data}|\text{Phase 1}) + P(\text{Phase 2})P(\text{data}|\text{Phase 2})$$

which in this case is equal to

$$P(\text{data}) = (0.5)[K\theta^4(1 - \theta)] + (0.5)[K\theta(1 - \theta)^4]$$

Because the likelihood is defined as $P(\text{data})$, we can set up a likelihood ratio test for linkage as

$$\Lambda = \frac{K\left[\dfrac{1}{2}\theta^4(1 - \theta) + \dfrac{1}{2}\theta(1 - \theta)^4\right]}{K\left[\dfrac{1}{2}(0.5)^4(0.5) + \dfrac{1}{2}(0.5)(0.5)^4\right]} = \frac{P(\text{data}|\theta)}{P(\text{data}|\theta = 0.5)} = \frac{L(\theta)}{L(\theta = 0.5)}$$

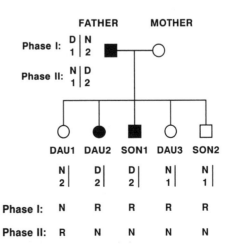

Figure 3–1. Linkage information contained in EX1.*

Because K can be factored out of both numerator and denominator, it is irrelevant for the likelihood ratio, and thus is typically ignored in all linkage analyses. Thus, in our family, the likelihood ratio reduces to

$$\Lambda = \frac{\frac{1}{2}\theta^4(1 - \theta) + \frac{1}{2}\theta(1 - \theta)^4}{0.5^5}$$

The lod score is then just the common logarithm of the likelihood ratio, and is equal to

$$Z(\theta) = \log_{10}(\Lambda) = \log_{10}\left[\frac{1}{2}(\theta^4(1 - \theta)) + \frac{1}{2}(\theta(1 - \theta)^4)\right] - 5\log_{10}(0.5)$$

The maximum of this lod score occurs at the same point as the maximum of the likelihood, so by maximizing the lod score over θ, we find the maximum likelihood estimate of the recombination fraction θ. In this case, the maximum occurs at approximately $\theta = 0.21$, with a corresponding lod score of

$$Z(0.21) = \log_{10}(\Lambda) = \log_{10}\left[\frac{1}{2}(0.21)^4(0.79) + \frac{1}{2}(0.21)(0.79)^4\right] - 5\log_{10}(0.5)$$

which equals $Z(\theta = 0.21) = 0.124929$.

3.2 MLINK

We have analytically derived the correct answer; now let us confirm our results by performing the same analysis with the LINKAGE programs. Let us first analyze our data using the MLINK program, which computes lod scores at a user-defined set of recombination fractions. In this example, let us compute the lod scores starting at $\theta = 0, 0.1, 0.2, 0.3, 0.4$, and 0.5. In other words, we start at $\theta = 0$ and calculate lod scores in steps of 0.1 until we get to $\theta = 0.5$. To do this we go back into PREPLINK and set up the parameter file to specify this analysis with the MLINK program.

First, enter *PREPLINK* on the command line, to activate the program. Next, choose option *(m) Read Datafile* and specify that the name of the datafile to be read is *EX1.DAT* (the file we created in the previous chapter). Now choose option *(i) Program Used*. This is where we can specify the analysis to be run by LINKAGE. You should see a menu of choices like the following:

```
*****************************
(a)    MLINK      : Y
(b)    ILINK      : N
(c)    LINKMAP    : N
(d)    RETURN TO MAIN MENU
*****************************
Use ILINK for CILINK or LODSCORE
Use LINKMAP for CMAP
enter letter to modify values
```

At this point, you should choose *(a)* to select the MLINK program, followed by *(d) RETURN TO MAIN MENU*.

Next we need to adjust the starting recombination value, by selecting choice *(j) Recombination values* from the main menu. You should then be prompted with

```
ENTER 1 NEW THETAS
```

to which you should respond *0*, because we wish to start calculating lod scores from $\theta = 0$. After entering this, you are automatically returned to the main menu of PREPLINK.

We need to tell the program one more thing: we wish to vary the recombination fraction in steps of 0.1 up to $\theta = 0.5$. To do this select option *(1) See or modify recombination to vary,* from the main menu. You should see a screen like the following:

```
*********************************
(a) RECOMBINATION TO VARY    : 1
(b) STARTING VALUE           : 0.0000
(c) INCREMENT                : 0.0100
(d) FINISHING VALUE          : 0.5000
(E) RETURN TO MAIN MENU
*********************************
enter letter to modify values
```

We now must set all of these values to specify our desired analysis. The first line, *(a) RECOMBINATION TO VARY,* may sound confusing. Here we are dealing with only a two-point analysis, so there is only one recombination fraction involved. However, if we are doing a multipoint analysis, there would be multiple interlocus recombination fractions, and MLINK can only vary one of them, hence you need to specify which one here. For our purposes, leave it at *1*. Now, you must set the *(b) STARTING VALUE* to *0.0000*, the *(c) INCREMENT* to *0.1000*, and the *(d) FINISHING VALUE* to *0.5000*. This should be clear, since we want to increment θ by steps of 0.1, stopping at $\theta = 0.5$. After making these adjustments, please enter *(e) RETURN TO MAIN MENU,* and *(n) Write Datafile,* calling it *EX1.DAT* (By the way, *YES* you *DO* want to overwrite the EX1.DAT file that exists, since you have just modified it, and no longer need the old one).

Now that we have fully prepared ourselves for the analysis, let us begin. The first thing you must do is to copy your pedigree file to a new name, PEDFILE.DAT, by typing

```
COPY EX1.PED PEDFILE.DAT
```

at the DOS prompt. Similarly, you need to copy the parameter file to DATAFILE.DAT, by typing

```
COPY EX1.DAT DATAFILE.DAT
```

This is required when the LINKAGE programs are run directly, though we'll be learning how to avoid all of this tedium in the next chapter.

We are now finally ready to do the linkage analysis. First, we must run the UNKNOWN program. This program is very important in eliminating impossible genotypes from consideration by the analysis programs. If you have a pedigree with a large number of individuals with unknown marker or disease genotypes, this program saves considerable time. It also checks for inconsistencies in your data. If you enter the data in such a way that a nonmendelian situation arises, the UNKNOWN program informs you of the error by saying *Incompatibility detected in this family at Locus 1,* or something like that. In any event, the LINKAGE programs are set up, on most computers, so that you *MUST* run the UNKNOWN program before the analysis programs, because it runs quickly, detects inconsistencies, and saves much time from the analysis programs in most situations. To run this program, type *UNKNOWN* at the DOS prompt. When the program has completed, type *DIR* to see that it has produced two new files: SPEEDFIL.DAT and IPEDFILE.DAT. In this case, because everybody is typed and all genotypes are uniquely determined, this file should be empty (i.e., the size should be 0 bytes). On the other hand, for the same reason, the IPEDFILE.DAT should be essentially identical in substance to the PEDFILE.DAT, with different spacings, and without the comments at the end of each line.

Now, you are finally ready to perform your first linkage analysis with the MLINK program. Enter *MLINK* at the DOS prompt, and the program begins to calculate lod scores for you. When the program is finished, new files are produced called OUTFILE.DAT and STREAM.DAT. For our present purposes, we ignore the STREAM.DAT file, though you'll see in later chapters why it is important. Now, look at the OUTFILE.DAT file in your word processor. It should resemble the following:

```
LINKAGE (V5.1) WITH 2-POINT AUTOSOMAL DATA
  ORDER OF LOCI:    1  2

_____

THETAS  0.500
_____

PEDIGREE | LN LIKE | LOG 10 LIKE
_____

       1   -19.830722      -8.612355
_____

TOTALS     -19.830722      -8.612355
-2 LN(LIKE) = 3.966144326368E+001 LOD SCORE =      0.000000
_____


_____

THETAS  0.000
_____

PEDIGREE | LN LIKE | LOG 10 LIKE
_____

       1-100000002004087734272.000000 -
43429358520716623872.000000
_____

TOTALS     -100000002004087734272.000000 -
43429358520716623872.000000
-2 LN(LIKE)  =  2.000000040082E+020 LOD SCORE
             = -43429358520716623872.000000
_____


_____

THETAS  0.100
_____

PEDIGREE | LN LIKE | LOG 10 LIKE
_____

       1   -19.780789      -8.590670
_____

TOTALS     -19.780789      -8.590670
-2 LN(LIKE) = 3.956157852618E+001 LOD SCORE  =      0.021685
_____


_____

THETAS  0.200
_____

PEDIGREE | LN LIKE | LOG 10 LIKE
_____

       1   -19.544641      -8.488112
_____

TOTALS     -19.544641      -8.488112
-2 LN(LIKE) = 3.908928168151E+001 LOD SCORE  =      0.124243
_____
```

```
THETAS  0.300

PEDIGREE │ LN LIKE │ LOG 10 LIKE

        1   -19.613033    -8.517814

TOTALS    -19.613033    -8.517814
-2 LN(LIKE)  =  3.922606586242E+001 LOD SCORE  =     0.094541


THETAS  0.400

PEDIGREE │ LN LIKE │ LOG 10 LIKE

        1   -19.758215    -8.580866

TOTALS    -19.758215    -8.580866
-2 LN(LIKE)  =  3.951642988211E+001 LOD SCORE  =     0.031489


THETAS  0.500

PEDIGREE │ LN LIKE │ LOG 10 LIKE

        1   -19.830722    -8.612355

TOTALS    -19.830722    -8.612355
-2 LN(LIKE)  =  3.966144326368E+001 LOD SCORE  =     0.000000
```

You should summarize this data, by extracting the important information and writing it in a little table. The most important pieces of information are the $\log_{10}$(likelihood), and the lod score at each theta. From this output file, you can extract the information shown in Table 3–1.

Essentially, the lod scores can be calculated as shown above, by subtracting the $\log_{10}$(likelihood) at $\theta = 0.5$ from each of the other likelihoods. You should try this by hand to verify this method of calculation. You may, moreover, wish to verify these lod scores by using the analytical formula we derived above and substituting in the appropriate values of θ to compute the lod scores. They should be identical. It should be apparent that from MLINK we not only get a good idea of where the maximum lod score occurs, but we get to see the whole lod score curve, which can provide information about how accurate the maximum likelihood estimate is. We'll pursue this point further in subsequent chapters. Notice that at $\theta = 0.20$ the lod score is 0.124243, very close to our theoretical maximum, for $\theta = 0.21$. As a test to verify our theoretical calculation, let's use the MLINK program to calculate the lod score at $\theta = 0.21$ to verify that we did it correctly by hand. Read your EX1.DAT file

Table 3–1. Analysis Results of EX1.PED; EX1.DAT

θ	Log_{10}(Likelihood)	Lod Score
0	$-\infty$	$-\infty$
0.1	-8.590670	0.021685
0.2	-8.488112	0.124243
0.3	-8.517814	0.094541
0.4	-8.580866	0.031489
0.5	-8.612355	0.000000

back in to PREPLINK and modify option *(1) See or modify recombination to vary*. This time set *(b) STARTING VALUE* to *0.21*, *(c) INCREMENT* to *0.1*, and *(d) FINISHING VALUE* to *0.22*. Then *(e) RETURN TO MAIN MENU*, write the new EX1.DAT file, and exit PREPLINK. Note that in the manner we set up our recombination to vary, it starts at $\theta = 0.21$ and moves in steps of 0.1 until $\theta > 0.22$, the finishing value. So, in this case, it only calculates the lod score at $\theta = 0.21$, because $0.21 + 0.1 = 0.31 > 0.22$. Now, copy the EX1.DAT file to DATAFILE.DAT, and we can begin the analysis (EX1.PED is unchanged, and still the same as our PEDFILE.DAT). Let's check it by running the UNKNOWN program again followed by the MLINK program, as outlined above. Your new OUTFILE.DAT file should look like this:

```
LINKAGE (V5.1) WITH 2-POINT AUTOSOMAL DATA
   ORDER OF LOCI:    1  2


_____

THETAS  0.500
_____

PEDIGREE | LN LIKE | LOG 10 LIKE
_____

       1  -19.830722     -8.612355
_____

TOTALS     -19.830722     -8.612355
-2 LN(LIKE) = 3.966144326368E+001 LOD SCORE =      0.000000
_____


THETAS  0.210
_____

PEDIGREE | LN LIKE | LOG 10 LIKE
_____

       1  -19.543061     -8.487426
_____

TOTALS     -19.543061     -8.487426
-2 LN(LIKE) = 3.908612143922E+001 LOD SCORE =      0.124929
```

Looking at this file, you can see that the lod score at $\theta = 0.21$ is 0.124929, both according to the MLINK program, and our theoretical analysis. You might have noticed that in this OUTFILE.DAT, the likelihoods and lod scores are given not only for $\theta = 0.21$, but also for $\theta = 0.5$. This was done because in order to compute a lod score, you need the likelihood at $\theta = 0.5$ as the denominator of the likelihood ratio. For this reason, no matter what θ's you want to compute lod scores for, the MLINK program always computes the likelihood at $\theta = 0.5$ first (*Note:* The lod score at this point is ALWAYS 0, because $L(0.5)/L(0.5) = 1$, and $\log_{10}(1) = 0$).

3.3 ILINK

We also frequently use the ILINK program for two-point analyses. This program doesn't give you the lod scores at predefined points, but rather attempts to maximize the likelihood numerically, and only returns the likelihoods at the maximum likelihood estimate of the iterated parameter (in this case, the recombination fraction). So, let's try to use this program to find the maximum likelihood estimate of θ. We know from our theoretical evaluation that the maximum is at approximately θ = 0.21. Let's see if ILINK returns a similar result.

Go back to PREPLINK, and set up the parameter file to do an ILINK analysis. First call up PREPLINK, and read in the EX1.DAT file. Then go back to option *(i) Program Used,* and select the *ILINK* program. Return to the main menu, and choose option *(1) See or modify iterated parameters.* Note that this is different from what option *(1)* said when we specified the MLINK program. Anyway, you should now see a menu like the following:

```
*****************************************************************
(a) RECOMBINATION VALUES TO BE ITERATED (1) OR FIXED (0) : 0
(b) LOCUS FOR WHICH VALUES MAY BE ITERATED               : 1
(c) RETURN TO MAIN MENU
*****************************************************************
NB : IF YOU WISH TO ITERATE OTHER PARAMETERS THE DATAFILE MUST BE
     MODIFIED AFTER EXITING FROM PREPLINK
enter letter to modify values
```

The first option *(a) RECOMBINATION VALUES TO BE ITERATED (1) OR FIXED (0)* is straightforward. In this case, there is only one recombination value, because we only have two loci. We merely need to tell the program whether it should try to maximize the likelihood with respect to this parameter or fix it at the specified value. To start out, let's use ILINK to find the maximum likelihood estimate of θ, so we should select option *(a),* and then enter a *1* to iterate the recombination value. Now we are confronted by the option *(b) LOCUS FOR WHICH VALUES MAY BE ITERATED.* The ILINK program can do more than just maximize the likelihood over recombination fractions. It can also estimate gene frequencies, penetrances, disequilibrium, and sex difference in recombination, among other things. For now, though, we are only going to be using it to estimate recombination fractions (which are not locus-specific values). Nevertheless, the program allocates memory as if it were going to maximize the likelihood over all of these parameters. For this reason one of the marker loci should be the locus for which values may be iterated, because there are fewer parameters at such a locus (no penetrances!). So, choose option *(b)* and locus *2* as the new locus for iterated values. Now return to the main menu. One more thing *must* be changed: option *(j) recombination values.* Because we are maximizing the likelihood over the recombination fraction, the value we enter here should be thought of as just a starting value for the maximization procedure. The closer it is to the maximum, the quicker the program converges to the estimate. Also, in some cases, different starting values may yield different estimates, because the algorithm can get trapped in a local maximum, or the program can stop for reasons other than the maximum was found. Also, you *cannot* start the iteration at θ = 0 because zero is a boundary value for θ, and the maximization algorithm used in ILINK does not work properly when started at a boundary. For this reason, one often starts at 0.1. Practically speaking, you may want to try multiple starting values, just to ensure they all end in roughly the same place. Anyhow, once this is changed, you can save the new EX1.DAT file and leave PREPLINK. Copy this file to DATAFILE.DAT and run the UNKNOWN program again. Now, instead of typing *MLINK* at the DOS prompt, type *ILINK* to run the ILINK program.

The ILINK program produces three output files: OUTFILE.DAT, FINAL.DAT, and STREAM.DAT. Again, we defer discussion of STREAM.

DAT to a later chapter. The most important output file from ILINK is the FINAL.DAT file, which should resemble the following:

```
CHROMOSOME ORDER OF LOCI :
  1  2
*********************** FINAL VALUES ********************
PROVIDED FOR LOCUS   2 (CHROMOSOME ORDER)
***********************************************************
GENE FREQUENCIES :
 0.500000 0.500000
***********************************************************
THETAS:
 0.212
***********************************************************
-2 LN(LIKE)  =  3.908608568137E+001
LOD SCORE  =  1.249370510945E-001
NUMBER OF ITERATIONS  =      4
NUMBER OF FUNCTION EVALUATIONS  =      12
PTG  =  -1.660797216309E-005
***********************************************************
***********************************************************
```

This gives us the final estimate of θ = 0.212 (pretty close to our approximate solution), with an associated lod score of 0.124937 (slightly larger than our value, because the program estimated θ to three decimal places, and we only did it to two). The gene frequencies are given for locus 2, which we specified as the locus at which parameters were to be estimated. They were not estimated, but because the program allows for this estimation, it outputs their final values. The -2ln(like) is given here, because it has a convenient statistical interpretation, being chi-square units asymptotically. (We'll be using this later.) The other values are not so important, but only specify how long the program took to converge and provide information about the gradient of the likelihood surface. Let us now look at the other output file, OUTFILE.DAT (remember that this was the name of the important file produced by MLINK). This should look like the following:

```
DIFFER INTER = 3.452668897808E-004 TRUNC UPPER
             = 1.858135866348E-002
ITERATION    1 T =      0.100 NFE =      2
F = 3.956157852618E+001
X=  1.000000000000E-001
G= -1.119885140454E+001
P=  1.119885140454E+001
TBND = 8.036538458179E-002 RESET T  = 4.015494478452E-002

ITERATION    2 T =      0.020 NFE =      5
F = 3.929637287819E+001
X=  3.248446298996E-001
G=  2.951007149097E+000
P= -4.689220798602E-002
FSMF = 2.652056479930E-001 PTG =-1.383792410037E-001 TMIN=
6.436095502122E-002
INITIAL T = 1.000000000000E+000
TBND = 6.927475669229E+000 RESET T  = 1.000000000000E+000

ITERATION    3 T =      2.000 NFE =      8
F = 3.909481766725E+001
X=  2.310602139275E-001
G=  8.576558660115E-001
```

```
P = -3.842391630530E-002
FSMF = 2.015552109388E-001 PTG = -3.295449721438E-002 TMIN =
5.586901493504E-002
INITIAL T = 1.000000000000E+000
TBND = 6.013447772779E+000 RESET T = 1.000000000000E+000

ITERATION    4 T =    0.500 NFE =    11
F = 3.908608568137E+001
X = 2.118482557749E-001
G = 2.680003275200E-002
P = -6.196996965180E-004
FSMF = 8.731985879677E-003 PTG = -1.660797216309E-005 TMIN =
5.586901493504E-002
EXIT CONDITION    5
Specified tolerance on normalized gradient met
```

Most of the information in this file is not of great importance to the user, with the exception of the final line, which indicates the exit condition: *"Specified tolerance on normalized gradient met."* This means the program converged to the maximum, within a predefined tolerance level. Sometimes, however, the program exits for other reasons, such as "Excessive cancellation in gradient," meaning that the final results obtained in the FINAL.DAT file are not really the maximum likelihood estimates, and perhaps the ILINK analysis should be restarted using the end points from FINAL.DAT as starting values.

Confirm that you have a maximum by starting ILINK using θ = 0.213 as the starting value and proceeding from there. To do this, read the EX1.DAT file back into PREPLINK, change the recombination value to 0.213, save the file EX1.DAT, copy it to DATAFILE.DAT, and rerun UNKNOWN and ILINK. The FINAL.DAT file should indicate that the new estimate of θ is 0.211 with a lod score of 0.124938, which is roughly the same as before, and only better in the sixth decimal place. Because this degree of precision is unimportant, we can stop here, satisfied that the best estimate of θ is approximately 0.21.

Again, we can also use ILINK to evaluate the lod score at the specific point θ = 0.21 to verify that ILINK computes the same lod score as MLINK and to confirm the lod score is identical to what we calculated by hand. To do this, read the EX1.DAT file into PREPLINK and set the recombination fraction to 0.21. Then, go to *(1) See or modify iterated parameters,* and set *(a) RECOMBINATION VALUES TO BE ITERATED (1) OR FIXED (0)* to *0,* because we now want to fix the recombination fraction and just calculate the lod score. Then write the new EX1.DAT file and exit PREPLINK. Now copy the EX1.DAT to DATAFILE.DAT as before and rerun UNKNOWN and ILINK; and this time, the FINAL.DAT file should indicate the lod score as 0.129429 to six decimal places.

In this chapter, we introduced the principles of basic two-point linkage analysis. Furthermore we calculated, theoretically, two-point lod scores for our sample pedigree and then introduced the UNKNOWN, MLINK, and ILINK programs of the LINKAGE package, and we used them to perform two-point analyses with our example pedigree. In the next chapter, we will see that there is an easier way.

□ **Exercise 3**

Analyze the example pedigree from Exercise 2. Try to analyze this pedigree analytically to get an idea of how very complicated and time-consuming it can be, then use the MLINK and ILINK programs to compute two-point lod scores as described in this chapter. Compute two-point lod scores for $\theta = 0$, 0.1, 0.2, 0.3, and 0.4 with MLINK (If you are running into problems, consult the answers given in Chapter 12 at the end of Part I). Then, do the same with ILINK (*Hint:* It takes five separate runs of ILINK.). Finally, find the best estimate of θ with ILINK, starting with a value of $\theta = 0.1$ and then refine the estimate by starting ILINK again from the value of θ given in the first FINAL.DAT file. Are you satisfied with this precision?

4.

Setting Up a Linkage Analysis Using LCP

In the previous chapter we learned how to use the LINKAGE programs to do a linkage analysis. Specifically, we learned how to manipulate the datafile for each different analysis we wanted to perform. The linkage control program (LCP) was written to make the whole process much simpler by allowing the user to specify any number of different analyses without modifying the parameter file each time by hand. The computer then does the analyses noninteractively (i.e., in *batch* mode), freeing up the researcher to do other things. In most situations, the LCP program is used to perform a linkage analysis, and we will be using it henceforward whenever we wish to use the LINKAGE programs (unless otherwise specified).

4.1 LCP

We now learn how to use LCP to set up an analysis of the data in EX1.PED and EX1.DAT. The LCP program is used to write a *batch file,* which contains a series of commands that define all of the steps involved in setting up and performing a set of linkage analyses.

First, start by typing *LCP* at the DOS prompt to activate the program. You are presented with a screen like the following:

```
COMMAND file name      [PEDIN.BAT] : PEDIN.BAT
LOG file name          [FINAL.OUT] : FINAL.OUT
STREAM file name       [STREAM.OUT] : STREAM.OUT
PEDIGREE file name     [PEDIN.DAT] : PEDIN.DAT
PARAMETER file name    [DATAIN.DAT] : DATAIN.DAT
Secondary PEDIGREE file name [ ]   :
Secondary PARAMETER file name [ ]  :
```

The COMMAND file name is the name of the batch file that LCP produces. The default name is PEDIN.BAT, and there is usually no reason to change it, unless you want to repeat the same analysis later for some reason. The LOG file, typically called FINAL.OUT, contains the results of all the analyses performed. Basically, this is a collection of the OUTFILE.DAT and FINAL.DAT files that we introduced in the previous chapter. Similarly, the

STREAM file is a collection of STREAM.DAT files, about which we defer discussion of until later. Finally, we need to indicate the PEDIGREE and PARAMETER files in which the data to be analyzed is stored. There is a very useful help screen available in LCP, which can be accessed at any time by hitting ⟨Ctrl-H⟩. Examine this to see a summary of the "control characters," which may be useful to you later.

At this point, we should adjust this first screen to correspond to our desired analysis. The only names we need to modify at this time are the PEDIGREE and PARAMETER files. Go to those lines, using the cursor keys and delete the file names currently shown (Use ⟨Ctrl-U⟩ to delete any entire line in LCP). Now, replace these names with your file names: *EX1.PED* for the PEDIGREE file and *EX1.DAT* for the PARAMETER file. Everything else on this screen is set up correctly, so you should now advance to the next screen by hitting the ⟨Page Down⟩ key. The next screen should look like this:

```
          General pedigrees :  <-
      Three-generation pedigrees :
  Experimental cross pedigrees :
```

The general version of the LINKAGE programs can be accessed through the *General pedigrees* option on this page. The *Three-generation pedigrees* option allows the user to choose one of the specialized versions of the LINKAGE programs designed to analyze codominant markers only in CEPH-type families, which are very specific types of three-generation pedigrees (discussed in detail in Part II). The *Experimental cross pedigrees* option allows the user to employ specific versions of the LINKAGE programs designed to analyze only animal crosses and is therefore not used in this book. For our purposes, we now choose the *General pedigrees* option from this menu and then hit the ⟨Page Down⟩ key again to move to the next page. Now, you have a list of the programs to choose from. Perform the same analysis as in the previous chapter, by first choosing the *MLINK* program from this menu, and hitting ⟨Page Down⟩. You should now see the following menu of choices:

```
        Specific evaluation :  <-
            Lod score table :
   Multiple pairwise lod table :
```

The *Specific evaluation* option is the one we used in the previous chapter, and the one we use now. However, in many situations, the *Lod score table* option may be more useful because it allows you to pick a set of recombination fractions at which to perform the lod score calculations, whereas under the *Specific evaluation* option, you must increment the steps by a constant factor, as we saw in the previous chapter. For now, choose the *Specific evaluation* option, and hit ⟨Page Down⟩. The next menu has only one choice (a limitation of LCP, not the analysis programs), for *No sex difference,* so hit ⟨Page Down⟩ again, and finally, you will see a menu of choices that should remind you of what we changed in PREPLINK in the previous chapter:

```
          Locus Order :
  Recombination Fractions : .1
     Recombination Varied : 1
          Increment Value : .1
              Stop Value : .5
```

Now, you should modify the *Locus order* to be *1 2* (or *2 1*, it makes no difference), with starting *Recombination fraction* of *0. Recombination varied,* as discussed in the previous chapter, remains at *1. Increment value* of *0.1,* and *Stop value* of *0.5* should be set. This, as you remember calculates the lod scores at θ = 0, 0.1, 0.2, 0.3, 0.4, and 0.5. Now *be sure to hit ⟨Page Down⟩* to write this analysis to the PEDIN.BAT file! There is no need to exit from the program at this point, however. In Chapter 3, we also analyzed the pedigree in question with the ILINK program. So, let us hit ⟨Page Up⟩ three times, to bring us back to the menu:

```
LODSCORE :
   ILINK :
 LINKMAP :
   MLINK :  <-
```

Now, move the arrow up to the *ILINK* program and hit ⟨Page Down⟩ to select it.

```
        Specific order :  <-
             All orders :
Inversions of adjacent loci :
```

Now, you see a screen that although meaningless in the context of two-point analysis is very important when you are trying to do a multipoint analysis, so we defer discussion of these until Part II. For now, just select Specific Order, and hit ⟨Page Down⟩. You should now see a selection of options regarding sex difference in recombination fractions. In this analysis, we assume there was no sex difference, so go to the *No sex difference* line, and hit ⟨Page Down⟩ again. Finally, you are presented with the screen on which you will select the analysis parameters:

```
        Locus order [ ] :
Recombination fractions :
```

Here, you should enter the *Locus order* of *1 2* (or equivalently, *2 1,* as above), and the starting value for the *Recombination fraction* should be set to *0.1,* as in the previous chapter. Now hit ⟨Page Down⟩ to enter this analysis, and we are then ready to exit the program and write the PEDIN.BAT file. Do this by entering ⟨Ctrl-Z⟩.

If you look at the file directory (by typing *DIR* at the DOS prompt), you should see a new file, PEDIN.BAT, which you just created with the LCP program. Feel free to look at it in your word processor. It is quite long and can be confusing to interpret, but it is basically instructing the computer how to perform all the cumbersome manipulations you had to do by hand in the previous chapter. Anyway, return to DOS, and type *PEDIN* to call this file. It then performs the analyses you requested. When it is finished, look at the FINAL.OUT file in your word processor. It should contain a brief summary of each analysis you requested, followed by the OUTFILE.DAT file (for the MLINK run) and then the FINAL.DAT file (for the ILINK run). These should contain the same lod scores as the analysis in the previous chapter. See how easy it is when LCP does all the hard work for you.

The following is a brief explanation of how this batch file works. The batch file uses another program, LSP (you'll see this again later), to modify the parameter files, replacing what you did with PREPLINK before, producing PEDFILE.DAT and DATAFILE.DAT files. LSP also writes a summary of the analysis, which is added to the FINAL.OUT file. Next, it calls the UN-KNOWN program and the desired analysis program (MLINK or ILINK). It then takes the appropriate output file, appends it to the FINAL.OUT file, and starts the process over for the next analysis, deleting all intermediate files in the process. It is really quite handy and efficient and much easier than doing the file manipulations by hand as in Chapter 3.

In this chapter, you learned how to use the linkage control program LCP to handle most of the drudgery of the linkage analysis process. You used this program to direct the computer efficiently through all of the required steps involved in using the LINKAGE programs in an automated manner.

☐ Exercise 4

Use LCP to perform the analyses you did in Exercise 3 and check that the results are, in fact, identical.

5.

Elementary Usage of the Affection Status Locus Type

In this chapter, you will be learning how to manipulate the affection status locus type to allow for autosomal dominant and autosomal recessive diseases. Furthermore, the concept of reduced penetrance is introduced on an elementary level. We also present some more example pedigrees to enter, giving you a chance to practice all of the skills you've learned thus far.

5.1 Autosomal Dominant Disease

The example pedigree we've been working on has been a phase–unknown pedigree with a dominant disease segregating. Now, let us suppose that we collect data on the parents of *father,* giving us the pedigree shown in Figure 5–1, with *fgrandpa* being unaffected (with *2/2* at the marker locus) and *fgrandma* affected (with *1/1* at the marker locus).

This information tells us that *father* must have received the disease and the *1* allele together from *fgrandma,* and the normal allele together with the *2* allele from *fgrandpa.* Thus, we know *father*'s phase with certainty to be $\underline{+\ 2}/D\ \underline{1}$. In this case, we can easily determine which children are recombinant and which are nonrecombinant. In this family, *dau1* is nonrecombinant, having received the $\underline{+\ 2}$ haplotype from *father,* and the others are all recombinant, having received the nonparental haplotypes $D\ \underline{2}$ (*dau2* and *son1*) or $\underline{+\ 1}$ (*dau3* and *son2*). The associated likelihood is then just $K\theta^4(1 - \theta)$, K being a constant, giving us a lod score of $\log_{10}[\theta^4(1 - \theta)/(0.5)^5]$, which equals $5\log_{10} 2 + 4\log_{10} \theta + \log_{10}(1 - \theta)$. This lod score function can be easily maximized by taking the first derivative with respect to θ as $dZ(\theta)/d\theta = 4/\theta - 1/(1 - \theta)$. Setting this equal to zero, and solving for θ yields a maximum likelihood estimate of $\hat{\theta} = 0.8$. Calculating the lod score at that point yields $Z(\theta = 0.8) = \log_{10}[(0.8)^4(0.2)/(0.5)^5] = 0.4185$. However, in human genetics, recombination fractions larger than 50% are meaningless, because when two genes are completely unlinked, the maximum possible recombination fraction is only 0.5. For this reason, the estimate is typically truncated to 0.5, given that the larger θ is meaningless. (An estimate of $\hat{\theta} > 0.5$ may also indicate that there is some data error, if the corresponding lod score is large.) In this case, therefore, our truncated MLE of θ is 0.5, with an associated lod score of 0.

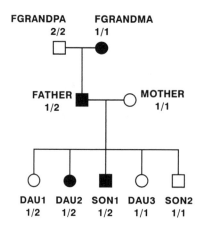

Figure 5–1. Phase-known Pedigree EX2.*

Create pedigree (EX2.PED) and parameter (EX2.DAT) files for this new pedigree. Make the disease autosomal dominant, as you did for the original pedigree (EX1.*). If you are unclear about how to do that, refer to Chapter 2. Give the disease locus gene frequencies of 0.99999 for the normal (wild type) allele, and 0.00001 for the disease allele. Then define an allele numbers locus with two equally frequent alleles. Now, use LCP to set up an analysis of this pedigree with the MLINK program, starting from $\theta = 0$ and proceeding in steps of 0.1 up to $\theta = 0.5$, and with the ILINK program, using a starting value of $\theta = 0.1$. After getting the first estimate of θ, restart the ILINK program to refine the estimate by setting up a further analysis with LCP. When these programs have run, you should interpret the output from FINAL.OUT and produce the results given in Table 5–1.

5.2 Autosomal Recessive Disease

Let us continue now by looking at an example of an autosomal *recessive* disease. Consider the family in Figure 5–2, showing grandparents, parents, and offspring.

Make a pedigree file corresponding to this pedigree, and name it EX3A.PRE. Process this file with MAKEPED as above (to make EX3A.PED) and create an appropriate parameter file (EX3.DAT) in PREPLINK as before,

Table 5–1. Analysis Results of EX2.PED; EX2.DAT

θ	Log_{10}(Likelihood)	Lod Score
0.0	$-\infty$	$-\infty$
0.1	-12.357079	-2.540602
0.2	-11.204114	-1.387637
0.3	-10.557742	-0.741265
0.4	-10.124935	-0.308458
0.5	-9.816477	0.000000

ILINK: $\hat{\theta} = 0.798$; $Z(\hat{\theta}) = 0.4185$.

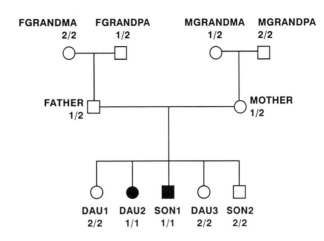

Figure 5–2. Recessive Pedigree EX3A.*

only this time specify the PENETRANCES for a recessive disease, which are as follows:

```
GENOTYPE   1 1 OLD PEN 0.000000
?
0
GENOTYPE   1 2 OLD PEN 0.000000
?
0
GENOTYPE   2 2 OLD PEN 1.000000
?
1
```

Again modify the gene frequencies to be 0.99999 and 0.00001, as in the previous dominant disease example. The marker should be a two-allele *Allele Numbers* type locus with equal gene frequency for the two alleles. Save this file as *EX3.DAT*.

Now analyze this family with MLINK and ILINK as you did above, and examine your output. It should correspond to the results given in Table 5–2.

Looking at this family, we can see that no information about linkage is obtained from the grandparents, since we have no way of knowing which grandparent was carrying the disease allele in each case. If you do not think this is correct, reanalyze this family, omitting *fgrandma, fgrandpa, mgrandpa,* and *mgrandma*. When you do this, the $\log_{10}$(likelihood)'s change, because there are fewer people in the family, but the lod scores remain identical. Make this new pedigree file *EX3B.PED* as above, and then use LCP to set up an analysis of this new family, using the same parameter file *EX3.DAT*. The resulting output should be as shown in Table 5–3.

Table 5–2. Analysis Results of EX3A.PED; EX3.DAT

θ	Log$_{10}$(Likelihood)	Lod Score
0	−15.418525	0.976874
0.1	−15.606399	0.789000
0.2	−15.824343	0.571056
0.3	−16.065391	0.330008
0.4	−16.291110	0.104290
0.5	−16.195199	0.000000

ILINK: $\hat{\theta} = 0.000$; $Z(\hat{\theta}) = 0.976874$.

Table 5–3. Analysis Results of EX3B.PED; EX3.DAT

θ	Log_{10}(Likelihood)	Lod Score
0	-13.612340	0.976874
0.1	-13.800214	0.789000
0.2	-14.018158	0.571056
0.3	-14.259206	0.330008
0.4	-14.484925	0.104290
0.5	-14.589214	0.000000

ILINK: $\hat{\theta} = 0.000$; $Z(\hat{\theta}) = 0.976874$.

Herein, you can see one fundamental difference between recessive and dominant disease analysis. In the dominant case we examined above, adding the grandparents helped to establish the phase in the parents, adding much additional information about linkage. In this recessive case, we added the grandparents, yet got absolutely no change in the lod scores. The grandparents contribute no phase information whatsoever, because we have no way of telling which unaffected grandparent was carrying the disease. In general, you can see that typing grandparents can be very useful in dominant diseases, but in recessive diseases it may be a waste of effort. Can you see how this might affect the experimental approach to mapping a disease, based on its mode of transmission?

This pedigree is more difficult to analyze by hand, as there are four possible phase combinations for the parents. We know that each parent is doubly heterozygous, giving two phase probabilities for each parent. Because the parents are independent, we have four combinations of phase at the two parents jointly. Fortunately, all of the children are homozygous, so we can tell with certainty what each parent transmitted to each child. The formal equations involved are therefore quite complex and not very illustrative, so we do not provide them here.

5.3 Incomplete Penetrance

So far we have spent most of this chapter learning how to model different modes of transmission of a disease using the affection status locus type. One other common complication in such modeling is that penetrance is not always complete. For many diseases, even if the individual has the disease predisposing genotype, he or she is not necessarily affected. In fact often, there are very complicated probability models for this phenomenon, as you will see in later chapters. For now, let us consider the simplest case, in which a random individual with the disease predisposing genotype has only a 50% chance of becoming affected. Let us go back to the phase-unknown example from files EX1.PED and EX1.DAT and modify EX1.DAT to allow for incomplete penetrance of this dominant disease. Read the file EX1.DAT back into PREP-LINK, then choose option *(k) See or modify locus parameters,* and *(a) SEE OR MODIFY A LOCUS,* specifying locus *1,* the disease. Now, modify the penetrances as follows:

```
GENOTYPE 1 1 OLD PEN 0.000000E+00
?
0
GENOTYPE 1 2 OLD PEN 1.000000E+00
?
0.5
```

```
GENOTYPE 2 2 OLD PEN 1.000000E+00
?
0.5
```

Then save the new parameter file as *INC.DAT* and reanalyze this pedigree with MLINK and ILINK, in the same way as before, and examine the new lod scores. The results are given in Table 5–4.

The estimate of θ is now 0 because the one likely recombinant is most likely assumed to be a case of nonpenetrance (i.e., the individual has the disease-predisposing genotype but did not express the disease for some reason). Let us take a look at this situation in a theoretical manner.

As we know from looking at this family in Chapter 3, there are two equally likely (a priori) phases for *father*. He can be either phase (1) *D1/+2* or he can be phase (2) *D2/+1*. Let us see what effect this reduced penetrance has on our analysis. First of all, because the disease gene frequency is so small, assume that *mother* is +/+ at the disease locus. Then, we know with certainty that *dau2* and *son1* have disease locus genotype *D/+*. However, *dau1*, *dau3*, and *son2* could each be either +/+ or *D/+*. Let us examine what happens under phase (1). In this case, first consider that *dau1* could have received + 2 from *father*. In this case, the probability of her being unaffected is 1 because her disease locus genotype is +/+. The probability of receiving the + 2 haplotype is $(1 - \theta)$. If she received D 2 from *father,* then she is unaffected with probability 0.5 because her disease locus genotype is D/+. Also, the probability of receiving this haplotype is θ because it is recombinant. Thus, the overall probability of observing *dau1*, and unaffected offspring with marker genotype *1/2* is $(1 - \theta) + 0.5(\theta) = 0.5(2 - \theta)$. Similarly, *dau3* and *son2*, who are identical phenotypically, can be shown to have a probability of $\theta + 0.5(1 - \theta) = 0.5(1 + \theta)$. Thus, the total probability of this family, assuming phase (1) is $[0.5(2 - \theta)][0.5(1 + \theta)]^2\theta^2$. Under phase (2) it can be shown to be $[0.5(2 - \theta)]^2[0.5(1 + \theta)][1 - \theta]^2$. Thus, the total likelihood of this family is

$$0.5\{[0.5(2 - \theta)][0.5(1 + \theta)]^2\theta^2 + [0.5(2 - \theta)]^2[0.5(1 + \theta)][1 - \theta]^2\}$$

which can be reduced to the following:

$$K\{(2 - \theta)(1 + \theta)[(1 + \theta)\theta^2 + (2 - \theta)(1 - \theta)^2]\}$$

The lod score can be represented then as

$$\log_{10}\left\{\frac{(2 - \theta)(1 + \theta)[(1 + \theta)\theta^2 + (2 - \theta)(1 - \theta)^2]}{\left(\frac{3}{2}\right)\left(\frac{3}{2}\right)\left[\left(\frac{3}{2}\right)\left(\frac{1}{2}\right)^2 + \left(\frac{3}{2}\right)\left(\frac{1}{2}\right)^2\right]}\right\}$$

Table 5–4. Analysis Results of EX1.PED; INC.DAT

θ	Log_{10}(Likelihood)	Lod Score	$Z(\theta)$ from EX1
0.0	−8.612351	0.374811	−∞
0.1	−8.703932	0.283230	0.021685
0.2	−8.800774	0.186388	0.124243
0.3	−8.892292	0.094870	0.094541
0.4	−8.961068	0.026094	0.031489
0.5	−8.987162	0.000000	0.000000

ILINK: $\hat{\theta} = 0$; $Z(\hat{\theta}) = 0.374811$.

Lod scores can then be computed as above. For example, if you substitute $\theta = 0$, you get

$$Z(\theta = 0) = \log_{10}\left(\frac{(2)(1)[0 + 2]}{\left[\left(\frac{3}{2}\right)^3\left(\frac{1}{2}\right)\right]}\right)$$

$$= \log_{10}\left(\frac{4}{\left(\frac{27}{16}\right)}\right)$$

$$= \log_{10}\left(\frac{64}{27}\right) = 0.37481$$

As you can see, the addition of incomplete penetrance makes it extremely difficult to compute lod scores analytically, making the computer programs much more important and useful. When you examine complicated pedigrees with complicated disease models, the process becomes even more intractable. Nevertheless, we can verify the results obtained with the LINKAGE programs by hand when we question the results.

In this chapter, we learned how to use the affection status locus type to specify various disease models, including simple applications of reduced penetrance.

□ **Exercise 5**

Reconsider the pedigree from Exercise 2 and analyze the pedigree assuming a penetrance of 75% for the dominant disease (in file USEREX5.DAT). How does this affect your results? Does it make sense to you? Try analyzing the disease assuming an autosomal recessive mode of inheritance with 70% penetrance. Does this result make sense? What happens if you reduce the penetrance to 30% in the dominant and recessive cases separately? Given that this disease is really autosomal dominant with full penetrance, do the results of this analysis make sense? What would you expect if the disease was really recessive and was analyzed as if it were dominant?

6.

Sex-linked Recessive Diseases

In this chapter, we introduce the concept of linkage analysis with sex-linked recessive diseases and the method for analyzing them in the LINKAGE programs. You will learn how to modify your parameter and pedigree files to enter such data and how to use the LINKAGE programs to analyze it. Because almost all sex-linked diseases are recessive, they are usually referred to simply as sex-linked.

6.1 Sex-linked Diseases

In humans, there are twenty-two pairs of homologous autosomal chromosomes. Each person receives one copy of each chromosome from the mother, and one from the father, thus explaining most observed patterns of inheritance. So far, we have only considered such autosomal loci. However, humans also have what we've described as *sex chromosomes,* which are responsible in part for determining the sex of an individual. In humans, these chromosomes are designated X and Y, with XX individuals being female, and XY individuals being male. Clearly, every person must receive one X chromosome from the two the mother can give, whereas fathers give their X chromosome to their daughters and their Y chromosome to their sons. On the sex chromosomes, recombination can only occur in females because they have two homologous X chromosomes, whereas men have the nonhomologous XY pair. Actually, two small regions of homology exist with recombination between X and Y, known as the *pseudoautosomal region,* in which loci behave as if they were autosomal. In general, though, it can be assumed that no recombination occurs on the X chromosome in males. Also, every male has only one allele at each X-chromosomal locus in the what is referred to as *hemizygous* state. This property establishes that if everyone in a pedigree is typed, we always know with certainty the phase in each individual, with the exception of female founders. That is to say, we know in each nonfounder female, which allele came from which parent (Males of course only receive X-chromosomal alleles from their mothers). This makes sex linkage very easy to analyze.

Many diseases in humans, such as hemophilia and some forms of retinitis pigmentosa, are known to be inherited as X-linked recessive diseases (Mc-Kusick, 1990). In fact, most of the known X-chromosomal diseases are fully penetrant recessives (sometimes with delayed age of onset) and are quite often lethal, for example, X-linked agammaglobulinemia (Kwan et al., 1990). These diseases will be discussed again in Part III. In recessive X-linked diseases, the only affected people are females who are homozygous for the disease allele and males who are hemizygous with the disease allele. The only way a female can be homozygous, however, is if she receives a disease allele from her affected father. Because many of these diseases are either lethal or cause an affected man to be unlikely to sire children, only males are usually affected. If the disease were not lethal, and the population gene frequency of the disease allele were, say, 0.01, the probability of a random male in the population to be affected would be 0.01, whereas the probability of a random female being affected would be $(0.01)^2 = 0.0001$. In any case, the majority of affected individuals are male (In this example, they are 100 times more likely to be affected. In Part III, you will see that for lethal diseases, it is virtually impossible for women to become affected). Similarly, if there were a disease gene on the Y chromosome, *only* males could be affected. In general, sex-linked diseases are characterized by this preponderance of males among affected individuals, and by the *absence of any male-to-male transmission* of the disease (because males can only get X chromosomes from their mothers!). Let us now examine how to analyze a sample pedigree segregating an X-linked recessive disease.

6.2 The Preparation of Pedigree and Parameter Files

Consider the pedigree shown in Figure 6–1. Enter this pedigree (EX4.PRE) in the standard LINKAGE format as you did in the previous autosomal examples. The only difference is that now, males have only one allele at each locus and females have two. We must code this in allele numbers format by entering the allele number twice in males, as if they were homozygous. That is to say, if a male has allele *2* at a locus, you enter his marker phenotype as *2 2*. This ensures that there are the same number of columns for males and females in the pedigree file at each locus. If you mistakenly enter a heterozygous genotype for any male in the pedigree file, the UNKNOWN program detects it as an inconsistency (because males can only have one allele per X-linked locus). The EX4.PRE file should be as follows:

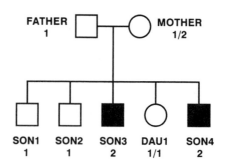

Figure 6–1. Sex-linked recessive pedigree EX4.*

```
ex4    father   0        0        1  1    1  1
ex4    mother   0        0        2  1    1  2
ex4    son1     father   mother   1  1    1  1
ex4    son2     father   mother   1  1    1  1
ex4    son3     father   mother   1  2    2  2
ex4    dau1     father   mother   2  1    1  1
ex4    son4     father   mother   1  2    2  2
[EOF]
```

Process this file with MAKEPED in exactly the same way as for autosomal traits, and save it as EX4.PED.

Now, you need to create a parameter file with the PREPLINK program. In this case, we have a fully penetrant sex-linked recessive disease with gene frequency of 0.01 for the disease allele, and an allele numbers type of marker locus with three equally frequent alleles. To make your EX4.DAT parameter file, call up the PREPLINK program. From the main menu, you first select the *(b) Sex-linked* option, to tell the program you are looking at a sex-linked disease and markers. This toggles the *N* in the row following *(b) Sex-linked* to a *Y,* meaning that from now on the program operates under the assumption that all loci are sex-linked. Next, you choose option *(k) See or modify locus description.* Change the first locus to affection status, as you did previously, and change the second locus to allele numbers. Then choose option *(a) SEE OR MODIFY A LOCUS,* specifying locus *1*. You should see a screen like the following:

```
*******************************
LOCUS NUMBER :              1
*******************************
(a) NUMBER OF ALLELES          :    2
(b) NUMBER OF LIABILITY CLASSES :    1
(c) PENETRANCES :
     MALES:
ALLELE 1 0.00000E+00
ALLELE 2 1.00000E+00
     FEMALES:
GENOTYPE   1 1 0.00000E+00
GENOTYPE   1 2 0.00000E+00
GENOTYPE   2 2 1.00000E+00
(d) GENE FREQUENCIES :
0.500000 0.500000
(e) EXIT
*******************************
enter letter to modify values
```

This is slightly different from what we saw in the autosomal case because we now must specify separate penetrances for males and females. Notice that for males, there are two penetrances, corresponding to the two possible hemizygous genotypes (alleles), whereas females have three, corresponding to the three possible two-allele genotypes. Looking at the indicated penetrance values closely, we can see that the default is for an X-linked recessive disease, with the disease-causing allele being allele *2*. As an exercise in entering the penetrances for a sex-linked disease, let us redefine the penetrances so we have a fully penetrant X-linked recessive disease, with the disease-causing allele being allele *1*. The results are identical! (If you don't believe this, try it both ways as an exercise.) Now enter the appropriate penetrances for our fully penetrant X-linked recessive disease, with option *(c) PENETRANCES.* You should adjust the values as follows:

```
ENTER NEW PENETRANCES
      MALES:
ALLELE  1 OLD PEN  0.00000E+00
?
1
ALLELE  2 OLD PEN  1.00000E+00
?
0
      FEMALES:
GENOTYPE  1 1 OLD PEN  0.00000E+00
?
1
GENOTYPE  1 2 OLD PEN  0.00000E+00
?
0
GENOTYPE  2 2 OLD PEN  1.00000E+00
?
0
```

In this case, we specified that all males hemizygous for allele *1* and all females homozygous for allele *1* are affected with probability 1, whereas all other individuals cannot be affected with the disease. In this example, we defined the penetrances such that allele *1* is the disease allele. To make this specification complete, you must modify the *(d) GENE FREQUENCIES* accordingly. Enter the new gene frequencies as follows:

```
ENTER 2 NEW GENE FREQUENCIES
0.01 0.99
```

Then, select *(e) EXIT* and *(a) SEE OR MODIFY A LOCUS,* specifying locus 2. At this allele numbers locus you can adjust the values just as you would for an autosomal locus, by setting the number of alleles to *3* and the gene frequencies to *0.33333, 0.33333,* and *0.33334* (so they sum to 1!). You already indicated that the analysis is to be done on sex-linked data, so the programs know that males must be hemizygous. Now, go back to the main menu and save the file as *EX4.DAT.*

6.3 Performing the Linkage Analysis

You already specified in the parameter file, EX4.DAT, that you are analyzing sex-linked data, so you needn't do anything different in LCP. Use LCP the same way you have been throughout the book, and specify that the program should do the analysis with MLINK, starting at $\theta = 0$, in steps of 0.05 this time, and stopping at $\theta = 0.45$ (We already know the lod score at $\theta = 0.5$ MUST be 0 by definition, and the likelihood is calculated as the first iteration in any case). Also specify an analysis with the ILINK program, with a starting value of $\theta = 0.2$ (for variety's sake). Now, exit LCP and do the linkage analysis. The results from the FINAL.OUT file are shown in Table 6–1.

Let us consider this example, analytically, trying to understand where this lod score came from. In this case, we know for a fact that the disease allele had to come from *mother* because *father* was unaffected, making him hemizygous normal. Furthermore, *mother* has to be heterozygous because she is unaffected herself, but has affected sons. We then know that *son1* and *son2* got the normal allele from *mother* together with the *1* allele at the marker

Table 6–1. Analysis Results of EX4.PED; EX4.DAT

θ	Log$_{10}$(Likelihood)	Lod Score
0.0	−4.644217	0.903088
0.05	−4.733319	0.813986
0.1	−4.827180	0.720125
0.15	−4.926119	0.621185
0.2	−5.030163	0.517142
0.25	−5.138642	0.408663
0.3	−5.249414	0.297891
0.35	−5.357506	0.189799
0.4	−5.453323	0.093982
0.45	−5.521958	0.025347
0.5	−5.547305	0.000000

ILINK: $\hat{\theta} = 0$; $Z(\hat{\theta}) = 0.903088$.

locus. Similarly, we know that *son3* and *son4* received the disease allele together with the *2* allele from *mother*. However, *dau1* could have received either the normal or disease allele from *mother,* because they are phenotypically indistinguishable. Hence, even though we know she received the *1* allele at the marker locus, we do not have any information about her disease locus genotype, so she is uninformative for linkage, and contributes nothing to the linkage analysis. To verify this, you should try analyzing the pedigree, leaving her out. The lod scores (but not the likelihoods) at every point are identical.

The result is essentially a phase-unknown situation, in which all the information comes from transmission from *mother* to *sons*. The analysis is then straightforward, as in the first example in the book. *Mother* is equally likely to have phase (1) d 1/+ 2 or phase (2) + 1/d 2. If she has phase (1), then all four offspring are obligate recombinants, with a probability of θ^4. If she has phase (2), they are all nonrecombinants, with a probability of $(1 - \theta)^4$. Hence, the overall likelihood of this pedigree as a function of θ is

$$K[0.5\theta^4 + 0.5(1 - \theta)^4] = K[\theta^4 + (1 - \theta)^4]$$

The lod score is then

$$\log_{10}\left\{\frac{\theta^4 + (1 - \theta)^4}{(0.5)^4 + (0.5)^4}\right\} = \log_{10}\{2^3[\theta^4 + (1 - \theta)^4]\}$$

If you substitute different values of θ, for example, $\theta = 0.05$, you should get a lod score of $\log_{10}\{2^3[(0.05)^4 + (0.95)^4]\} = 0.81399$, which is the same as you calculated with the LINKAGE programs above.

Females are not always uninformative for linkage. Assume that in the pedigree we analyzed above, *dau1* married *husband,* who is unaffected, and has marker locus allele 3, and had a child, *gson,* who was affected with marker locus allele 1 (of course, because *dau1* is homozygous for the *1* allele.), as shown in Figure 6–2.

In this case, we cannot tell whether a recombination occurred from *dau1* to *gson,* since *dau1* is homozygous at the marker locus. However, the fact that *gson* is affected forces *dau1* to be heterozygous at the disease locus, telling us that she received the *1* allele together with the disease allele from her mother. This has a significant effect on the linkage analysis. Add this information to the pedigree in file EX4.PRE (saving it again as *EX4.PRE*), process the file with MAKEPED (saving it as *EX4.PED*), and reanalyze this pedigree, using the same command file (*PEDIN.BAT*) as before (It is not

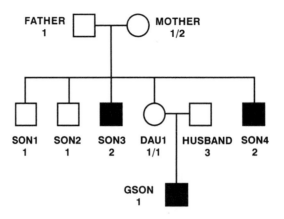

Figure 6–2. Extension of pedigree EX4.*

necessary to rerun LCP because we are going to do the same analyses involving files with the same names as before). Just type *PEDIN* to analyze this new pedigree. The results should be as shown in Table 6–2.

Do you notice anything interesting about these lod scores? If you look at the lod scores obtained in the first example in the book, the phase-unknown family with five offspring (EX1.*), you notice that they are identical. To understand why, look again at the analytical computation of the lod score. Using the notation above, if *mother* has phase (1), the four *son*s are recombinants, but *dau1*, who received a <u>d 1</u> haplotype from *mother*, is a nonrecombinant, with a likelihood of $K\theta^4(1 - \theta)$. Similarly under phase (2), the four boys represent nonrecombinants, and *dau1* must have received a recombinant haplotype from *mother*, so the likelihood is $K\theta(1 - \theta)^4$. The overall likelihood of the pedigree is $K[\theta^4(1 - \theta) + \theta(1 - \theta)^4]$, for a lod score of

$$\log_{10}\left\{\frac{\theta^4(1 - \theta) + \theta(1 - \theta)^4}{(0.5)^4(0.5) + (0.5)(0.5)^4}\right\} = \log_{10}\{2^4[\theta^4(1 - \theta) + \theta(1 - \theta)^4]\}$$

which is identical to the lod score computed for files EX1.*, with the phase-unknown family from chapter 3.

In this chapter, we learned how to analyze a sex-linked disease in the LINKAGE programs, and saw how to do it analytically for some simple examples. Different properties of sex-linked traits were introduced, especially

Table 6–2. Analysis Results of Modified EX4.PED; EX4.DAT

θ	$\text{Log}_{10}(\text{Likelihood})$	Lod Score
0.0	$-\infty$	$-\infty$
0.05	-6.816792	-0.185952
0.1	-6.609155	0.021685
0.15	-6.530573	0.100267
0.2	-6.506597	0.124243
0.25	-6.512741	0.118099
0.3	-6.536299	0.094951
0.35	-6.567995	0.062845
0.4	-6.599351	0.031489
0.45	-6.622368	0.025347
0.5	-6.630840	0.000000

ILINK: $\hat{\theta} = 0.211$; $Z(\hat{\theta}) = 0.124938$.

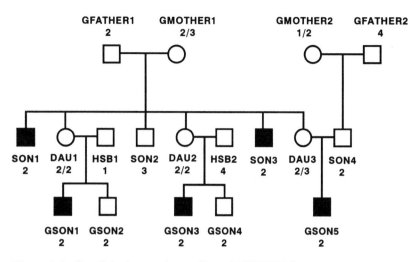

Figure 6-3. Sex-linked recessive pedigree USEREX6.*

the concept of hemizygosity and its effects on linkage analysis. Furthermore, we saw that if we change our pedigree file (or parameter file) without changing its name, we can rerun an analysis without going through LCP again, by calling the same PEDIN.BAT file as that used in the previous analysis. Note that to do this, all file names must be unchanged, and the same analysis must be performed (i.e., MLINK starting from θ = 0, through θ = 0.45, in steps of 0.5, ILINK with starting recombination value of 0.2 in our example).

□ **Exercise 6**

Analyze the pedigree in Figure 6-3, assuming an X-linked, fully penetrant, recessive disease; with a gene frequency of 0.01; and a marker with four equally frequent alleles (in files USEREX6.*). Examine this family both analytically and using the LINKAGE programs MLINK and ILINK, at the same points as the analysis detailed above in this chapter. Exactly what is going on at the genotype level, and which meioses are informative for linkage? Find the equation for the lod score in this family. Compare the results with what was obtained from the LINKAGE programs. They should be the same.

7.□

Loops

In this chapter you will learn what *loops* are and how to deal with them in the LINKAGE programs. We introduce the concept of *consanguinity* loops and *marriage* loops and their ramifications in a linkage analysis. Further, you will learn how to deal with these in the LINKAGE programs, and finally, we briefly introduce a utility program called *LOOPS,* which is designed to detect the presence of unbroken loops in a LINKAGE pedigree file and is automatically run every time MAKEPED is used to process a pedigree file. For the first time, we analyze more than one pedigree in a single pedigree file; most real linkage studies have multiple pedigrees.

In the few very simple examples we've looked at of analytical calculation of likelihoods, you saw how complicated it can be, even in small nuclear families. In more complex pedigrees, analysis by hand quickly becomes intractable. It also quickly becomes apparent that designing a computer program to handle any general pedigree structure in a theoretically justifiable manner is anything but straightforward. The *Elston-Stewart algorithm* provides a way of calculating the likelihood in a recursive manner, allowing for the possibility of computer-based linkage analyses in general pedigrees. One of the main features of this algorithm is its dependence on *clipping* (or *peeling*). In the process of clipping, small nuclear families within a larger pedigree are analyzed, and all of the information is collapsed on to one of the parents (or other relatives), whose own sibship is analyzed next, and so on, until all of the information is collapsed onto one final person, the proband (For a detailed description, please consult Ott, 1991, 169–172). This method is pretty straightforward unless there is a loop in the pedigree. A loop is present in a pedigree when it is possible to start at any individual in a pedigree drawing and draw a connected sequence of lines ending up back at the original individual, without retracing your steps. If a loop exists in a pedigree, the process of collapsing circles around and around in the connected series of individuals, catching the algorithm in an infinite loop.

To circumvent this problem, the LINKAGE programs require that in each loop, one individual who is both an offspring and a parent must be *"doubled."* This effectively *"breaks"* the loop because the program considers these two doubled individuals to be genotypically identical (including phase), but still separate individuals. This allows the breaking of the infinite loop described above and permits the likelihood to be computed, albeit slowly. The most efficient persons to double in any given pedigree are those members of the loop with the greatest amount of known genotypic information, including phase. This greatly reduces the computational time, as explained in Ott (1991).

There are two primary types of loops: consanguinity loops, and marriage loops. In a consanguinity loop, inbreeding is present. In other words, the parents of a given individual must be related. In a pure marriage loop, no inbreeding occurs, yet a completed pedigree circuit is created nevertheless. An example is two brothers who are married to two sisters, as you will see below. The distinction is immaterial for the LINKAGE programs and is only important in that it points out the possibility of having loops in a pedigree without inbreeding!

7.1 Consanguinity Loops

Let us consider again the recessive disease pedigree from EX3A.PED and EX3.DAT, which you analyzed in Chapter 5. Suppose that we went out and collected more data on that extended family, only to learn that there was a consanguinity loop, as indicated in Figure 7–1.

Clearly this relatedness has a major effect on the linkage information in the pedigree. Given the very small gene frequency of the disease allele, it is most likely that the disease allele was present in only one of the founders (persons with no parents in the pedigree). Hence, that makes *fgrandpa* and *mgrandma* the most likely carriers of the disease allele. Also, it adds considerable linkage information, as you will see. So, let us analyze this new pedigree with the LINKAGE programs, as before. You can use the same parameter file, EX3.DAT, because nothing needs to be changed there. The only difference is in the pedigree file, so enter the pedigree in the figure into a new file, EX5.PRE, in the same format as before (with pedigree identifier *ex5*), and then call up the MAKEPED program to process the pedigree file. Proceed in

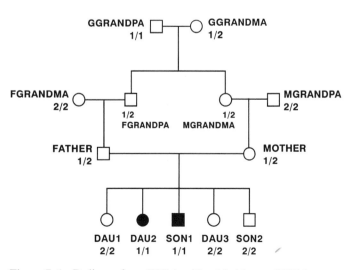

Figure 7–1. Pedigree from EX3A with added loop—EX5.*

the MAKEPED program exactly as before, only when the program prompts you with the following:

```
Does your pedigree file contain any loops?  (y/n)?   ->
```

Respond *Y*, after which you will be asked if you have a file of loop assignments. The answer is *No*. A file of loop assignments is another file that indicates at which individual in which pedigree you can break the loop(s). You do not have one, and generally will not. Next, you are asked the following:

```
Enter identifiers for each pedigree and person . . .
Enter pedigree 0 when finished.
   Pedigree  ->      ex5
   Person       ->   father
```

In this case, you could break the loop at *father, mother, fgrandpa,* or *mgrandma.* You may wonder how to decide where to break it. Although it makes no difference in the results where you break the loop, it may affect the computing time greatly. You should always break the loop at the individual with the least ambiguity in genotype. In this case, *father* and *mother* must be heterozygous at the disease locus, so you know their genotypes more exactly than the grandparents, because the disease allele doesn't have to come from a specific grandparent. So in this case, let's break the loop at *father.* Then type *0* when prompted with

```
Pedigree  ->
```

to continue. You are next asked:

```
Do you want these selections saved for later use?  (y/n)   ->
```

Respond *n*, because "saving" them only creates a file of loop assignments like the one you were asked for above, and does not affect the final *.PED file in any way. It is generally of little use to you to make a file of loop assignments. Next, have the program select all probands automatically, as before, to complete the processing of your file EX5.PED. Now analyze this pedigree with MLINK and ILINK as before, using the same parameter file (EX3.DAT), through the LCP program, and compare your results to those in Table 7–1.

Compare these values with those obtained in the prior analysis, in which your maximum lod score was only about half as large. In the absence of recombination, every phase-known meiosis contributes roughly 0.3 units of lod score. In this case, adding this consanguinity (two additional individuals typed), the additional information is roughly equivalent to three new phase-known meioses. Why is this the case? The fact that both affected individuals are homozygous for the *1* allele, suggests that the disease is probably segregating together with the *1* allele throughout the pedigree from a common ancestor. The concept of homozygosity mapping (Smith, 1953; Lander and

Table 7–1. Analysis Results of EX5.PED; EX3.DAT

θ	$\text{Log}_{10}(\text{Likelihood})$	Lod Score
0	−11.622653	1.879919
0.1	−11.901587	1.600985
0.2	−12.221869	1.280703
0.3	−12.591054	0.911518
0.4	−13.015882	0.486690
0.5	−13.502572	0.000000

ILINK: $\hat{\theta} = 0.001$; $Z(\hat{\theta}) = 1.878120$.

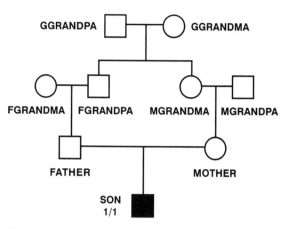

Figure 7–2. Homozygosity mapping pedigree.

Botstein, 1987) is based on this idea, that homozygous affected individuals, whose parents are related, most likely received a common haplotype without recombination from a single founder, allowing us to gain linkage information from all presumed nonrecombinant meioses from the original founder haplotype to the affected children. In recessive disease pedigrees, there is often a good deal of inbreeding. One reason marriages between closely related individuals is illegal is this increased propensity for recessive genetic disease among their offspring. However, for linkage analysis, these families are a godsend. Consider a family with the same structure as above, with only one affected child, with marker genotype *1 1*. Consider everyone else in the pedigree to be untyped at the marker locus and unaffected. Then analyze this pedigree with the LINKAGE programs, assuming that the gene frequency of the *1* allele is 0.01, and there are two alleles at the marker locus (the disease is as defined for the previous example). Analyze this family (shown in Figure 7–2) with LINKAGE as you have learned to do. From only one typed individual who is affected and homozygous for this rare allele, you get a maximum lod score at $\theta = 0$, of 1.14.

This result occurs because both the disease allele and the marker are so rare that they most likely entered the pedigree only once. Further, if they are both known to be present in the affected child, then he or she must have received them together without recombination from a common ancestor, assuming each allele entered the pedigree only once. The fact that we do not know which ancestor carried the disease allele, nor do we know which one carried the *1* allele adds noise to our analysis, but when one has a recessive disease, you can gain more linkage information per individual typed with inbred families in many situations, especially when you have a marker locus with a great many rare alleles. It is important to consider, however, that although inbred families make a linkage analysis more cost-effective in terms of the number of people you need to type, there is a large cost in computer time. In fact, the time it takes to complete a likelihood calculation in a pedigree increases exponentially with the number of loops in the pedigree.

7.2 Marriage Loops

Consider the case in which two pedigrees must be analyzed at the same time. This can be done quite simply by including both pedigrees in the same pedi-

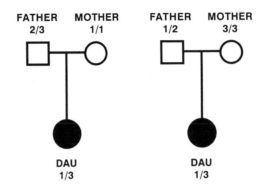

Figure 7–3. Two nuclear pedigrees—no loop—EX6A.*

gree file with different pedigree names. At present, analyze two nuclear families with one affected offspring each, as shown in Figure 7–3. Create a single pedigree file containing both pedigrees, and name the pedigrees *ex61* and *ex62*.

Name these pedigree files *EX6A.PRE* and then *EX6A.PED*. Make a parameter file as before with the PREPLINK program, specifying the disease to be recessive, with gene frequency of 0.00001 for the disease allele, as before. At the marker locus, however, allow for three alleles, with gene frequencies of 0.25, 0.40, and 0.35. Call this file *EX6.DAT*. Now analyze these families with MLINK and ILINK as before. As expected, there is no information in these pedigrees because they are phase-unknown matings with only one offspring, and no linkage disequilibrium. However, for interest's sake, take note of the magnitude of the log likelihoods. You should find lod scores of 0 everywhere.

Note, however, that you discovered a relationship between these two pedigrees: they are actually two siblings marrying two other siblings, as shown in Figure 7–4. This marriage creates a loop in the pedigree, because you can start from *fathera,* and connect him to himself through the route *fathera–motherb–daub–fatherb–mothera–daua–fathera.* This is a loop that must be broken before you can analyze this pedigree in the LINKAGE programs, as outlined above. Enter this combined pedigree as one large pedigree and name this file *EX6B.PRE.* Call MAKEPED, and specify that there is indeed a loop in this

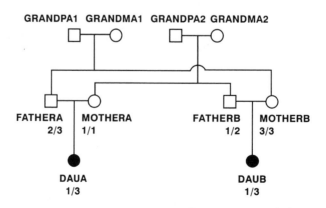

Figure 7–4. Same two nuclear pedigrees connected via marriage loop— EX6B.*

pedigree, a marriage loop, which can be broken at either of the four parents. You must break a loop at an individual in the loop who is an offspring and a parent. The best strategy is to select one such individual about whom the most complete genotypic information, including phase, is known. In this example, we know that each of the parents are carriers, but the parents who are heterozygous at the marker locus carry somewhat less phase information. Clearly the homozygous parents are uninformative for linkage, and we know that in *motherb* the disease and normal alleles are each on a haplotype with a *3* allele. So, in this example, it may be slightly more economical to break the loop at either *mothera* or *motherb* because they are homozygous at the marker locus, whereas the *father*s are heterozygous and phase-unknown. Proceed as in the previous example and analyze the family with MLINK and ILINK. Output is given in Table 7–2.

Again, the addition of the information on the relatedness of these two pedigrees has taken two completely uninformative nuclear families, and given us one larger informative family with positive lod scores. Can you see why? Are the log likelihoods different from the combined family and the two smaller ones? Can you explain the magnitude of the difference?

The answers to all of these questions center on the fact that four independent disease alleles segregate when you have two separate nuclear families. These alleles each have frequency of 0.00001, so the probability of observing four separate such alleles is $(0.00001)^4$. Clearly, once we add the relationships in, we only need two such disease alleles to explain the pedigree as observed. If one member of each grandparental pair is a carrier, then all of the parents can be carriers. The chance to observe two independent realizations of the disease allele is much larger, at $(0.00001)^2$, which is 10^{10} times more likely. Hence, the likelihoods are much larger in the second pedigree than in the other two combined. As for the linkage information, again we obtain the additional information from the same phenomenon that characterized homozygosity mapping. Here, we have two first cousins who are both affected, and who have the same marker locus genotype. Furthermore, we can tell that the daughters both received a *1* allele and a disease allele from either *grandma2* or *grandpa2*. Further, the *3* allele came from the other grandparental pair together with an additional disease allele. Because both grandparental pairs contributed an identical haplotype to their grandchildren, there is some linkage information present. This information is limited, however, because each child has one homozygous parent, further diluting the information present in this family. As an analogous case to the homozygosity mapping example, consider this same pedigree, only make everyone unknown at the marker locus except the two daughters. Then, alter the parameter file so that the gene frequencies of the three marker locus alleles are 0.01, 0.98, and 0.01. In this way,

Table 7–2. Analysis Results of EX6B.PED; EX6.DAT

θ	Log_{10}(Likelihood)	Lod Score
0	−14.718037	0.374809
0.1	−14.901117	0.191729
0.2	−15.023110	0.069736
0.3	−15.082021	0.010825
0.4	−15.095476	−0.002630
0.5	−15.092846	0.000000

ILINK: $\hat{\theta} = 0.001$; $Z(\hat{\theta}) = 0.373373$.

we force the *1* and *3* alleles to occur only once each in this pedigree (most likely). Then rerun the analysis with the MLINK and ILINK programs as you have been doing. The maximum lod score from having typed only these two affected cousins is now 1.18, all of the linkage information coming from the loop, and the observed alleles being so rare as to have most likely occurred only once in the pedigree.

7.3 The LOOPS Program

Xie and Ott (1992) wrote a computer program to detect the presence of unbroken loops in pedigree files after they've been processed by the MAKEPED program. This program uses concepts of graph theory to detect connected graphs in the pedigree. Essentially, each individual is a node, and each marriage point is a node. If any unbroken path can be traced between nodes of the graph, from one individual back to himself without retracing, then the program informs you that an unbroken loop still exists, and it gives you a list of the nodes involved in the connected graph. Reprocess the files *EX5.PRE* and *EX6B.PRE* with MAKEPED, specifying that there are no loops. When MAKEPED calls the LOOPS program, it tells you that a loop has been detected, and it gives you a listing of the nodes of the connected graph, in the file *LOOPS.OUT*. Then you can go back and reprocess the file in MAKEPED, breaking the indicated loop. After breaking the loops, the LOOPS program should tell you that there are no loops detected in the pedigree. This program is now automatically run after MAKEPED to detect any undeclared loops you may have overlooked. Also, if there are no loops, but you made data entry errors resulting in a loop, LOOPS helps you catch them. It is possible to use MAKEPED without using the LOOPS program (by typing *MAKEPED1* instead of *MAKEPED*), but as a safeguard you should always use the LOOPS program.

In this chapter, you learned about loops, and why they are useful in a linkage analysis. You also saw how to analyze pedigrees with loops in the LINKAGE programs. In addition, you were introduced to the method for ana-

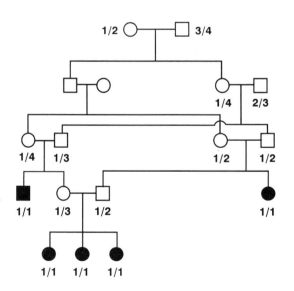

Figure 7–5. Complicated pedigree with multiple loops—USEREX7.*

lyzing multiple pedigrees at the same time, and were shown how to use the LOOPS program to detect any loops that may be present in a pedigree. It should be emphasized that although analyzing pedigrees with loops may be more cost-effective for the molecular biologist, they can be very time-consuming to analyze. You will see just how time-consuming when you try to solve Exercise 7.

☐ **Exercise 7**

This problem involves the identification and breaking of consanguinity, marriage loops, or both in pedigree data. Look at the pedigree drawn in Figure 7–5. Make a pre-MAKEPED pedigree file and a parameter file for this pedigree (USEREX7.*). In this case, we are analyzing a fully penetrant, recessive disease with gene frequency of 0.001 and a four-allele, codominant allele, numbers type of marker with equal gene frequencies for each allele. Remember that you should always break loops at an individual with the least genotypic ambiguity. How many loops are there in this pedigree? Where is the best place to break them? Check your processed file with the LOOPS program to ensure that you've broken them all!

Try to solve this on your own. Answers are given in chapter 10, but try to think it through yourself. If you are unsure how to break loops, reread the sections on consanguinity and marriage loops. Then analyze this family with the MLINK and ILINK programs in the same manner as in Exercise 4. If you get the wrong answers, check to verify that you've correctly broken each and every loop present in the family. Also, be sure you haven't broken too many loops.

8.

Locus Types I: Allele Numbers and Binary Factors

In this chapter, you will be introduced to the *binary factors* locus type, which is perhaps the most basic way of inputting data into the LINKAGE programs. You will also see the relationship between binary factors and the allele numbers locus type. In addition we present a simple way to use this locus type to code the ABO blood group, and for the first time, we show you how to use LCP to analyze a subset of the total number of loci present in a given data set.

8.1 Codominance

In a binary factors type of locus, a phenotype consists of the presence or absence of a number of *factors*. At a given locus, each allele is presumed to cause the presence of a different subset of the total number of factors codable by the sum of all alleles at that locus. Understand that every allele has its own binary factors notation, and the *OR* of any two alleles occurring in a genotype yields the notation for the corresponding phenotype. As a simple example, consider a locus with two codominant alleles (*1 = 2*, read *1* "is codominant with" *2*). The first allele is assumed to cause the presence of one factor, and the second allele is assumed to cause the presence of another. In this case, the factor may be the presence of a given band on a Southern blot, corresponding to the allele in question, or it may refer to the observation at the phenotypic level of the presence of the same allele. The factor needn't have any real phenotypically meaningful interpretation—just assume that our locus can cause either of two factors to be observed. Alleles are coded by a sequence of 0's and 1's. For each factor at a given locus, we must enter one column in our data file, consisting of either a *0* (if the factor is not present) or a *1* (if the factor is present). In this case, our allele *1* would be *1 0*, because the first factor (presence of allele *1*) is present and the second factor is absent (allele *2* is of course not present in allele *1*). Analogously, allele *2* is *0 1* at this locus. However, what we observe in an individual are phenotypes, which are determined by combinations of two alleles. Clearly in our codominant locus, we can have three genotypes, *1 1, 1 2,* and *2 2* (in allele numbers format), each of which corresponds to a unique phenotype, because the locus is codominant. How do we combine alleles in this locus type? It is basically a logical OR operation. If any factor is present in *either* the maternally or paternally derived allele, then it is present in the combined phenotype, much like the OR operation on a computer. Therefore, genotype *1/1* is 1 0/1 0 in binary factors. If we perform this logical OR operation we get 1 0 OR 1 0 = 1 0. The first factor is present in either the first or the second allele (in this case, in both), and the second factor is absent from *both* alleles. Hence, the phenotype is 1 0. For genotype *1/2,* we now have binary factors genotype 1 0/0 1, which corresponds to a phenotype of 1 0 OR 0 1 = 1 1, because factor 1 is present in the first allele, and factor 2 is present in the second allele. Similarly, genotype *2/2* corresponds to a binary factors phenotype of 0 1. Note also that in binary factor notation in the LINKAGE programs, a phenotype of 0 0 does *not* mean absence of both markers (which does not make sense here), but rather is the code for unknown (i.e., untyped) phenotypes. The entire situation is summarized in Table 8–1.

This table shows how to code such a codominant system as a binary factors type of locus with two alleles and two sample coded factors. This simplest application of the binary factors locus type has been implemented in the LINKAGE programs in a more user-friendly way, through the allele numbers locus type, which you have been using throughout this book. The simple correspondence between allele numbers and binary factors is illustrated in Table 8–1. As an exercise, go back to the original phase-unknown pedigree from Chapter 2, which you entered in the files EX1.DAT and EX1.PED. At this point, add a third locus to the pedigree file (EX1.PRE) in binary factors format, which should be the binary factors equivalent of the allele numbers marker locus already entered in this file. Put these new phenotypes directly after the allele numbers phenotypes on each line, using the format shown in Table 8–1. Your file should eventually look like the following:

```
ex1    father   0        0        1  2  1  2  1  1
ex1    mother   0        0        2  1  1  1  1  0
ex1    dau1     father   mother   2  1  1  2  1  1
ex1    dau2     father   mother   2  2  1  2  1  1
ex1    son1     father   mother   1  2  1  2  1  1
ex1    dau3     father   mother   2  1  1  1  1  0
ex1    son2     father   mother   1  1  1  1  1  0
[EOF]
```

Save this file as *EX7.PRE,* and process it with MAKEPED to produce a pedigree file called *EX7.PED.* Next, we must modify our parameter file to indicate

Table 8–1. Binary Factors Representation of Codominant Locus with Two Alleles and Two Factors

Real		Binary Factor Genotype	Factor Status		Binary Factors Phenotype
Genotype	Phenotype		Factor 1	Factor 2	
1/1	1 1	1 0/1 0	Present	Absent	1 0
1/2	1 2	1 0/0 1	Present	Present	1 1
2/2	2 2	0 1/0 1	Absent	Present	0 1
Unknown	0 0	Unknown	Unknown	Unknown	0 0

the addition of a new locus. Read the *EX1.DAT* file into the PREPLINK program by typing the following at the DOS prompt:

```
PREPLINK EX1.DAT
```

Now, from the main menu, select option *(k) See or modify loci description*, and from the subsequent menu, choose option *(c) ADD LOCUS*. You are returned to the same menu again, only with an additional locus indicated at the top of the screen. Now we first need to *(e) CHANGE LOCUS TYPE*, specifying locus *3* and changing it to *(a) BINARY FACTORS*. Next, you should *(a) SEE OR MODIFY A LOCUS*, specifying locus *3*. You see a screen like the following:

```
****************************************
LOCUS NUMBER:              3
****************************************
(a) NUMBER OF ALLELES                :    2
(b) NUMBER OF FACTORS                :    2
(c) FACTORS PRESENT (1) OR ABSENT (0) FOR EACH ALLELE :
1 0
0 1
(d) GENE FREQUENCIES :
  0.500000 0.500000
(e) EXIT
****************************************
enter letter to modify values
```

Disregard what is already there, and set up this locus as discussed above. First set the number of alleles by choosing option *(a) NUMBER OF ALLELES* and specifying that there are *2* alleles. Then, specify the *(b) NUMBER OF FACTORS* as *2* also, as explained above. Now, choose option *(c) FACTORS PRESENT*. You should respond to the questions as follows:

```
ENTER NEW FACTORS.  1 = PRESENT 0 = ABSENT
LEAVE A SPACE BETWEEN FACTORS
ALLELE 1
1 0
ALLELE 2
0 1
```

This is also as we discussed above. Now, the gene frequencies should be set equal for the two alleles, as in EX1.DAT. Go back to the main menu, and save this new file as *EX7.DAT*. We are now ready to analyze this family with the LINKAGE programs.

Call up the LCP program, specifying, as the pedigree file *EX7.PED* and *EX7.DAT* as the parameter file. Proceed as in previous examples, by selecting the MLINK program. This time you want to do the same analyses as before, starting from $\theta = 0$, in steps of 0.1, stopping at $\theta = 0.4$ (Remember that $\theta = 0.5$ always gives a lod score of 0 by definition.). However, this time, after specifying that the analysis be performed between locus 1 and 2 (the disease and the allele numbers locus), specify a further analysis with locus order = *1 3* (the disease and the new binary factors locus). To do this, hit ⟨Page Down⟩ after entering the analysis parameters for 1 versus 2 and then return to the same screen, only modifying the first line to read *Locus Order 1 3*, followed by ⟨Page Down⟩. Then go back, and as before specify the same analyses with ILINK, again first stipulating 1 versus 2, hitting ⟨Page Down⟩, and repeating the analysis with 1 versus 3. Then exit LCP with ⟨Ctrl-Z⟩, and perform the analysis by typing *PEDIN* at the DOS prompt. Examine the FINAL.OUT file in your word processor when the analysis is finished, and compare the likelihoods and lod scores for the two analyses: 1 versus 2 , and 1 versus 3. Notice that everything is equal, because loci *2* and *3* represent exactly the same locus, entered in a different format. If they are not always equal, then recheck your pedigree and parameter files for possible errors!

8.2 Multiple Factors: Two Alleles (the CEPH Database)

There is a large data bank for human genetics at the CEPH (Centre d'Étude du Polymorphisme Humain) in Paris (Dausset et al., 1990). In this data base, much of the phenotypic data has been entered in this binary factors format, because historically, this was the first data entry format available. However, situations frequently arise in which there are two-allele codominant systems with multiple factors. Many of these systems contain additional constituently present factors, for example, constant bands on a Southern blot. These add no additional genetic information, but many investigators thought it was more meaningful to include full banding patterns in the input files, for future reference. As an example of this, consider a two-allele codominant situation with five factors; of which factors 1, 3, and 4 are constituently present. Now, allele *1* is coded as *1 1 1 1 0* (factors 1–4 present, factor 5 absent), and allele *2* is coded as *1 0 1 1 1* (factors 1, 3, 4, and 5 present, factor 2 absent). In this case, the same logical OR operation can determine our phenotypic correspondence. This situation is summarized in Table 8–2.

As you can see, this is essentially the same as the two-factor situation we used above, for if the constituently present factors, 1, 3, and 4 are eliminated, the result is exactly the same binary phenotypes we had before. Nevertheless, for practice in using this form of the binary factors locus type, which is common in the CEPH data base, go back to the last example, files *EX7.PED* and *EX7.DAT,* and add a new locus, of the binary factors type with two alleles and five factors as described in Table 8–2. Make this locus identical in genetic information to loci 2 and 3 in this file. Save the new pedigree *(EX8.PED)* and parameter files *(EX8.DAT)*. Then, analyze the disease versus locus 4, to ensure that the likelihoods and lod scores are all identical with the ones you obtained from analyzing loci 1 versus 2, and 1 versus 3.

8.3 Dominance and Recessivity

For the next extension, consider how to use the binary factors locus type in situations in which the allele numbers locus type cannot be used. One such case occurs when we wish to analyze a fully penetrant dominant locus. As-

Table 8–2. Alternative Binary Factors Representation of Codominant Locus with Two Alleles and Five Factors

Real		Binary Factors	
Genotype	Phenotype	Genotype	Phenotype
1/1	1 1	1 1 1 1 0 / 1 1 1 1 0	1 1 1 1 0
1/2	1 2	1 1 1 1 0 / 1 0 1 1 1	1 1 1 1 1
2/2	2 2	1 0 1 1 1 / 1 0 1 1 1	1 0 1 1 1
Unknown	0 0	Unknown	0 0 0 0 0

Table 8–3. Incorrect Attempt at Characterizing a Dominant Trait in Binary Factors Notation with One Factor

| | Binary Factors | |
Genotype	Genotype	Phenotype
1/1	1/1	1
1/2	1/0	1
2/2	0/0	0
Unknown	Unknown	0

sume that we have a two-allele locus, which determines a dominant trait, and allele *1* is dominant over allele *2 (1 > 2)*. This can be visualized by assuming that allele *1* produces some protein, and allele *2* produces nothing. In addition, the protein is produced equally effectively with one or two copies of allele *1*. An intuitive way of coding this is to specify one factor, the protein in question, and have allele *1* be *1* (for factor 1 present: i.e., the protein is produced), and allele *2* be *0* (for factor 1 absent: i.e., no protein produced). If this were the case, we would have a genotype–phenotype relationship as outlined in Table 8–3.

This wouldn't be a problem, except that unknown individuals as well as *2/2* individuals would be coded as 0. This is unacceptable, so we need to add an additional factor that is constituently present, for example, a factor "typed" with an intuitive meaning such that if the individual is typed at the locus, this factor is present, and if the individual is not typed, the factor is absent. This factor must behave much like the functionless factors added in EX8.PRE; only now, having the additional function of discriminating between *2/2* individuals and unknown individuals, as shown in Table 8–4.

Return to this same example (EX8.*) and recode the fully penetrant disease as if it were a binary factors locus type, keeping the gene frequencies the same. Then check it by comparing an analysis of locus 1 versus 2 with that of locus 5 (the new binary factors representation of the disease) versus locus 2. They *must* be identical as well.

A recessive condition is also immediately specified, because whenever a dominance relationship exists there is an accompanying recessive relationship. In this case we had *1 > 2* (allele *1* is dominant over allele *2*), which means that *2 < 1* (allele *2* is recessive to allele *1*), because it is required for there to be two copies of the nonprotein-producing allele, in this example, for the "absence of protein" phenotype to be observed. This is the definition of recessivity. Thus, we can use the same coding scheme as above to code a recessive system, only being sure to specify allele *2* as the recessive disease-predisposing allele!

Table 8–4. Correct Representation of a Dominant Trait in Binary Factors Notation with Two Factors

| | Binary Factors | |
Genotype	Genotype	Phenotype
1/1	1 1/1 1	1 1
1/2	1 1/0 1	1 1
2/2	0 1/0 1	0 1
Unknown	Unknown	0 0

Table 8–5. Incorrect Representation of ABO Blood Group in Binary Factors Format with Two Factors

ABO		Binary Factors	
Phenotype	Genotype	Genotype	Phenotype
A	*A/A*	1 0/1 0	1 0
	A/O	1 0/0 0	1 0
B	*B/B*	0 1/0 1	0 1
	B/O	0 1/0 0	0 1
AB	*A/B*	1 0/0 1	1 1
O	*O/O*	0 0/0 0	0 0
Unknown	Unknown	Unknown	0 0

8.4 Systems with Dominance and Codominance: The ABO Blood Group

More complicated dominance–codominance relationships can be specified as well with the binary factors notational system. Consider the ABO blood group. To this point, we have not learned any way of coding this in a LINK-AGE input file, even though it is among the most basic loci in humans. In fact, many early linkage studies were done with this very locus, and we do not yet know how to use this kind of data. These relationships can, however, be easily coded for in the LINKAGE programs as a binary factors locus. Think about this for a while on your own. If you cannot figure it out, then go on to read the following section.

In the ABO blood group, it is well known that there are three alleles, *A*, *B*, and *O*. The *A* allele causes, among other things, the production of a certain cell-surface antigen "A." Similarly, the *B* allele produces cell-surface antigen "B." The *O* allele, however, produces *no* cell-surface antigens. The actions of these three alleles in the production of cell-surface antigens are independent, so it can be clearly seen that the dominance relationship can be summarized as follows: $(A = B) > O$ (*A* and *B* are codominant, and both are dominant over the *O* allele). We know how to code the codominance, and we know how to code the dominance, but how can we combine the two phenomena in the same locus? Let us begin by considering that the cell-surface antigens A and B can be considered as binary factors. If this were the case, allele *A* is *1 0*, allele *B* is *0 1*, and allele *O* is *0 0*. This locus is summarized as in Table 8–5.

Table 8–6. Correct Representation of ABO Blood Group in Binary Factors Notation with Three Alleles

ABO		Binary Factors	
Phenotype	Genotype	Genotype	Phenotype
A	*A/A*	1 0 1/1 0 1	1 0 1
	A/O	1 0 1/0 0 1	1 0 1
B	*B/B*	0 1 1/0 1 1	0 1 1
	B/O	0 1 1/0 0 1	0 1 1
AB	*A/B*	1 0 1/0 1 1	1 1 1
O	*O/O*	0 0 1/0 0 1	0 0 1
Unknown	Unknown	Unknown	0 0 0

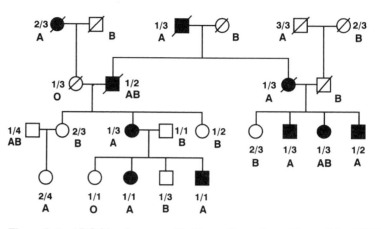

Figure 8–1. ABO blood group added to pedigree from Figure 2-3—USEREX8.*

This is an intuitively satisfying approach, except that now O blood type individuals are indistinguishable from unknown individuals in terms of their binary factors phenotypes. Disregarding the *O* allele completely, however, we see a straightforward codominance relationship between *A* and *B* alleles. Further, disregarding the *A* allele, we can see a straight dominance relationship specified with *B* > *O*. The same holds for *A* > *O*. Thus, our dominance relationships are correct, and we merely need to allow the program to distinguish O phenotypes from unknown individuals. This is the same situation we encountered in the straight dominance example above. To remedy this situation, add an additional constituently present factor to allow for this discrimination, as shown in Table 8–6.

In this chapter, you learned about the binary factors locus type and how to use it to enter phenotypic data under codominance, dominance, recessivity, and any combination thereof. We also studied the relationship between the binary factors and allele numbers locus types, and learned that the allele numbers locus type is just a shorthand form for entering codominant binary factors data. Additionally, for the first time, you used LCP to extract subsets of loci from a pedigree and parameter file to perform analyses on various subsets of the loci in these files.

☐ Exercise 8

Go back and reenter the data from all previous exercises, adding binary factors representations of all allele numbers locus types, and fully penetrant diseases. Compare the results to ensure they are compatible.

Add the ABO blood group data to the pedigree in Exercise 2, as shown in Figure 8–1 (Make new files USEREX8.*, containing the disease and both loci). Use gene frequencies of 0.28 for the *A* allele, 0.06 for the *B* allele, and 0.66 for the *O* allele (Cavalli-Sforza and Bodmer, 1971). Analyze those data in two-point analysis, disease versus ABO, and marker 1 versus ABO. Are these results consistent? Why or why not?

9.

Advanced Applications of Affection Status I: Incomplete Penetrance Revisited

In this chapter we use the affection status locus type to allow for various penetrance models which are sometimes quite complicated. We review the basics of incomplete penetrance, and learn how to allow for age-dependent penetrance through the use of *liability classes,* while allowing for phenocopies in a possibly age-dependent manner.

9.1 Age-dependent Penetrance

One potential problem in a linkage analysis is the presence of incomplete penetrance. In Chapter 5, we saw how to allow for constant reduced penetrance. However, in most cases, the penetrance reduction is not constant, but is rather dependent on age. Let us return to the pedigree EX1.PED, from Chapter 2, and reanalyze it under the assumption of age-dependent penetrance. In this case, we assume that the penetrance is 0 for persons up to 10 years of age, and then age of onset is uniformly distributed, with a maximum penetrance of 1 at age 20. This age-of-onset function means that given the susceptible genotype, everyone becomes affected at some point between age 10 and 20, with onset at each age being equally likely. The density function and corresponding distribution function are shown graphically in Figure 9–1.

To incorporate such an *age-of-onset* function in the LINKAGE programs, you need to use what are known as liability classes in conjunction with the affection status locus type. In this case, we can have separate penetrance definitions for persons of each age from age ≤ 10 (penetrance $= 0$), through age ≥ 20 (penetrance $= 1$) as follows: Read the file INC.DAT into the PREP-LINK program. Then select options *(k) See or modify loci description* and *(a) SEE OR MODIFY A LOCUS,* for locus *1,* the disease. Now, we want to define the age-of-onset penetrances by using liability classes, but how many liability classes do we need? To determine this, we need to know the ages of the persons in the pedigree *(current age,* or *age last seen).* The ages are as follows: *father* $= 50$, *mother* $= 45$, *dau1* $= 8$, *dau2* $= 13$, *son1* $= 16$, *dau3* $= 17$, *son2* $= 22$. The penetrances for each of them are easily computed, given our assumptions about age-dependent penetrance. For simplicity, and

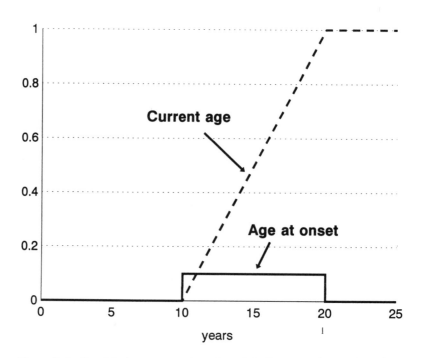

Figure 9–1. Graphical representation of straight line age-of-onset functions

since we have only information about current age, and not age of onset, we use the distribution function of the age of onset as our penetrance function, that is,

$$\text{Penetrance} = P(\text{Becoming affected at or before}$$

$$\text{the current age} \mid \text{Genotype})$$

For persons aged 10 and under, the penetrance is 0; for persons 20 and over, the penetrance is 1; and for persons between 10 and 20, the penetrance is just $0.10 \times (\text{age} - 10)$, which is the equation of the distribution function, in other words, the line between coordinates (age = 10, penetrance = 0) and (age = 20, penetrance = 1). Therefore, the penetrances for each person in the pedigree are as follows: *father* = 1, *mother* = 1, *dau1* = 0, *dau2* = 0.3, *son1* = 0.6, *dau3* = 0.7, *son2* = 1. Because there are five different penetrance classes needed to specify the penetrances for all the persons in this pedigree, we need to use PREPLINK now, to change option *(b) NUMBER OF LIABILITY CLASSES* to 5. Then, you must modify the penetrances for each of the five liability classes in the following manner. Select *(c) PENETRANCES:*, and modify the penetrances, letting liability class 1 be for persons aged less than 10 years (*dau1*, for example). The new penetrances should be entered as follows:

```
LIABILITY CLASS: 1
GENOTYPE  1 1    OLD PEN   0.000000
?
0
GENOTYPE  1 2    OLD PEN   1.000000
?
0
GENOTYPE  2 2    OLD PEN   1.000000
?
0
```

This is because the probability of being affected is 0 for all genotypes in this age class. Next you are asked to provide penetrances for liability class 2, which, for convenience sake, should be the next largest penetrance value, which occurs for the 13-year-old *dau2*, who has penetrance of 0.3. Because this disease is still assumed to be autosomal dominant with reduced penetrance, the value 0.3 should be given for both susceptible genotypes, *1 2*, and *2 2* (*2* being the disease allele) as follows:

```
LIABILITY CLASS  :  2
GENOTYPE  1 1    OLD PEN    0.000000
?
0
GENOTYPE  1 2    OLD PEN    0.000000
?
0.3
GENOTYPE  1 2    OLD PEN    0.000000
?
0.3
```

Continue to enter penetrances for the remaining liability classes as indicated in Table 9–1.

After you enter these penetrances, return to the main menu, and save this file as INC2.DAT. Next, copy the file EX1.PRE to INC2.PRE, and read it into your word processor. You must now modify the phenotypes given for the affection status locus by adding an extra column, indicating the liability class for each individual. In this case, you can determine which liability class goes with each individual by consulting Table 9–1. Please add an extra column after the affection status (1 = unaffected, 2 = affected), with the appropriate liability class number. One important thing to note, which is different from all other locus types, is that when an individual is unknown at an affection status locus with multiple liability classes, you must specify the individual as being 0 (Unknown), in any liability class. Which liability class you use is immaterial, but this second column *must* be nonzero. A safe way of coding this information is to put the individual in the appropriate liability class, based on his age, in case you go back to add new phenotypic information later, although using 0 1 as the code for unknowns gives appropriate results for *all* unknowns as well! The final pedigree file (INC2.PRE) should look like the following:

```
ex1   father  0        0        1  2 5  1 2
ex1   mother  0        0        2  1 5  1 1
ex1   dau1    father   mother   2  1 1  1 2
ex1   dau2    father   mother   2  2 2  1 2
ex1   son1    father   mother   1  2 3  1 2
ex1   dau3    father   mother   2  1 4  1 1
ex1   son2    father   mother   1  1 5  1 1
[EOF]
```

Table 9–1. Penetrance Class Definitions for INC2.PED; INC2.DAT

| Liability Class | Age | Penetrances for Genotypes | | | Relevant Individuals |
		1 1	*1 2*	*2 2*	
1	<10	0	0	0	*dau1*
2	13	0	0.3	0.3	*dau2*
3	16	0	0.6	0.6	*son1*
4	17	0	0.7	0.7	*dau3*
5	>20	0	1	1	*father, mother, son2*

Table 9–2. Analysis Results of INC2.PED; INC2.DAT

θ	Log$_{10}$ Likelihood	Lod Score
0.0	−8.152963	0.789145
0.1	−8.321516	0.620593
0.2	−8.505736	0.436372
0.3	−8.698514	0.243595
0.4	−8.868216	0.073893
0.5	−8.942108	0.000000

ILINK: $\hat{\theta} = 0.000$; $Z(\hat{\theta}) = 0.789145$.

Now, process the file with MAKEPED to produce pedigree file INC2.PED, and analyze the pedigree with MLINK and ILINK through the LCP shell program, as you have been doing throughout the book. The output is presented in Table 9–2.

Can you understand why these results are so different from those we obtained when we allowed for complete penetrance in Chapter 3, and from the simple incomplete penetrance model used in Chapter 5? The individual *dau1* was the individual who was a likely recombinant if penetrance was complete, but when one allows for the fact that at her young age, she had no possibility of being affected, regardless of her genotype, all the evidence for a recombination disappears.

If there is full penetrance in reality, though, and you model the disease as having reduced penetrance, you tend to lose information, as you will see in the next example. Please go back to the example of a known, fully penetrant, recessive disease we analyzed in Chapter 5 (files EX3.*). Let us model this disease as if it were autosomal recessive with constant reduced penetrance of 50%. Modify the penetrances for the affection status locus in the parameter file, EX3.DAT, by the same method as in the dominant disease above. This time, however, change the penetrances to fit an autosomal recessive trait with 50% penetrance.

Then, save this file as INCREC.DAT, and reanalyze the pedigree in EX3.PED. The lod scores obtained are shown in Table 9–3.

Go back to the example in Chapter 5 where we analyzed this pedigree under the model of complete penetrance and see that the maximum lod score was 0.976874. So, information was lost by specifying the reduced penetrance model. Whereas all unaffected persons were previously known not to be homozygous for the disease, under this model it is possible for any of the unaffected individuals to have the disease-susceptibility genotype. Hence, it is not clear whether or not they represent recombinants. Here, there is a lowering of the lod score from allowing for reduced penetrance, whereas in our

Table 9–3. Analysis Results of EX3.PED; INCREC.DAT

θ	Log$_{10}$ Likelihood	Lod Score
0.0	−16.020575	0.776033
0.1	−16.200742	0.595866
0.2	−16.391282	0.405326
0.3	−16.579914	0.216694
0.4	−16.733805	0.062803
0.5	−16.796608	0.000000

ILINK: $\hat{\theta} = 0.000$; $Z(\hat{\theta}) = 0.776033$.

previous example, the lod score rose substantially from such allowances. There are situations when a wrong model may give a higher lod score than the true model, but under the true genetic model, your power will be higher, in general.

9.2 Distribution Functions versus Density Functions

It is important to delineate exactly what age it is that you are reporting as part of a phenotype. If the individual concerned is affected with the disease, then there are two different types of age observation possible. If it is known at what age the person became affected with the disease, then report this age of onset for the disease. Sometimes, however, it is not known at what age an individual became affected, and is merely known that they are currently affected with the disease, in which case the current age (or age of last examination) should be reported in the phenotype. If the age of onset is only approximately known, it may still be useful to incorporate such information in the analysis. These two situations require very different penetrance definitions. If you are using current age, then all you know is that at some point before the current age, the person became affected. Hence, the probability we are interested in is

P(affected *before* current age)

which is a cumulative distribution function. This is analogous to the age-of-onset distribution applied in the first example in this chapter. If the data are available on age of onset, however, it is imperative to consider something a little bit different

P(affected *at* age of onset)

which can be taken more accurately from the probability density function, not the distribution function. This difference is very subtle, but can be of major importance. For unaffected individuals, of course, there is no such thing as an age of onset, but merely the age of last exam (or current age). In this situation, we are interested in

P(not affected before age of last exam) = 1 − *P*(affected before age of last exam)

Therefore, this is also based on the distribution function described above.

Consider the simple case of a dominant disease. For any given individual, the penetrances *f* for the three genotypes are as follows:

$$P(\text{aff} \mid DD) = P(\text{aff} \mid Dd) = f(\text{age}); P(\text{aff} \mid dd) = 0.$$

For any affected individual, therefore, genotype *dd* is impossible, and the other two genotypes have equal penetrance, so the only discriminatory power comes from the elimination of genotype *dd*. In this case, you can see that the likelihood of any affected individual may be written as

$$f(\text{age})P(DD) + f(\text{age})P(Dd) + 0 \times P(dd) = f(\text{age})[P(DD) + P(Dd)]$$

If *P(DD)* is a function of θ, then the likelihood ratio is

$$\frac{f(\text{age}) [P(Dd;\theta) + P(DD;\theta)]}{f(\text{age}) [P(Dd;\theta = 0.5) + P(DD;\theta = 0.5)]}$$

The numerical value of *f*(age) is unimportant, therefore, because it only acts as a constant multiplier of the likelihood in both numerator and denominator of the likelihood ratio and factors out of the lod score equation. So, in the absence of phenocopies, the numerical value of the penetrance is immaterial for affected individuals. However, for unaffected individuals, the corresponding penetrances are as follows:

$$P(\text{Not aff.} \mid DD) = P(\text{Not aff.} \mid Dd) = 1 - f(\text{age})$$
$$P(\text{Not aff.} \mid dd) = 1$$

In this case, the numerical value of $f(\text{age})$ is important in discriminating between genotypes, because there is no longer this equal weighting factor. The likelihood of any unaffected individual is thus

$$[1 - f(\text{age})]*[P(Dd;\theta) + P(DD;\theta)] + P(dd;\theta)$$

There is no longer a common factor to cancel in numerator and denominator, and thus the numerical value of the penetrance is crucial to the analysis.

9.3 Phenocopies

The situation is much more complicated, however, when the presence of *phenocopies* is allowed for. If there are separate age distributions for phenocopies and genetic cases, then rather complicated situations can arise. For unaffected individuals, the distribution function must be used for both penetrances, for the same reasons outlined above. However, for affected persons, the distinction between density and distribution function can be crucial. Consider that if $f(\text{age})$ is the penetrance for genetic cases, and $f_p(\text{age})$ is the penetrance for phenocopies, then the likelihood of any affected individual is

$$f(\text{age}) [P(DD) + P(Dd)] + f_p(\text{age})P(dd)$$

No longer is there a common factor that can factor out of numerator and denominator in the likelihood ratio. Therefore, special attention must be paid to the numerical value of the penetrances. Consider the extreme case of a genetic disease with age-dependent penetrance according to a straight-line, age-of-onset distribution function, on the range of 10 years to 20 years, with the penetrance for individuals at age 20 or above being full. Similarly, let the phenocopies follow a similar straight-line distribution function, starting from 0 up to age 15 and rising to 10% at age 30. It is significant that in general using a uniform distribution is far from ideal because its density function is either 0 or a fixed larger value. In general, it is wiser to use a lognormal or normal age-of-onset density function because these allow age to be a greater discriminatory factor in interpreting the genotypic background, given the phenotypes. The distribution functions and densities corresponding to our uniform distributions are outlined in Table 9–4.

Table 9–4. Uniform Distribution and Density Functions Shown for Phenocopies and Genetic Cases

| Age | Phenocopies | | Genetic Cases | |
	Distribution	*Density*	*Distribution*	*Density*
0–10	0	0	0	0
10–15	0	0	0.1 (age − 10)	0.1
15–20	0.0067 (age − 15)	0.0067	0.1 (age − 10)	0.1
20–30	0.0067 (age − 15)	0.0067	1	0
30–	0.1	0	1	0

Table 9–5. Values of f_p (age)/f (age) for Each Age Group

Age	Distribution	Density
0–10	Undefined	Undefined
10–15	0	0
15–20	0.067 (age − 15)/(age − 10)	0.067
20–30	0.0067 (age − 15)	∞
30–	0.1	Undefined

If we think of the likelihood of an individual

$$f(\text{age}) \,[P(DD) + P(Dd)] + f_p(\text{age})P(dd)$$

as being a function of the ratio of phenocopies to genetic cases, then we can parametrize it as

$$f(\text{age})[P(DD) + P(Dd)] + kf(\text{age})[P(dd)$$
$$= f(\text{age})[P(DD) + P(Dd) + kP(dd)]$$

where $k = f_p(\text{age})/f(\text{age})$. In this representation, $f(\text{age})$ is now equal in numerator and denominator and is factored out of the likelihood ratio. Therefore, the entire amount of information available from the penetrances comes from the ratio $f_p(\text{age})/f(\text{age})$. Values of $f_p(\text{age})/f(\text{age})$ are shown in Table 9–5 for all age ranges.

The ratios are extremely different between the groups, as you can see. Consider an individual with onset at age 25. If we were to use the density functions, we would see that it was impossible for him to have been a genetic case, so he would definitely have been interpreted as a phenocopy. However, based on the distribution function, the ratio would be only 0.067. The interpretations are highly different, because the latter does not give much discriminatory power, and might favor the genetic causes, but the former implies that it was definitely a phenocopy. These ratios are the most important factor in any penetrance model. Clearly, when the ratio is 1:1, there is no phenotypic basis for discriminating between the possible genotypes, and the situation is analogous to that in which the true phenotype is unknown. The more deviant this ratio is from 1, the greater the power to discriminate between genotypes based on phenotype.

In selecting a model, it is important to select a phenocopy probability that makes sense on a population level. If the population prevalence of a disease ϕ is known, then it is imperative that the disease gene frequency p and penetrances f satisfy

$$\phi = f_{DD}p^2 + 2f_{Dd}p(1 - p) + f_{dd}(1 - p)^2$$

Assuming a dominant disease in the extreme case for $p = 0$, clearly $\phi = f_{dd}$, because all cases are nongenetic, so it is clear that $f_{dd} \le \phi$ in all cases. Analogously, for a sex-linked recessive disease, the situation is that only males can be affected, so that effectively $\phi = pf_D + (1-p)f_+$. In this situation, again $f_+ \le \phi$, and all penetrances must be selected such that the prevalence equations are satisfied.

☐ **Exercise 9**

Again, using the same family as in Exercise 8 (files USEREX8.*), assume that there is now incomplete penetrance following a straight-line age-of-onset

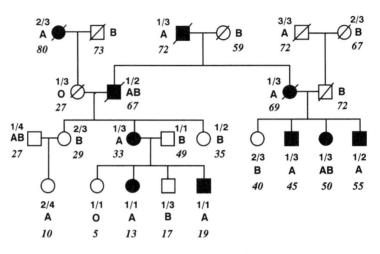

Figure 9–2. Ages added to pedigree from Figure 2–3—USEREX9.*

curve starting from 0.1 at ages less than 10 up to 0.9 at ages 60 and above, where the current ages are given in Figure 9–2 (for more information, consult Ott (1991), p. 160). Please divide your pedigree members into appropriate age classes, and define liability classes containing the penetrances for individuals in each age class. For simplicity's sake, we recommend using age classes as follows (0–9), (10–19), (20–29), . . . Use the midpoint of each age class as the basis for determining the penetrances for people in that class, for example, use age 15 to calculate penetrances for people in the age class (10–19). Analyze the pedigree data starting from $\theta = 0$ up through $\theta = 0.5$ in steps of 0.1 with MLINK, and also analyze the data with ILINK, as you have done throughout this chapter. Please consider both disease versus marker 1, and disease versus ABO.

10.

Advanced Applications of the Affection Status Locus Type II

In this chapter, we explain how to use the affection status locus type to allow for nonstandard situations. We consider complicated dominance relationships, including allowing the identification of obligate carriers. Then, we see how to include data about loci for which only partial information is available. Along the same lines, we discuss elementary approaches to modeling errors in marker typings, and diagnostic uncertainty.

10.1 Generalized Definition of the 2 Phenotype

The fact that a locus is coded as an "affection status" does not in any way imply that the locus must be a disease locus. It merely defines the way the data are entered in the pedigree and parameter files for the analysis. Further, it is an unfortunate convention that people think of the phenotype 2 as affected, and of the phenotype 1 as unaffected at this type of locus. Although this may typically be the case in any given analysis with a disease, in reality the phenotype 2 really indicates the presence of a given phenotype defined by the penetrances given in the parameter file. Further, the phenotype 1 really represents the absence of the phenotype defined by the penetrances given in the parameter file. This may sound confusing, but it really is only an unfortunate historical consequence. You see, this locus type was originally formulated with the idea that it would be used only for diseases. Its full potential was apparently not realized at that time. In the case of a disease, the 2 phenotype indicates the presence of the phenotype "affected with the disease" defined by the penetrances in the parameter file, and the 1 phenotype represents the absence of that phenotype defined by the same penetrances. However, in no way does the program assume anything regarding the biological meaning of the 2 phenotype. As an extreme case, in a recessive disease, the trait "unaffected" is dominant over the "affected" trait. One could use an affection status locus to code the trait "normal" by defining penetrances corresponding to a fully penetrant dominant trait, with gene frequency of the trait allele being very high. Then, the phenotype 2 corresponds to the presence of the "unaffected" phenotype, and 1 means the absence of the "unaffected" phenotype (or, simply affected with the disease). As an additional example, reconsider the fully penetrant dominant disease data from files EX8.*. Add a fifth locus to this pedigree. First read the parameter file EX8.DAT into PREP-LINK, and add an additional locus to the file, as you have already learned to do. At this additional locus, our goal is to set up the penetrances such that the 2 phenotype corresponds to the absence of disease. In other words, our phenotype in this case is "absence of disease." We have already seen that recessivity and dominance are the same thing, meaning that when (*1* > *2*), clearly (*2* < *1*). So in our fully penetrant dominant disease, (*disease* > *nondisease*), so (*nondisease* < *disease*). Thus, we set up this new locus to represent a fully penetrant recessive condition.

Change the newly added locus in the parameter file to an affection status locus type, and set up the penetrances to correspond to a fully penetrant recessive condition, with penetrances as follows:

```
ENTER NEW PENETRANCES
GENOTYPE   1 1 OLD PEN   0.00000E + 00
?
0
GENOTYPE   1 2 OLD PEN   0.00000E + 00
?
0
GENOTYPE   2 2 OLD PEN   1.00000E + 00
?
1
```

The only thing we need to be careful about now is our gene frequency representation. Clearly, the recessive allele is the nondisease allele, so it must get the corresponding gene frequency of 0.99999. In this representation, the nondisease allele is allele number *2*, so you must modify the gene frequencies, such that allele *1* has frequency of 0.00001, and allele *2* has frequency of 0.99999. Finally, save this new file as EX9.DAT.

Now, go back to the pedigree file EX9.PRE and add the new affection status phenotypes at the end of each line (after the two binary factors loci). Be sure to code all diseased individuals as 1, and all normal individuals as 2. This should be exactly the opposite of the first locus, in the sense that all individuals who were coded as 2 at locus 1, should now be coded as 1 at locus 5, and vice versa. Please analyze locus 5 versus 2, by setting up the MLINK and ILINK analyses in LCP in the same manner as you have been doing throughout the book. The results should be identical to the lod scores and likelihoods obtained in the original analysis of this pedigree in Chapter 3. Now, you should be able to clearly see that the 2 phenotype does not necessarily mean affected but has a biological meaning only in accordance with how you defined the penetrances in the parameter file.

10.2 Codominant Marker Loci

We continue this chapter by pointing out that you can code markers as affection status loci as well, if you wish to. Reconsider the same pedigree from files EX9.*, with the fully penetrant autosomal disease. We shall now add a sixth locus to this pedigree, in which we recode the codominant allele numbers locus as an affection status locus type. For our example, we merely want to define a simple codominant marker as an affection status locus to show the

Table 10–1. Affection Status Representation of Two-allele Codominant System

| Liability Class | Allele Numbers | Penetrances for Genotypes | | | Affection Status Coded as |
		1 2	*1 2*	*2 2*	
1	*1 1*	1	0	0	2 1
2	*1 2*	0	1	0	2 2
3	*2 2*	0	0	1	2 3

potential equivalence of locus types; so for the marker we've been looking at in this example, the penetrances are presented in Table 10–1.

Now you see the penetrance relationship between genotypes and phenotypes, where penetrance is defined as P(phenotype | genotype). So, in row 1, you see the probability of phenotype 1 1 given genotype *1 1* is 1, and the probability of phenotype 1 1 given genotype *1 2* or *2 2* is 0. This is just a straight codominant locus. The last column is the affection status notation by which you define each phenotype. The first 2 means presence of some phenotype for which penetrances are defined, and the second number indicates which liability class the appropriate penetrances are given in. If the phenotype is 2 in liability class 1, it means that at the locus in question, the penetrances in liability class 1 are the probabilities of the observed phenotype (whatever that may be) given each of the possible genotypes. So you know that the person has probability 1 of having this phenotype if he has marker genotype *1 1,* and probability 0 of having this phenotype if he has genotype *1 2* or *2 2.* Thus, you know this person has genotype *1 1.*

However, you can also assign the phenotype 1 in liability class 1, in which case the penetrances for the individual's phenotype are 1 minus the penetrances given in liability class 1. In other words a person with phenotype 1 in liability class 1 has the given phenotype with probability 0 for genotype *1 1,* and with probability 1 for genotype *1 2* or *2 2.* Therefore, all you know about this individual is that he is definitely not a *1 1,* but he could be either *1 2* or *2 2.* This is one way of coding a dominance relationship. But for our purposes, we want to code a codominance relationship, so we give everyone phenotype 2, with the appropriate liability class assigned to each phenotype. Now, following the scheme in the last column of Table 10–1, please add a sixth column to EX9.PRE, corresponding to the marker type of each individual in affection status notation. Then save it as EX10.PRE, and process it with MAKEPED to make a file EX10.PED. Now, call up the PREPLINK program, read in EX9.DAT, and add a sixth locus, this time of affection status type. Then, make the screen, under see or modify locus 6, look like the following:

```
*****************************************
(a) NUMBER OF ALLELES          :2
(b) NUMBER OF LIABILITY CLASSES  :3
(c) PENETRANCES:
LIABILITY CLASS  : 1
GENOTYPE    1 1  1.00000E + 00
GENOTYPE    1 2  0.00000E + 00
GENOTYPE    2 2  0.00000E + 00
LIABILITY CLASS  : 2
GENOTYPE    1 1  0.00000E + 00
GENOTYPE    1 2  1.00000E + 00
GENOTYPE    2 2  0.00000E + 00
LIABILITY CLASS  : 3
```

```
GENOTYPE   1 1  0.00000E + 00
GENOTYPE   1 2  0.00000E + 00
GENOTYPE   2 2  1.00000E + 00
(d) GENE FREQUENCIES :
0.500000 0.500000
(e) EXIT
*****************************************
```

Then, save the new file as EX10.DAT. Invoke LCP to use MLINK to analyze loci 1 and 6, and compare this with an analysis of loci 5 and 2, in the manner described above. Then compare the results again. Of course, they should again be identical, or else you should recheck your input files, and reconsider the logic of your model.

10.3 Carrier Status

There are frequently recessive diseases for which some carriers of the disease allele (heterozygotes) show some mild phenotypic effect that distinguishes them from homozygous normal individuals. In such cases, it may be useful to incorporate this information in the linkage analysis. However, it is very important to point out that if the only reason for calling an individual an obligate carrier is genetic (i.e., because he has affected children), it is *not* in principle a good idea to tell the program this individual is a carrier. If this person is an obligate carrier, the programs determine that themselves, although at some minor expense in computing time. Further, when you add this kind of information, errors are more likely, and occasionally can be based on unwarranted assumptions. Therefore, indicate that a person is an obligate carrier only for phenotypic reasons. If all carriers are recognizable, then the disease is essentially codominant, with each genotype corresponding to a unique phenotype ($+/+$ = Unaffected, $+/d$ = Carrier, d/d = Affected). Then, the disease can be coded in the same manner as the codominant marker system in the previous example. Let us return to the recessive disease pedigree we analyzed in Chapter 5 (files EX3.*). This time, we assume that we know that the following unaffected people are carriers: *fgrandpa, mgrandma, father, mother*. Similarly, *fgrandma, mgrandma, dau1, dau3,* and *son2* are phenotypically determined to be homozygous unaffected individuals. Now, enter this new third locus at the end of each line of the data file. You can use the same penetrance scheme as explained for codominant marker loci, assigning the *2* allele, for example, as the disease-causing allele. Please make the appropriate modifications to the pedigree and parameter files, and save them as EX11.*. Then analyze them as usual with MLINK and ILINK. The solutions are given in Table 10–2.

In this example, our lod score tripled from 0.98 to 3.01, due to the phenotypic information we used to distinguish carriers from homozygous normal individuals. Of course, if there were no linkage, we would expect that adding the additional information would likely make the lod scores significantly smaller. This example shows how much more information we can get from a codominant locus versus a recessive locus in the same family. Now, every meiosis is phase-known and informative, from *mother* and *father* to their children. These 10 phase-known nonrecombinants give us a lod score of $\log_{10}[(1 - \theta)^{10}/(0.5)^{10}]$, which is maximized at $\theta = 0$, to give us $\log_{10}[2^{10}] = 10 \log_{10}[2] = 3.010$. When the disease is recessive with no phenotypic means

Table 10–2. Analysis Results for EX11.PED; EX11.DAT

θ	Log₁₀(Likelihood)	Lod Score
0.0	−15.418534	3.010294
0.1	−15.876108	2.552720
0.2	−16.387632	2.041196
0.3	−16.967550	1.461277
0.4	−17.637017	0.791811
0.5	−18.428828	0.000000

ILINK: $\hat{\theta} = 0.000$; $Z(\hat{\theta}) = 3.010294$.

to discriminate carriers from homozygous normal individuals, much less phase and genotype information is available, causing the observed drastic reduction in lod score.

10.4 Diagnostic Uncertainty

Now, consider a situation in which you do not know whether someone is truly affected, but a clinician can assign the individual a probability of being affected *(based on nongenetic reasons!)*. How can we use the LINKAGE programs to allow for such diagnostic uncertainty? It is possible to model such diagnostic uncertainty in the affection status locus type by using liability classes to define penetrances for each such degree of uncertainty. Ott (1991) described a method whereby the penetrances can be generated for individuals who have a given uncertainty of diagnosis by forming a weighted average of the penetrances for unaffected and affected phenotypes. Essentially if we know the probability p of being affected with a disease, then we can compute the penetrance given genotype *1/1* as

$$p(P(\text{affected} \mid 1/1)) + (1-p)(P(\text{unaffected} \mid 1/1))$$

and so on for the other genotypes. The justification for such an ad hoc approach is discussed in detail in Ott (1991).

Let us assume, for example, that the disease you wish to analyze is inherited as an autosomal dominant disorder. You need to have a certain degree of uncertainty in the diagnosis. Let us assume that you have the four following different observed phenotypes at the disease locus: (1) Definitely affected; (2) Definitely unaffected; (3) Affected with 80% certainty; (4) Unaffected with 80% certainty. Assuming the disease to be fully penetrant, and using the affection status locus type, devise a method of using all of this information in your analysis. Enter the data from Figure 10–1, in which the values under each person in the drawing correspond to the age of the individual, his or her diagnostic class (as defined above), and his or her ABO blood type.

Please enter all the necessary information about this pedigree in LINKAGE format (files EX12.PED; EX12.DAT), with gene frequency for the disease allele of 0.1, and at ABO, use binary factors notation, and gene frequencies of .26 for the A allele, 0.06 for the B allele, and 0.68 for the O allele. Then run MLINK and ILINK on this family in the manner you have been doing throughout the book. (This problem is further developed in Exercise 10.)

For individuals in diagnostic class 3, the penetrance for AA or Aa individuals is $(0.8) \times (1) + (0.2) \times (0) = 0.8$, and that for people with aa genotype

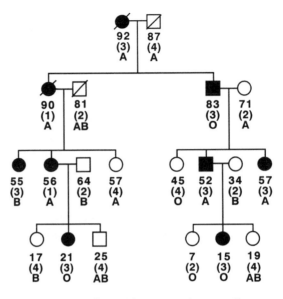

Figure 10–1. Diagnostic uncertainty pedigree—EX12.*

is $(0.8) \times (0) + (0.2) \times (1) = 0.2$. In essence, we can code our four phenotypes with the following penetrance classes:

	AA	Aa	aa
(1)	1	1	0
(2)	0	0	1
(3)	0.8	0.8	0.2
(4)	0.2	0.2	0.8

In this simple case, the penetrances for phenotype 2 are equal to 1 minus the penetrance for phenotype 1, and the same relationship applies between phenotypes 3 and 4. Therefore, we need only two liability classes, corresponding to phenotypes 1 and 3. Then individuals in class 2 are coded as 1 in the liability class for phenotype 1, and class 4 individuals are coded as 1 in the liability class for phenotype 3. In essence we need the following two liability classes:

Class 1	1	1	0
Class 2	0.8	0.8	0.2

Table 10–3. Analysis Results for EX12.PED; EX12.DAT

θ	$\text{Log}_{10}(\text{Likelihood})$	Lod Score
0.0	−17.663268	−0.208789
0.1	−17.357955	0.096524
0.2	−17.317604	0.136875
0.3	−17.347853	0.106626
0.4	−17.397023	0.057456
0.5	−17.454479	0.000000

ILINK: $\hat{\theta} = 0.186$; $Z(\hat{\theta}) = 0.137380$.

And, the codes for the four phenotypic classes are as follows: Class 1 = 2 1 Class 2 = 1 1, Class 3 = 2 2, Class 4 = 1 2, Unknown = 0 1 or 0 2, with no difference.

MLINK results are given in Table 10–3.

10.5 ABO Blood Group Revisited

In Chapter 8, we learned how to code the ABO blood group as a binary factors type of locus. Now that you have a basic idea about binary factors loci, we discuss another important application of affection status loci. This application is sometimes useful if there are complicated dominance relationships at your marker locus, as there are at the ABO blood group. This only means that you must define the penetrances for each phenotype in separate liability classes. The penetrances for the ABO blood group phenotypes are shown in Table 10–4.

In this example, you can see how the affection status locus type can be used to specify complicated dominance relationships.

In summary, in this chapter we saw that the affection status locus type can be used to characterize any type of mendelian inheritance and is not limited to disease traits. In fact, a more appropriate name for this locus type is *dichotomous locus type*. We saw earlier that the allele numbers locus type can handle a subset of all possible binary factors in a simpler notation. Similarly, in this chapter, we saw that the binary factors locus type can code a small subset of all possible modes of inheritance codable under an affection status locus type. Any phenotype–genotype equivalence that can be described with the allele numbers or binary factors notation can also be handled in an affection status. Plus, the affection status has the additional advantage of allowing for penetrance values other than 0 or 1, making it even more flexible than the other locus types. It is possible to perform all linkage-analyses with the LINKAGE programs without ever using any allele numbers or binary factors loci, but as we have seen, they provide convenient shorthand notations for simple, fully penetrant genetic loci.

□ Exercise 10

Go back to the second part of Exercise 8 (files USEREX8.*), and recode the ABO blood group as an affection status locus in the manner described above. Then, perform the same analyses as you did in Exercise 8 with ABO, replacing the binary factors representation of it with the new affection status representation. The results of the analysis will be identical, unless you have made

Table 10–4. Affection Status Representation of ABO Blood Group

Liability Class	Phenotype	Penetrances for Genotypes						Affection Status Coded as
		AA	AB	AO	BB	BO	OO	
1	A	1	0	1	0	0	0	2 1
2	B	0	0	0	1	1	0	2 2
3	AB	0	1	0	0	0	0	2 3
4	O	0	0	0	0	0	1	2 4

errors. Also, recode the disease from that exercise as a recessive trait (In this case, the 2 phenotype represents "normal"). Finally, recode the codominant marker locus from this example as an affection status locus. Reanalyze the pedigree with these new affection status loci, and compare the results. They should be identical to the results obtained from the earlier allele numbers and binary factors representations.

Reconsider the example from this chapter's text (EX9.*), with the 80% diagnostic certainty. Assume that that disease has constant 70% penetrance, instead of the full penetrance you previously assumed. Analyze the pedigree with MLINK and ILINK.

Next, go back and insert the 0.5% phenocopy rate in the analysis, along with the diagnostic uncertainty and reduced penetrance models. Reanalyze the pedigree with MLINK and ILINK.

Next, assume that the disease is also inherited with reduced penetrance following a straight-line, age-of-onset curve. In this case the penetrances for the susceptible genotypes range from 10% for those younger than age 10 up to 90% for those older than 50, and the penetrance curve for those with non-susceptible genotypes (phenocopy rate) also follows a straight-line, age-of-onset curve, with penetrances ranging from 0.2% younger than age 20, rising to 1% for those older than age 60. Now define a liability class notation for this locus by dividing the population into six age classes as follows (0–9), (10–19), (20–34), (35–49), (50–59), (60–100), calculating penetrance values for the median age of each group (e.g., (0–9) : use age 5; (20–34): use age 27). Note that you now need many liability classes. Because not all of them are used in this specific pedigree, you can recode the locus to include only the liability classes you do need for this analysis, based on the diagnostic class–age combinations appearing in this pedigree.

Let us assume now that it is possible for some individuals to be (1) either type A or AB; (2) type B or AB; (3) A or O; or (4) B or O. In other words, the blood types are not uniquely determined, but some information was obtained from a partial test. In this pedigree, now assume that the 56-year-old mother of three in the third generation has type (1) above, the probably affected 15-year-old girl in the fourth generation has type (2) above, the 57-year-old probably affected female on the extreme right of the drawing in the third generation has type (3) above, and the 17-year-old probably unaffected female in the fourth generation on the extreme left of the drawing has type (4) above. Now recode your pedigree file, and reanalyze the family.

11 □

The LIPED Program

LIPED (for LIkelihoods in PEDigrees) was the first generally available program for linkage analysis (Ott, 1974). It has changed little since it was extended to handle general pedigrees (Ott, 1976), except that age-of-onset functions were later incorporated. It contained one error relating to the likelihood of qualitative traits; fortunately, that mistake was caught by Dr. Robert Elston soon after the program was distributed. The fact that is has been bug-free ever since is probably the main reason it is still being used and is considered by many people to be the gold standard for such programs. Below we give you a general description of the LIPED program and provide an example of how to use it.

11.1 Characteristics of LIPED

LIPED is written in FORTRAN 77 and runs almost unmodified on most computers. Many researchers have adapted it to their computers and have made various modifications to it. We support only its PC version, which currently is compiled with Microsoft FORTRAN 5.1. It is distributed with various sample input files and an extensive documentation. Also, batch files are included that provide the commands necessary for compiling it under DOS and OS/2.

Only two loci can be handled by LIPED at any one time, but the program is set up to carry out various two-point analyses in a single run. All preprocessing steps, such as the ones carried out by the MAKEPED program, are incorporated in a single program. Below, the main similarities and differences between LIPED and LINKAGE are pointed out.

As in the LINKAGE programs, the likelihood is calculated recursively by the use of the Elston-Stewart algorithm, but no iterative parameter estimation is possible as in the ILINK program. In both LIPED and LINKAGE, program constants are set for maximum number of alleles, loops, and so on, and new values of these constants require recompilation of the programs.

LIPED calculates lod scores for a sequence of recombination fractions or a sequence of points of male (θ_m) and female (θ_f) recombination fractions, which are displayed in a rectangular coordinate system with axes of θ_m and θ_f.

Five locus types (selected through a variable called KONT) are distinguished in LIPED:

1. Qualitative phenotypes with penetrances of 0 or 1
2. Qualitative phenotypes with any penetrances
3. Quantitative phenotypes following a normal distribution
4. Disease phenotypes (affected/unaffected) with age of onset following a lognormal distribution
5. Disease phenotypes with age of onset following a straight-line penetrance curve.

The last two locus types make it very easy to handle age-dependent penetrance because the different cases of age-of-onset known or unknown are allowed for through their appropriate density or distribution function. In the LINKAGE programs, properly allowing for age-dependent penetrance can require the setting up of many liability classes.

LIPED cannot directly handle the situation in which both parents in a pedigree have parents in the same pedigree. Such a situation must be accommodated by doubling one of the parents, similar to breaking a loop (see the example below). This requirement is a consequence of the fact that only peeling of the Elston-Stewart type (going up through pedigrees) is incorporated in LIPED, not more general pedigree-traversing algorithms.

For the analysis of a given two-locus problem, LIPED is generally somewhat slower than MLINK, particularly, of course, when upwards branching is present requiring the doubling of individuals in LIPED but not in MLINK.

11.2 An Example: Monozygotic Twins

Several examples are provided in the LIPED documentation so it is not necessary for us to give extensive details here on using the program. Only one example is outlined here, which also demonstrates how monozygotic twins should be handled by LIPED. This example can be calculated in pretty much the same way by MLINK and is thus not specific to LIPED.

Figure 11–1 shows a small three-generation pedigree in which a dominant disease is segregating together with a marker locus with three alleles. Penetrance is incomplete (90%), but no phenocopies occur. Individuals 3.4 and 3.5 are monozygotic twins; that is, they represent two phenotypic expressions of the same genotype. Therefore, for linkage analysis purposes, these two individuals must be represented as a single individual (here denoted by 345). In addition, the penetrances for that single individual must be the squares of the penetrances appropriate for one of the two twins. For example, given the genotype *D/D*, the penetrance for the affected phenotype is 0.90 and that for the unaffected phenotype (the case of our two twins) is 0.10. Thus, the penetrance for the single individual representing the two monozygotic twins must be $(0.10)^2 = 0.01$. To allow for this different set of penetrances, a separate phenotype (liability class) is introduced, here denoted by the symbol MT. Incidentally, no such extra liability class is required in the MENDEL program because it directly provides for the presence of monozygotic twins.

The left side of Figure 11–1 shows the original pedigree, and the pedigree manipulated for input to LIPED is displayed on the right side (note that one of the parents must be doubled). The input file appropriate for this problem is shown below. Comments to the right of ← are optional and are given here only for better clarity.

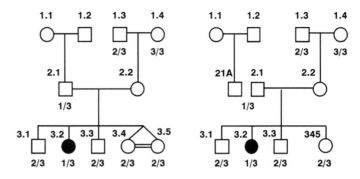

Figure 11–1. Pedigree with monozygotic twins—LIPED

```
1 0000                  Correct analysis
(20A4)
(2A4,21F4.0)
(20A4)
                  m                 ←symbol for unknown (here blank), male (here m)
   2  3                             ←number of alleles at loci 1, 2,. . .
   3  6                             ←number of phenotypes
  −1  0                             ←locus types
   2                                ←output option
 Dis    D    +  AF   NA   MT ←locus name, allele symbols, phenotype symbols
    0.001    0.999                  ←allele frequencies (d = recessive disease allele)
      D    D  .9  .1   .01          ←genotype and penetrances
      D    +  .9  .1   .01
      +    +   0   1    1
 S61    1    2   3  1/1 1/2 1/3 2/2 2/3 3/3 ←allele and phenotype sym-
bols
        .2       .5        .3
   1    1   1
   1    2   0   1
   1    3   0   0    1
   2    2   0   0    0   1
   2    3   0   0    0   0   1
   3    3   0   0    0   0   0   1
   11    1Pedigree with monozygotic twins
  1.1               f   NA
  1.2               m   AF
  21A 1.1 1.2       m   NA 1/3
  1.3               m   NA 2/3
  1.4               f   NA 3/3
  2.2 1.3 1.4       f   NA
  2.1               m   NA 1/3
  3.1 2.1 2.2       m   NA 2/3
  3.2 2.1 2.2       f   AF 1/3
  3.3 2.1 2.2       m   NA 2/3
  345 2.1 2.2       m   MT 2/3
  2.1 21A               ← This line identifies the doubled individual
 9000                   ← Stop value
```

The 1 and 0's on the first input line indicate the presence of a single marker locus, autosomal inheritance, gene frequencies (as opposed to haplotype frequencies), and no mutation. The next three lines contain FORTRAN format statements by which the user can specify the widths (number of spaces) for various input quantities; that is, symbols for loci, alleles, and phenotypes, and the penetrance values. Here, all these quantities are expected to occupy four spaces at most and should be right justified. The following five lines define the symbols for unknown parent (here blank), male sex (here m), and unknown phenotypes (here blank); numbers of alleles, numbers of phenotypes, and locus type for the different loci; and an output option (2 specifies equal male and female recombination fractions with values as shown in the output below).

Next, a group of input lines is reserved for each locus. In each group, the first line specifies the locus symbol, allele symbols for use in the few lines immediately below, and phenotype symbols used in the pedigree data. The next line furnishes the allele frequencies in fixed format F8.4, that is, at most eight spaces are allowed for each of these values. After that, as many lines as there are genotypes are expected, each line defining a genotype and the associated penetrances for each phenotype (blank instead of a number is interpreted by FORTRAN as zero). Be aware that here the penetrances are the conditional probabilities with respect to the phenotypes listed on the first line in each group, whereas in LINKAGE penetrances refer to the 2 phenotype. Because the monozygotic twins are unaffected (phenotype MT), the penetrances for genotypes D/D and $D/+$ are small.

To beak a loop or one of two inheritance lines ascending from two parents, a suitable individual must be doubled. The principle is the same as in the LINKAGE programs, except that here it is the user who must carry out the doubling: One of the two doubles must be coded as an offspring and the other as a mate without parents. The two are later identified as representing the same individual.

On line 23 the first number (here m = 11, right justified in columns 1–4) specifies the number of family members to follow, and the second number (in columns 5–8) denotes the number of pairs of doubled individuals present. The comment (starting in column 9) following the two numbers is optional and appears on the output. The next m lines describe the pedigree data: in each line a unique individual ID, parents' ID's, sex, and phenotypes are needed. After the m-th line, for each pair of doubled individuals, the ID's of the two doubles are listed on one line. Finally, a code consisting of four digits directs the LIPED program to take further actions as indicated by input lines following that code. Here, a stop code *(9000)* is provided.

To run this input file, invoke the program by typing *LIPED*. It then asks for a buffer size to which you give a default response by simply pressing the ⟨Enter⟩ key. Next, LIPED asks for the name of the input file and an output file name (the latter is optional); pressing the ⟨Enter⟩ key only displays the results on the screen. Part of the output resulting from the input shown above is as follows:

```
PROBLEM  1    Correct analysis
**********
(autosomal linkage)

Pedigree     1  Pedigree with monozygotic twins
_____

                           11 individuals

LOCUS  0    Dis    VS.    LOCUS  1    S61
_____

GENE FREQUENCIES FOR  0    Dis    .0010    .9990
GENE FREQUENCIES FOR  1    S61    .2000    .5000    .3000

R MALE    R FEM.    LOG10[L(R)]    LOD-SCORE
.5000    .5000    -10.40960        .000
.4000    .4000    -10.33163        .078
```

.3000	.3000	−10.15452	.255
.2000	.2000	−9.95545	.454
.1000	.1000	−9.76631	.643
.0500	.0500	−9.67790	.732
.0010	.0010	−9.59526	.814
.0000	.0000	−9.59361	.816

As these results show, the maximum lod score (at $\hat{\theta} = 0$) is 0.816. If the two twins are replaced by a single person with unmodified penetrance (here of 0.10), the resulting lod score is 0.779, which in this case is smaller than the correct lod score of 0.816. On the other hand, if the two twins are treated as regular twins (each with penetrance of 0.10), a maximum lod score of 1.039 is obtained, which is clearly higher than the correct lod score. Generally, treating monozygotic twins as fraternal twins tends to have the same effect as duplicating an offspring, that is, "inventing" data for one additional individual. In the long run, this does not introduce a bias in the recombination fraction estimate, but it tends to inflate the lod score and increase the type I error rate, although, in any specific case, the lod score may also be decreased (when the twins represent recombinants).

☐ **Exercise 11**

Modify the input to LIPED shown above to verify that falsely replacing the twins by a single individual with penetrance as for any unaffected phenotype results in a maximum lod score of 0.779. Why is the lod score now smaller?

Similarly, prepare the input so the twins appear as fraternal siblings, leading to a lod score of 1.039. You may have to consult the LIPED manual if you experience problems. Interpret the result.

12.

Solutions to the Exercises in Part I

□ **Exercise 2**

The pre-MAKEPED file USEREX2.PRE should be as follows:

```
userex2    1    0    0    2    2    2 3
userex2    2    0    0    1    1    0 0
userex2    3    0    0    1    2    1 3
userex2    4    0    0    2    1    0 0
userex2    5    0    0    1    1    3 3
userex2    6    0    0    2    1    2 3
userex2    7    2    1    2    1    1 3
userex2    8    3    4    1    2    1 2
userex2    9    3    4    2    2    1 3
userex2   10    5    6    1    1    0 0
userex2   11    8    7    2    1    2 3
userex2   12    0    0    1    1    1 4
userex2   13    8    7    2    2    1 3
userex2   14    0    0    1    1    1 1
userex2   15    8    7    2    1    1 2
userex2   16   10    9    2    1    2 3
userex2   17   10    9    1    2    1 3
userex2   18   10    9    2    2    1 3
userex2   19   10    9    1    2    1 2
userex2   20   12   11    2    1    2 4
userex2   21   14   13    2    1    1 1
userex2   22   14   13    2    2    1 1
userex2   23   14   13    1    1    1 3
userex2   24   14   13    1    2    1 1
[EOF]
```

This is not the only acceptable method for identifying individuals. You can just as easily name individuals in the pedigree with character ID's, but in this case we decided to identify each individual by a number. On processing this file with MAKEPED, the following USEREX2.PED file should result:

```
1    1    0    0    7    0    0   20    2    2 3    Ped:    userex2    Per:    1
1    2    0    0    7    0    0   11    1    0 0    Ped:    userex2    Per:    2
1    3    0    0    8    0    0   10    2    1 3    Ped:    userex2    Per:    3
```

1	4	0	0	8	0	0	2 0	1	0 0	Ped:	userex2	Per:	4
1	5	0	0	10	0	0	1 0	1	3 3	Ped:	userex2	Per:	5
1	6	0	0	10	0	0	2 0	1	2 3	Ped:	userex2	Per:	6
1	7	2	1	11	0	0	2 0	1	1 3	Ped:	userex2	Per:	7
1	8	3	4	11	9	9	1 0	2	1 2	Ped:	userex2	Per:	8
1	9	3	4	16	0	0	2 0	2	1 3	Ped:	userex2	Per:	9
1	10	5	6	16	0	0	1 0	1	0 0	Ped:	userex2	Per:	10
1	11	8	7	20	13	13	2 0	1	2 3	Ped:	userex2	Per:	11
1	12	0	0	20	0	0	1 0	1	1 4	Ped:	userex2	Per:	12
1	13	8	7	21	15	15	2 0	2	1 3	Ped:	userex2	Per:	13
1	14	0	0	21	0	0	1 0	1	1 1	Ped:	userex2	Per:	14
1	15	8	7	0	0	0	2 0	1	1 2	Ped:	userex2	Per:	15
1	16	10	9	0	17	17	2 0	1	2 3	Ped:	userex2	Per:	16
1	17	10	9	0	18	18	1 0	2	1 3	Ped:	userex2	Per:	17
1	18	10	9	0	19	19	2 0	2	1 3	Ped:	userex2	Per:	18
1	19	10	9	0	0	0	1 0	2	1 2	Ped:	userex2	Per:	19
1	20	12	11	0	0	0	2 0	1	2 4	Ped:	userex2	Per:	20
1	21	14	13	0	22	22	2 0	1	1 1	Ped:	userex2	Per:	21
1	22	14	13	0	23	23	2 0	2	1 1	Ped:	userex2	Per:	22
1	23	14	13	0	24	24	1 0	1	1 3	Ped:	userex2	Per:	23
1	24	14	13	0	0	0	1 0	2	1 1	Ped:	userex2	Per:	24

In this file, the additional pointers were added, as explained in Chapter 2. The parameter file USEREX2.DAT should look like the following (after PREPLINK):

```
2 0 0 5  << NO. OF LOCI, RISK LOCUS, SEXLINKED (IF 1) PROGRAM
 0 0.0 0 0.0 0 << MUT LOCUS, MUT RATE, HAPLOTYPE FREQUENCIES (IF 1)
  1 2
1 2  << AFFECTION, NO. OF ALLELES
 0.999990 0.000010  << GENE FREQUENCIES
 1 << NO. OF LIABILITY CLASSES
 0.0000 1.0000 1.0000 << PENETRANCES
3 3  << ALLELE NUMBERS, NO. OF ALLELES
 0.333330 0.333330 0.333330  << GENE FREQUENCIES
 0 0  << SEX DIFFERENCE, INTERFERENCE (IF 1 OR 2)
 0.10000 << RECOMBINATION VALUES
 1 0.10000 0.45000 << REC VARIED, INCREMENT, FINISHING VALUE
```

Depending on the version of PREPLINK you are using, there may be some differences in the number of decimal places in the output files, but the format for this example should be the same as that indicated above.

□ Exercise 3

The analytic solution in this pedigree is extremely complicated and involves a large number of difficult formulas. For this reason, most pedigrees need to be analyzed with computer programs like LINKAGE. In this case, however, we can get some idea of what the recombination fraction should be from examining the most likely situation in this pedigree. The disease appears to be segregating with the *1* allele in this pedigree. If the disease is actually segregating with the *1* allele, there is one obligate recombinant in the unaffected female in the bottom generation with marker genotype *1 1*. Otherwise, there are 12 meioses informative for the disease, in which there are no obligate recombination events. So, we guess that the recombination fraction estimate should be somewhere around 1/13 = 0.077. Of course, the actual estimate is not exactly equal to this because the pedigree is phase-unknown in the upper branches and because there are a few untyped individuals.

When you call up the UNKNOWN program, it gives you the following message:

ERROR: Incompatibility detected in this family for locus 2

This message typically implies there is some error in the input files. First, you should look over the pedigree to ensure that there are no mendelian inconsistencies (i.e., a *1/1* father and a *2/2* mother having a *2/2* child is inconsistent with mendelian inheritance). However, unless you made a typing error when entering the data, this should not be the case. The next thing to investigate is the description of the loci in the parameter file. It seems that the parameter file created in Exercise 2 is compatible with the description of the loci given in that exercise. However, on closer scrutiny of the pedigree, it is clear that although the marker locus was entered as a three-allele system, in the third generation a man married into the pedigree with genotype *1/4,* which is impossible at a three-allele locus. Hence, we need to recode this locus in PREP-LINK to allow for four alleles instead of three. For now, let us assume the four alleles are equally frequent, with gene frequency 0.25 for each allele. Later, in Part III, we will learn more appropriate ways of dealing with gene frequency estimation; we defer further discussion of it until then. Now, when you run the analysis you should get the results shown in Table 12–1. Notice how close the estimated recombination fraction of 0.079 was to our approximation of 1/13 = 0.077. Perhaps we should try and modify our DATA-FILE.DAT file, so that we use a starting value of 0.079 for the recombination fraction (in the ILINK analysis), and see if we can refine this estimate of θ further. When you do this, your new estimate should be $\hat{\theta} = 0.077$, which is exactly 1/13, with $Z(\hat{\theta}) = 1.783275$. Running the ILINK analysis at each recombination fraction (as can be easily done in MLINK) is accomplished by modifying the bottom three lines of your data file. Initially they should look like this:

```
0.10000 << RECOMBINATION VALUES
0 << THIS LOCUS MAY HAVE ITERATED PARS
1
```

This causes the ILINK program to start at $\theta = 0.10000$ and then iterate (since the last line contains a 1) the recombination fraction until the MLE is found. To compute the likelihood at $\theta = 0.10000$, you need to modify the bottom line of the parameter file by replacing the 1 (iterate recombination fraction) with a 0 (fix the recombination fraction). Then you specify the desired recombination fraction on the third line from the bottom of the file. Every time you wish to compute the lod score for a different θ, alter the third line from the bottom and run the ILINK program again. The results will be exactly the same as those shown in Table 12–1).

Table 12–1. Analysis Results from USEREX2.* with MLINK and ILINK

θ	Log_{10}(Likelihood)	Lod Score
0.0	$-\infty$	$-\infty$
0.1	-26.896276	1.767576
0.2	-27.187291	1.476561
0.3	-27.650514	1.013338
0.4	-28.180207	0.483646
0.5	-28.663852	0.000000

ILINK: $\hat{\theta} = 0.079$; $Z(\hat{\theta}) = 1.783267$.

☐ **Exercise 4**

Using LCP, you should specify the values on the first screen as follows:

```
       COMMAND file name [PEDIN.BAT] : PEDIN.BAT
           LOG file name [FINAL.OUT] : FINAL.OUT
        STREAM file name [STREAM.OUT] : STREAM.OUT
      PEDIGREE file name [PEDIN.DAT] : USEREX2.PED
     PARAMETER file name [DATAIN.DAT] : USEREX2.DAT
     Secondary PEDIGREE file name [] :
     Secondary PARAMETER file name [] :
```

Then, after selecting the *MLINK* program, with the *Specific Evaluations,* and *No sex difference* options, you should complete the *MLINK–Lod Score Specification* screen as follows:

```
                     Locus order [  ] : 1 2
     Recombination fractions [.1] : 0
        Recombination varied [1] : 1
           Increment varied [.1] : 0.1
                 Stop value [.5] : 0.4
```

Then, go back and select the *ILINK* program, with the *Specific order,* and *No sex difference* options, and set up the *ILINK–Locus Order Specifications* screen as follows:

```
                     Locus order [  ] : 1 2
     Recombination fractions [.1] : 0.1
```

Then, hit ⟨Page Down⟩ to save this analysis, and hit ⟨Ctrl-Z⟩ to exit. Type *PEDIN* at the DOS prompt, and then examine the FINAL.OUT file. The results contained within this file should be identical to those in Table 12–1.

☐ **Exercise 5**

The results of the analysis of the USEREX2.PED pedigree under 75% penetrance (autosomal dominant) are presented in Table 12–2. Note that in this analysis, the estimated recombination fraction was *0*. This is because it was more likely that the "obligate recombinant" individual in the pedigree was nonpenetrant than a recombinant, when both options were allowed for. The lod score also jumped by about 0.4 units, owing largely to the decreased estimate of θ. With the same amount of data, the smaller the estimated recombination fraction, the stronger the evidence for linkage (this makes sense because the fewer recombinants observed in a fixed sample, the greater the likelihood that the two loci are linked).

Table 12–2. Analysis Results from USEREX2.PED with Autosomal Dominant Model with 75% Penetrance

θ	Log_{10}(Likelihood)	Lod Score
0.0	−27.197236	2.209401
0.1	−27.583813	1.822823
0.2	−28.029907	1.376729
0.3	−28.519204	0.887432
0.4	−29.006410	0.400227
0.5	−29.406636	0.000000

ILINK: $\hat{\theta} = 0.001$; $Z(\hat{\theta}) = 2.206964$.

The analysis of this pedigree under the autosomal recessive model with 75% penetrance is presented in Table 12–3. Note that now the lod scores are almost all uniformly negative. This makes sense, because now all of the affected individuals are forced to be homozygous for the disease allele and thus uninformative for linkage. The unaffected individuals (who did not carry the disease allele under the dominant model) are now forced to be carriers of the disease allele in at least one copy if they have affected children (who must also be homozygous for the disease allele). Thus, all of the information is coming from the individuals who were uninformative in the dominant analysis. If the disease truly were dominant, you would expect these (actual homozygous normal) individuals to transmit either allele to their affected children with equal probability, and therefore, the expected estimate of θ should be 0.5 in these situations.

The results of the same analyses when only 30% penetrance is allowed for are presented in Table 12–4 for the dominant case, and Table 12–5 for the recessive case. From these results, you can see the general effect of lowering the penetrance is to flatten the lod score curve. The magnitudes (positive and negative) are reduced significantly when the penetrance is reduced because the ability to discriminate genotypes among the unaffected individuals is severely limited. When there is 70% penetrance, the unaffected persons have penetrances 1 for $+/+$ genotypes, and 0.3 for $+/D$ or D/D genotypes (assuming a dominant disease). The ratio of penetrances is thus 10/3, or about 3.33:1. However, when the penetrance is reduced to 30%, the ratio of penetrances is reduced to 10/7, or about 1.4:1. When you consider that a penetrance ratio of 1:1 implies an inability to distinguish between genotypes based on a given phenotype, then you can see that a ratio of 1.4:1 isn't much different from calling the unaffected individuals unknown in phenotype, and so you are losing information. Of course, when penetrance is complete, the penetrances for unaffected persons are 1 for $+/+$ genotypes, and 0 for $+/D$ or D/D genotypes, for a penetrance ratio of 1:0 or infinity, because all unaffected individuals must have genotype $+/+$. This is the reason reducing the penetrance has such a major effect on the analysis, and it points out that the effect is due to increased uncertainty about the genotypes of unaffected individuals. Of course, for affected individuals, the penetrance ratio is always $0/f = 0$, whatever the value of f (the penetrance). Hence, the ability to discriminate the genotypes of affected individuals is not altered, unless you are allowing for phenocopies as shown in Chapter 9.

If the disease were actually recessive, and you analyzed it as a dominant disease, you would expect quite a different result. First of all, you would probably have to assume reduced penetrance for the disease, because in a recessive disease parents are typically unaffected. Because in a recessive disease

Table 12–3. Analysis Results from USEREX2.PED with Autosomal Recessive Model with 70% Penetrance

θ	Log$_{10}$(Likelihood)	Lod Score
0.0	−64.367120	−10.326114
0.1	−54.633665	−0.592695
0.2	−54.195452	−0.154446
0.3	−54.031058	0.009948
0.4	−53.993094	0.047912
0.5	−54.041006	0.000000

ILINK: $\hat{\theta} = 0.389$; $Z(\hat{\theta}) = 0.0482982$.

Table 12–4. Analysis Results from USEREX2.PED with Autosomal Dominant Model with 30% Penetrance

θ	Log$_{10}$(Likelihood)	Lod Score
0.0	−30.608103	1.805107
0.1	−30.984986	1.428225
0.2	−31.384362	1.028849
0.3	−31.790104	0.623107
0.4	−32.155375	0.257836
0.5	−32.413210	0.000000

ILINK: $\hat{\theta} = 0.001$; $Z(\hat{\theta}) = 1.802592$.

both parents contribute one disease allele to affected children, if you are looking at a linked marker, it would have to show linkage in both parental meioses. If you were to analyze the disease as if it were dominant, then you would only be considering segregation of the disease from one of the parents, with the other parent typically considered to be homozygous normal. Thus, you would be throwing away half of your truly informative meioses for the disease and marker. Still, you are retaining roughly half of the meioses, in which the marker is, of course, still cosegregating with the linked disease allele. Therefore, you would in general still expect to find positive lod scores and reasonable estimates of the recombination fraction, although your power should be roughly half.

☐ Exercise 6

Looking closely at this pedigree, it is clear that the information for linkage can be collapsed into what is shown in Figure 12–1. Clearly, *GMOTHER2* and *GFATHER2* contribute no information about linkage because they have only one son and did not transmit the disease allele. Hence, they can be left out. Similarly, *GSON1* and *GSON2* merely serve to identify *DAU1* as a carrier of the disease allele, but because she is a homozygote at the marker locus, they provide no other information about linkage. The same holds for *GSON3* and *GSON4*, who only tell us that *DAU2* is a carrier of the disease allele. On the other hand, *GSON5* does provide evidence for linkage. Clearly, the fact that he is affected tells us that his mother, *DAU3*, is a carrier of the disease allele. Furthermore, she is a heterozygote, who received both the disease and the *3* allele from *GMOTHER1*. Because she then transmitted the *2* allele with the disease allele to *GSON5*, there was an obligate recombination event. We also know the phase in each of the six children in this collapsed nuclear family, as

Table 12–5. Analysis Results from USEREX2.PED with Autosomal Recessive Model with 30% Penetrance

θ	Log$_{10}$(Likelihood)	Lod Score
0.0	−66.341955	−9.203737
0.1	−57.732587	−0.594369
0.2	−57.299879	−0.161660
0.3	−57.133608	0.004611
0.4	−57.091982	0.046237
0.5	−57.138219	0.000000

ILINK: $\hat{\theta} = 0.394$; $Z(\hat{\theta}) = 0.046381$.

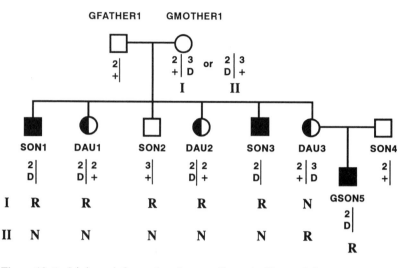

Figure 12–1. Linkage information from pedigree in Figure 6–3

indicated in Figure 12–1. However, we do not know the phase in *GMOTHER1*. Because each of the two phases have equal probability, we can compute the likelihood of this nuclear family from counting recombinants and nonrecombinants under each phase as $\frac{1}{2}[\theta^5(1 - \theta)] + \frac{1}{2}[(1 - \theta)^5\theta]$. Because there is one additional obligate recombinant from *DAU3* to *GSON5*, this whole likelihood should be multiplied by θ to obtain the likelihood for the entire pedigree. The likelihood ratio, therefore, is

$$\{\theta[\theta^5(1 - \theta) + (1 - \theta)^5\theta]\}/(0.5)^6$$

and the lod score, accordingly is

$$6 \log_{10}(2) + \log_{10}(\theta) + \log_{10}[\theta^5(1 - \theta) + (1 - \theta)^5\theta]$$

The results of the analysis of this example with MLINK and ILINK are shown in Table 12–6. To confirm that your analytical result is compatible with the computer analysis, compute the numerical value of the lod score from the formula above at $\theta = 0.10$. From the formula above

$$Z(0.10) = 6 \log_{10}(2) + \log_{10}(0.10) + \log_{10}[(0.10)^5(0.90) + (0.90)^5(0.10)]$$

$$= 1.80618 - 1 - 1.22872 = -0.42254$$

which is exactly what was found with the MLINK program. To further confirm the reduction of the data into the genotypic information contained in Figure 12–1, please enter the pedigree shown in that figure in LINKAGE pedigree and parameter files, coding the disease locus as an allele numbers locus, with the + allele being coded as *1* and the disease allele coded as *2*. Assume gene frequency of 0.01 for the *2* allele at this locus. Leave the second locus as a four-allele allele numbers locus, and analyze this reduced pedigree (remember, the reason for using an allele numbers locus is to allow carriers [*1 2*] to be distinguished from homozygous normal individuals [*1 1*]). When you analyze this new pedigree, the lod scores should be identical to those in Table 12–6, although the likelihoods will be much larger because the pedigree is much smaller.

Table 12–6. Analysis Results from USEREX6.*

θ	Log$_{10}$(Likelihood)	Lod Score
0.0	$-\infty$	$-\infty$
0.05	-12.566381	-0.907257
0.10	-12.081665	-0.422540
0.15	-11.853246	-0.194121
0.20	-11.733741	-0.074617
0.25	-11.676429	-0.017305
0.30	-11.658802	0.000322
0.35	-11.665186	-0.006062
0.40	-11.679781	-0.020657
0.45	-11.683900	-0.024775
0.50	-11.659124	0.000000

ILINK: $\hat{\theta} = 0.857$; $Z(\hat{\theta}) = 0.559736$.

□ **Exercise 7**

If you run the MAKEPED program without declaring any loops, the LOOPS program reports that *Loop(s) present in Family 1*. The LOOPS.OUT file should look like the following:

```
Program LOOPS version 1.17
Programmed by Xiaoli Xie July 1992
Design: Jurg Ott and Xiaoli Xie
Loop(s) in family 1!
Individuals in parentheses are married
The individuals and/or marriages involved are:
Loop 1: 3-(3,4)-7-8-(6,5)-5-(1,2)-3
Loop 2: 7-8-(5,6)-10-9-(3,4)-7
Loop 3: 8-(5,6)-10-(10,9)-13-12-(7,8)-8
Note: ID numbers are as assigned by MAKEPED
```

Thus, the program reports having found three loops in this pedigree: the first being a consanguinity loop connecting the first set of first cousins who married (the first two people in the third generation); the second being a marriage loop with the two brothers in the third generation marrying two sisters; and the third being a consanguinity loop between the two cousins who married in the fourth generation of the pedigree, with the three affected sons. Of course, it is possible to list other loops, such as the consanguinity between the second couple who married in generation 2, and so forth. But the program is saying that if you break the three loops it outlined, no further loops would occur in the pedigree. To see this, go through the pedigree and break one loop at a time. It is important to remember that you need to break the loops by doubling the individuals about whom there is the least amount of genotypic ambiguity (including phase). Begin by breaking the first loop discovered by the LOOPS program by doubling the *1/3* unaffected male in the third generation. The resulting pedigree looks like Figure 12–2. Of course, there are still loops left in this pedigree, so we next decide to break another loop in this pedigree. Run the MAKEPED program and break this one loop, having the LOOPS program identify the remaining loops. In this case, after running the LOOPS program, the first loop detected involves the two cousins who married in the fourth generation. By looking at the pedigree you can see that this loop is still present, even after breaking the first loop. Proceed to break this loop at the unaffected mother of the three affected girls in the fourth generation (the twelfth individual in the pedigree) as shown in Figure 12–3. By looking at this figure,

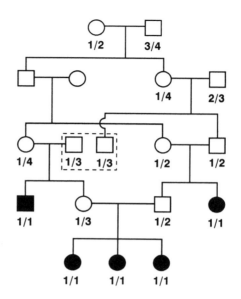

Figure 12–2. Pedigree from Figure 7–5 with one loop broken

however, you can see that at least one loop remains because there is still a first-cousin marriage in the second generation. If you run MAKEPED to break the two loops as we did, the LOOPS program again detects a loop, indicated in the LOOPS.OUT file as the first-cousin marriage in the third generation. If we break this loop by doubling the unaffected male with *1/2* genotype in the third generation (he has the most genotypic information because his parents are typed, and he has to be a carrier of the disease), we are left with the pedigree in Figure 12–4. From examination of this pedigree, no loops seem to remain, as can be more clearly seen if we redraw the pedigree, separating the doubled individuals in such a way that the absence of loops is more apparent, as shown in Figure 12–5. Clearly when the pedigree is redrawn like this, the

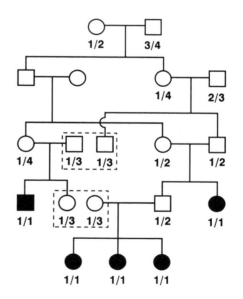

Figure 12–3. Pedigree from Figure 7–5 with two loops broken

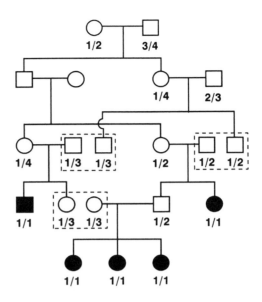

Figure 12–4. Pedigree from Figure 7–5 with three loops broken

absence of remaining loops is apparent. If you now run the MAKEPED program and break the loops in the places we did, the LOOPS program should report *No loop detected in Family 1*, confirming what we see in Figure 12–5.

Of course, we did not select the only possible individuals at which to break the loops. They could just as easily have been broken elsewhere, but it is important to remember that the best strategy (as far as computer time is concerned) is to break all loops at the individuals with the minimum amount of genotypic ambiguity (including phase), because the computing time increases exponentially with the number of possible genotypes for the doubled individual.

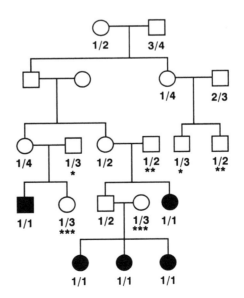

Figure 12–5. Summary of broken loops from pedigree from Figure 7–5

Table 12–7. Analysis Results from USEREX7.*

θ	Log$_{10}$(Likelihood)	Lod Score
0.00	−43.319936	3.131127
0.05	−43.714184	2.736879
0.10	−44.113965	2.337099
0.15	−44.516191	1.934873
0.20	−44.915445	1.535618
0.25	−45.301537	1.149526
0.30	−45.656453	0.794610
0.35	−45.955451	0.495613
0.40	−46.180268	0.270795
0.45	−46.336644	0.114420
0.50	−46.451063	0.000000

ILINK: $\hat{\theta} = 0.001$; $Z(\hat{\theta}) = 3.125729$.

The results of the linkage analysis with this pedigree are shown in Table 12–7. Because of the intense level of consanguinity in this one small pedigree, there is enough evidence for linkage to have a significant test result, with $Z(\hat{\theta}) > 3$. Because we have a significant test result for linkage in this case, it is for the first time meaningful to construct a 3-unit-lod-score support interval around this maximum to give us some idea of the accuracy of our estimate of $\hat{\theta} = 0$. In this case, our support interval covers all values of θ with $Z(\theta) \in [0.13, 3.13]$, which in this example means our support interval for $\hat{\theta}$ extends throughout the interval [0, 0.45). So, although our test of linkage is significant, we have little ability in this small data set to estimate the recombination fraction accurately. Obviously, in a real life situation, the solution is to collect more families or to type more markers and do a multipoint analysis, which will be discussed in Part II.

□ Exercise 8

The results from the binary factors representations of all markers in all previous user exercises should be identical to the results obtained originally when the allele numbers representations of those loci were used. They are not, therefore, repeated here.

For the pedigree USEREX8.PED with the four-allele marker and the ABO blood group markers, you were supposed to do linkage analyses between the two markers and between ABO and the disease. If you remember, the analysis of disease versus marker 1 was done in Exercise 3 (the results are shown in Table 12–1), with $\hat{\theta} = 0.077$ $\{Z(\hat{\theta}) = 1.78\}$, after further refinement of the estimate in the table of 0.079. The results of disease versus ABO are presented

Table 12–8. Analysis of Disease versus ABO in USEREX8.*

θ	Log$_{10}$(Likelihood)	Lod Score
0.00	−25.714063	3.499118
0.10	−26.276072	2.937108
0.20	−26.890589	2.322592
0.30	−27.569724	1.643457
0.40	−28.332891	0.880289
0.50	−29.213181	0.000000

ILINK: $\hat{\theta} = 0.001$; $Z(\hat{\theta}) = 3.495397$.

Table 12–9. Analysis of Marker 1 versus ABO in USEREX8.*

θ	Log$_{10}$(Likelihood)	Lod Score
0.00	$-\infty$	$-\infty$
0.10	-30.341911	0.310354
0.20	-29.883658	0.768607
0.30	-29.974499	0.677766
0.40	-30.289189	0.363077
0.50	-30.652265	0.000000

ILINK: $\hat{\theta} = 0.220$; $Z(\hat{\theta}) = 0.778700$.

in Table 12–8, and the results of the analysis of ABO versus marker 1 are given in Table 12–9. The recombination fraction between the disease and marker 1 was estimated at 0.077, and the recombination fraction between the disease and ABO was estimated to be 0. However, the recombination fraction between marker 1 and ABO was estimated to be 0.220. How can this be consistent? If you examine the pedigree closely, it is clear that for a large number of meioses the disease is not informative, but the ABO and marker 1 are informative. In these meioses, a large number of obligate recombinants appear between ABO and the marker. Remember that when the penetrance of the disease is lowered to 75%, the recombination fraction estimate between marker 1 and the disease is 0. Analyze the disease versus ABO, assuming 75% penetrance for the disease. The results of this analysis are presented in Table 12–10. Now, we have a situation in which both markers show 0% recombination with the disease in this pedigree, and yet the two markers show about 22% recombination between themselves. This causes even more confusion. Consider the fate of the unaffected child in the last generation with marker type *1 1*, and ABO type *O*. When the analysis is done with marker 1, the most likely scenario has this child carrying the disease allele, but being nonpenetrant. Yet, when the analysis is done with the ABO blood group, this child is most likely not carrying the disease allele, because recombination is estimated to be 0%, and the disease allele is segregating with the *A* allele, yet this child received the *O* allele from his mother. This apparent discrepancy can be dealt with by doing a multipoint analysis, which will be discussed in Part II.

☐ Exercise 9

The formula for the penetrance for each age class is obtained as follows: Clearly for individuals younger than 10, the penetrance is 0.1, and for individuals older than 60, the penetrance is 0.9. For individuals in the middle, we

Table 12–10. Analysis of Disease versus ABO in USEREX8.* with 75% Penetrance for the Autosomal Dominant Disease

θ	Log$_{10}$(Likelihood)	Lod Score
0.00	-26.944701	3.011264
0.10	-27.446887	2.509077
0.20	-27.990525	1.965439
0.30	-28.583064	1.372901
0.40	-29.234883	0.721082
0.50	-29.955965	0.000000

ILINK: $\hat{\theta} = 0.001$; $Z(\hat{\theta}) = 3.007926$.

Table 12–11. Penetrances for Individuals in Different Age Classes According to the Age-of-Onset Function Defined in Exercise 9

Liability Class	Age Range	Penetrances for Genotypes		
		$+/+$	$+/D$	D/D
1	<10	0	0.10	0.10
2	10–19	0	0.18	0.18
3	20–29	0	0.34	0.34
4	30–39	0	0.50	0.50
5	40–49	0	0.66	0.66
6	50–59	0	0.82	0.82
7	≥ 60	0	0.90	0.90

need to determine the formula for the line connecting the points (10, 0.1) and (60, 0.9), which is (age − 10)[0.8/50] + 0.10. If we then divide our set into age classes, the appropriate penetrances are given in Table 12–11. After making the appropriate modifications to the pedigree and parameter files, you should get the results shown in Table 12–12 from the analysis of disease versus marker 1, and those in Table 12–13 from the analysis of disease versus ABO.

□ **Exercise 10**

To determine the penetrance values of a disease with 80% diagnostic certainty and 70% penetrance, apply the formula given in Chapter 10,

$$pP(\text{affected} \mid \text{genotype}) + (1 - p)P(\text{unaffected} \mid \text{genotype})$$

where p is the probability of the individual being affected (the diagnostic certainty). In this case then, the penetrances for people with genotype AA or Aa with a diagnostic certainty of 80% (notation from Chapter 10) are $(0.8)(0.7) + (0.2)(0.3) = 0.62$, and for people with genotype aa are $(0.8)(0) + (0.2)(1) = 0.2$. Thus the penetrance classes with the disease being 70% penetrant are as follows:

```
       AA      Aa      aa
   1.  0.7     0.7     0
   2.  0.62    0.62    0.20
```

Thus, in this case, very little genotype discrimination is possible for the affected with 80% certainty liability class, because the penetrance ratio is only 0.62/0.20 = 3.1:1, which is much smaller than 0.7/0 = ∞. The results of the analysis of the pedigree under this model are given in Table 12–14.

Table 12–12. Results of Analysis of Disease versus Marker 1 in Files USEREX8.*

θ	Log$_{10}$(Likelihood)	Lod Score
0.0	−27.591976	1.982445
0.1	−27.995795	1.578626
0.2	−28.426063	1.148357
0.3	−28.869965	0.704456
0.4	−29.280893	0.293528
0.5	−29.574421	0.000000

ILINK: $\hat{\theta} = 0.001$; $Z(\hat{\theta}) = 1.979753$.

Table 12–13. Result of Analysis of Disease versus ABO in Files USEREX8.*

θ	Log$_{10}$(Likelihood)	Lod Score
0.0	−27.912368	2.211381
0.1	−28.308307	1.815443
0.2	−28.727879	1.395871
0.3	−29.171507	0.952243
0.4	−29.638251	0.485498
0.5	−30.123749	0.000000

ILINK: $\hat{\theta}$ = 0.001; $Z(\hat{\theta})$ = 2.208726.

Inserting the phenocopy penetrance of 0.005 is relatively straightforward. We go back to the formula above and substitute the new values, so the new penetrance for *AA* and *Aa* individuals with 80% diagnostic uncertainty is now 0.8*0.7 + 0.2*0.3 = 0.62 (the same as above), and the penetrance for *aa* individuals is now 0.8*0.005 + 0.2* 0.995 = 0.203. Using this information now defines our liability classes as follows:

```
        AA      Aa      aa
   1.   0.7     0.7     0.005
   2.   0.62    0.62    0.203
```

The results of the analysis under this model are given in Table 12–15.

When we allow for the age-dependant penetrance, we can compute the penetrances as (age − 10)[0.8/40] + 0.10 for genotypes *AA* and *Aa* and for individuals between age 10 and 50. For genotype *aa*, the penetrance can be computed as (age − 20)[0.008/40] + 0.002 for individuals between age 20 and 60. Because we are provided with information about current age, we are only able to use the distribution functions for the age-dependent penetrance calculations. The penetrances are given in Table 12–16 for the age classes specified in the exercise. In this pedigree, however, 3 of these 12 possible age and diagnosis combinations are never used, 100% diagnostic certainty in classes (10–19) and (35–49), and 80% diagnostic certainty in class (< 10). To make the program more efficient, allow for only the necessary nine liability classes in your analysis. The results of your analysis should match up with those in Table 12–17.

To allow for uncertainty of phenotype at the ABO blood group locus, we first have to recode the ABO blood group phenotypes as an affection status locus. Then, we can allow for the ambiguity in genotype as shown in Table 12–18. As you can see in this table, the phenotype A or AB is exactly complementary to the phenotype B or O, in terms of penetrance, so it is possible to use one additional liability class to code for both of these options as shown

Table 12–14. Result of Analysis of Pedigree with Diagnostic Certainty of 80%, and Penetrance of 70%

θ	Log$_{10}$(Likelihood)	Lod Score
0.0	−17.296418	0.437915
0.1	−17.399164	0.335169
0.2	−17.505815	0.228518
0.3	−17.600109	0.134224
0.4	−17.674374	0.059959
0.5	−17.734333	0.000000

ILINK: $\hat{\theta}$ = 0.001; $Z(\hat{\theta})$ = 0.437261.

Table 12–15. Result of Analysis of Pedigree with Diagnostic Uncertainty of 80%, Penetrance of 70%, and Penetrance for Homozygous Normal Individuals of 0.5%

θ	Log$_{10}$(Likelihood)	Lod Score
0.0	−17.306317	0.431483
0.1	−17.408201	0.329599
0.2	−17.513479	0.224322
0.3	−17.606208	0.131592
0.4	−17.679049	0.058751
0.5	−17.737800	0.000000

ILINK: $\hat{\theta} = 0.001$; $Z(\hat{\theta}) = 0.430832$.

Table 12–16. Age-dependent Penetrance Distribution with and without Diagnostic Uncertainty for Exercise 10

	Penetrances for Genotypes					
	Diagnostic Class 1			*Diagnostic Class 3*		
Age Class	*AA*	*Aa*	*aa*	*AA*	*Aa*	*aa*
<10	0.1	0.1	0.002	0.26	0.26	0.201
10–19	0.2	0.2	0.002	0.32	0.32	0.201
20–34	0.44	0.44	0.0034	0.464	0.464	0.202
35–49	0.74	0.74	0.0064	0.644	0.644	0.204
50–59	0.90	0.90	0.009	0.74	0.74	0.205
≥60	0.90	0.90	0.01	0.74	0.74	0.206

Table 12–17. Results of Analysis Using the Age-dependent Scheme Outlined in Table 12–16

θ	Log$_{10}$(Likelihood)	Lod Score
0.0	−16.576215	0.656951
0.1	−16.758859	0.474307
0.2	−16.926905	0.306261
0.3	−17.065199	0.167967
0.4	−17.165189	0.067976
0.5	−17.233166	0.000000

ILINK: $\hat{\theta} = 0.001$; $Z(\hat{\theta}) = 0.655672$.

Table 12–18. Penetrances for ABO Blood Group, Including Uncertain Phenotype Allocations

	Penetrances for Genotypes						
Phenotype	*AA*	*AB*	*AO*	*BB*	*BO*	*OO*	Coded as
A	1	0	1	0	0	0	2 1
B	0	0	0	1	1	0	2 2
AB	0	1	0	0	0	0	2 3
O	0	0	0	0	0	1	2 4
A or AB	1	1	1	0	0	0	2 5
B or AB	0	1	0	1	1	0	2 6
A or O	1	0	1	0	0	1	1 6 or 2 7
B or O	0	0	0	1	1	1	1 5 or 2 8

Table 12–19. Results of Analysis with Age-dependent Penetrance Scheme Outlined in Table 12–16 and ABO Blood Group Uncertainty of Phenotype Scheme Outlined in Table 12–18

θ	Log_{10}(Likelihood)	Lod Score
0.0	− 15.742181	0.587896
0.1	− 15.910975	0.419103
0.2	− 16.065113	0.264965
0.3	− 16.189603	0.140475
0.4	− 16.275887	0.054190
0.5	− 16.330077	0.000000

ILINK: $\hat{\theta} = 0.001$; $Z(\hat{\theta}) = 0.586712$.

in Table 12–18. The same relation applies to B or AB and A or O. To make things most efficient, use the minimal six liability classes, instead of eight, as outlined in the table. The results of your analysis should match those in Table 12–19.

□ **Exercise 11**

To accommodate monozygotic twins in a linkage analysis, it is often recommended that the two twins be replaced by a single individual because the two individuals represent two identical copies of the same genetic material. This works fine with full penetrance because $1^2 = 1$. With incomplete penetrance, however, treating the two twins as a single individual with penetrance as for any individual with the same phenotype represents an error that could possibly result in a change of lod score. The direction of the lod score change depends on the phenotype and whether that phenotype is indicative of a recombinant or nonrecombinant. To represent the twin pair as a single individual with penetrance as for any unaffected sibling, in the input line for individual 345 (third line from the bottom), we replace MT by NA. This changes the penetrance from 0.01 to 0.10. Consequently, the penetrance ratio for genetic versus nongenetic cases changes from $0.01/1 = 0.01$ to 0.10, that is, it is now (falsely) closer to 1 so that the phenotype of the single twin has less weight than the phenotypes of the two twins jointly. An unaffected individual with marker type 2/3 in the given sibship appears to be a nonrecombinant. Because nonrecombinants increase the lod score and recombinants decrease it, in this case bringing the penetrance ratio closer to 1 (giving the phenotype less weight) decreases the lod score.

To make the monozygotic twins appear as fraternal siblings, we replace the single line for the 345 individual by two lines corresponding to two offspring: 3.4 and 3.5. Each of these two individuals has phenotype NA. As outlined above, this deviation from the correct analysis amounts to adding nonexistent linkage information. Because the added information is in the direction of a nonrecombination, the resulting lod score turns out to be inflated.

PART II

Multipoint Linkage Analysis with the LINKAGE Package

13 □

Gene Mapping in CEPH Families

In this chapter, we introduce a specialized set of linkage analysis programs designed for use in three-generation CEPH-type pedigrees. For reasons to be outlined in this chapter, always type new markers in the CEPH pedigrees and do the analysis with these programs when constructing a genetic map of a given chromosomal region.

13.1 What Is CEPH?

Centre d'Étude du Polymorphisme Humain (CEPH) is a center for genetic studies in Paris. Researchers at CEPH and at the University of Utah in Salt Lake City have assembled a large homogeneous panel of families for use in making maps of genetic markers. These families all consist of nuclear pedigrees with many offspring and, in most cases, the grandparents. This basic three-generation pedigree structure has come to be known as *CEPH-type* pedigrees and is illustrated in Figure 13–1. The standard family set comprises 40 families, with an extended family set of 64 families (Dausset et al., 1990).

Blood from each member of this panel is stored at CEPH and can be made available to researchers around the world who wish to type a new marker against the panel. In this way, each time a new marker is generated, it is typed throughout this panel, adding to the CEPH data base. This data base, consisting of all the published markers typed in the panel, can then be accessed by linkage analysts for the purpose of generating good genetic maps and determining the map locations of all newly generated markers based on the information on other markers in the data base. Whenever generating a new marker for use in a genetic analysis, its location should always be mapped using the CEPH panel rather than using the disease pedigrees.

13.2 Why Use the CEPH Panel?

Why should you take the time, expense, and trouble to type a new marker throughout this data set? To generate accurate and reliable marker maps requires enormous data sets. The CEPH panel has enough markers typed

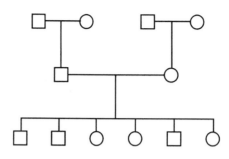

Figure 13-1. Example of CEPH-pedigree structure

through it that not only is it large, but many markers near any new marker have typically already been well mapped, making the process of mapping a new marker much more efficient, simpler, and more accurate. Furthermore, it is not clear how the presence of various disease-inducing mutations may affect recombination rates in the immediate region surrounding them. For example, if the mutation causing the disease of interest is a chromosomal inversion, the frequency of recombination may be reduced, due to lack of homology. Similarly, if a large deletion exists it appears to make more distantly spaced markers appear closer together. Other mutations can induce hot-spots of recombination, and so forth. So, for these regions, it is desirable to do all marker mapping in the same genetically healthy pedigree set. Be cautioned, however, that rather large error rates have appeared in the marker typings seen in the CEPH pedigrees in the past (Brzustowicz et al., 1993), so if you want to generate a very high resolution map, it is advisable to check the marker typings at neighboring loci, especially if you observe double recombinants over a very short region.

13.3 CLINKAGE

A set of specialized linkage analysis programs were written especially to analyze the CEPH pedigrees, which use very efficient computational algorithms specific to the analysis of pedigrees with the CEPH structure. As was mentioned above, CEPH-type pedigrees consist of a nuclear family with up to four grandparents.

Due to memory constraints in the normal LINKAGE programs, there are very strict limitations about the number of loci and number of alleles per locus that can be analyzed. However, the CLINKAGE programs have many fewer of these constraints and, as such, can analyze many loci at a time with many alleles at each locus. Further, these analyses are incredibly rapid relative to very small analyses produced with the more general LINKAGE programs. There are severe restrictions, however, in the applicability of these programs. First of all, they can only be used to analyze codominant marker loci of the allele numbers or binary factors type, so no trait loci or quantitative variables can be used. Secondly, the only parameters that can be varied are the recombination fractions and female-to-male map distance ratios; these programs cannot be used to estimate linkage disequilibrium, gene frequencies, or interference. So, although these programs are incredibly fast, and efficient for generating genetic maps of codominant loci and ordering a set of loci relative to one another, they are limited to these applications. Of course, the restriction on pedigree structure limits these programs' usefulness primarily to analyzing large sets of codominant loci typed against the CEPH panel. We will be investigating each of these programs and doing some sample exercises with them in the next few chapters.

13.4 General Strategies for Map Construction

To order a number n of marker loci and estimate the lengths of the $n - 1$ intervals between adjacent markers, ideally the maximum likelihood strategy should be applied. This amounts to computing the likelihood for each possible order; then the order with the highest associated likelihood is the best estimated order of loci. Depending on the amount of data, for numbers of loci as small as six or seven this approach is often feasible. However, for a large number of loci, the sheer number of possible orders ($n!/2$) and the length of time it takes to calculate pedigree likelihoods prohibit considering all orders, and alternative methods of map construction must be employed.

One approach might be to evaluate all orders but to calculate a simple, approximate measure for the plausibility of the data under each order. Several such measures have been proposed, for example, the sum of adjacent recombination fractions (SARF, the smaller the better), which is obtained by adding the recombination fraction estimates in each interval. Another measure is the sum of two-point lod scores for all pairs of adjacent loci (SAL, large values are good). An overview of these methods is found in Weeks (1991). Our limited experience with these methods leads us to conclude that they do not work very well with real data; as a matter of fact, hardly anyone in the gene-mapping field uses them.

The most popular strategy in current use is to calculate exact (or almost exact) likelihoods for only a limited number of markers at a time. Therefore, rules are required by which to select an initial set of markers for building a "trial map" and build on it by adding new markers. The MAPMAKER and CRI-MAP programs have built-in rules for iterative map construction. Of course, the final map resulting from such a procedure is not guaranteed to be the overall best map (by the rigorous likelihood criterion), so various ways of corroborating the proposed best map are needed. Also, MAPMAKER and CRI-MAP make some approximations in the likelihood calculations although such approximations do not seem to have a major effect. For references to these programs, see Appendix C. Below, we sketch some basic steps in map construction. For more detailed information, you may want to consult some of the recent chromosome map reports (e.g., Mills et al., 1992; Petrukhin et al., 1993).

If you do not want to rely on automatic map building using one of these programs, another strategy is to use only the most informative markers to construct a "skeletal" map whose order can be established unequivocally. The informativeness of a marker in a particular set of data may be assessed by computing the lod score at $\theta = 0$ of this marker against itself; those markers with the highest lod scores are most informative (Mills et al., 1992). Additional markers are then "dropped" into each interval of this map, in which case all map distances are recalculated each time. If likelihood calculation with all markers is not possible, then only a subset of markers in the vicinity of the position of the new markers are used.

The final 5 to 10 best map orders should then be scrutinized carefully. A common strategy for corroborating a given map is to invert pairs of adjacent loci one at a time (or to evaluate all orders for any triple of adjacent loci), recalculating the likelihood each time. Also, map building is usually carried out assuming equal male and female recombination rates. This restriction must be relaxed and map distances reestimated allowing for sex-dependent recombination rates. Because the programs used in the map-building phase generally calculate approximate likelihoods, it is recommended that the likelihoods for the best maps be recalculated by the CILINK program as it carries out exact likelihood calculations. For each of the best maps, three assumptions on female-to-male map distance ratio $R = x_f/x_m$ should be evaluated: (1) $R = 1$ throughout the map, (2) $R \neq 1$ but constant in each interval, and (3) $R \neq 1$ and possibly different in each interval. The hypothesis with a significant maximum likelihood is retained, in which significance is assessed by chi-square tests as outlined in Chapter 18.

An important component of map construction is error detection. Apart from retyping everyone and applying specialized statistical methods to pinpoint pedigree errors (e.g., Ott, 1993a; Brzustowicz et al., 1993; Haines, 1992), marker errors are typically recognized by the occurrence of double crossovers over a short map distance. Because this strategy requires the assumption of a locus order, the following two steps are generally repeated as often as necessary: (1) Build a map using one of the techniques incorporated in the MAPMAKER or CRI-MAP programs, and (2) follow up on individuals in whom multiple crossovers occur within, say, 30 cM (the CHROMPICS option of CRI-MAP is most useful at this stage). Each occurrence of such multiple crossovers is followed up, perhaps by retyping individuals in the lab, to correct any errors.

14.

The Locus-Ordering Problem: CILINK

In this chapter, you learn how to use CILINK of the CLINKAGE package in locus-ordering problems. Locus ordering is of critical importance in any multipoint linkage analysis. For a multipoint linkage analysis of a disease to be meaningful an accurate map is required. For this reason, the locus-ordering problem is one of the most significant and troublesome topics in all of linkage analysis.

14.1 How to Order a Set of Loci

One of the crucial problems in linkage analysis is the ordering of sets of closely linked markers. Once a positive test of linkage is achieved (i.e., $Z > 3$), the location of this linked gene needs to be found. For example, if we have a known map of markers and find that a new one is linked to this set of markers, we need to find out exactly where along this map the new marker falls. Another possible situation is that you know that a set of three genes are linked to each other, but you have no idea of their relative orientation. You then need to order the three loci in question. So, the question remains, how can we determine the order of a series of loci from pedigree analysis?

Consider the case of three loci known to be linked to one another. Further assume that for each meiosis in our sample, we can determine whether alleles at any pair of the two loci are cosegregating or not. In other words, we can determine for any meiosis whether or not a recombination event occurred between any pair of the loci. Consider that we have loci A, B, and C. Four meiosis types are possible, as indicated in Table 14–1.

Other combinations are not possible, because what happens between markers A and B and markers A and C uniquely determines what happened between markers B and C, irrespective of true locus order. Now, we can reformulate the four meiosis types indicated above into a 2 × 2 table for any particular locus order, as in Table 14–2.

The specific locus orders possible for this experiment are ABC, ACB, and BAC. The corresponding 2 × 2 tables are shown in Table 14–3 (where roman numerals refer to meiosis type).

Table 14–1. Four Possible Meiotic Three-locus Recombination Events, Irrespective of Locus Order

	Interval		
Meiosis	*AB*	*AC*	*BC*
Type I	R	R	N
Type II	R	N	R
Type III	N	R	R
Type IV	N	N	N

Clearly, one way to choose which order is best, is to pick the one that requires the fewest number of double recombinants, because these are necessarily rare events, with a frequency of $\theta_1\theta_2$, or less if there is positive interference (cf. Chapter 19). In this example if 100 informative meioses are collected and 90 Type IV meioses, 6 Type III meioses, 3 Type II meioses, and 1 Type I meiosis are found, the results are shown in Table 14–4.

On inspection, locus order BAC seems to be the best because it has the minimum number of double recombinants. Assuming no interference (an assumption routinely made by the LINKAGE programs), the recombination fractions are independent, so the rows and columns of the 2 × 2 tables in Table 14–3 are as close as possible to independent. One measure of the deviation from such independence is a simple chi-square test of independence on each of these tables. If you use the linkage utility program, CONTING, you can calculate these chi-square values. Further information about the CONTING program will be given in Part III. For the data in Table 14–4, the corresponding chi-square values are: ABC - 22.16, ACB - 54.09, BAC - 2.07 (Using a Yates correction, the corresponding values of χ^2 are 14.56, 44.48, and 0.19, respectively). This seems to indicate that order BAC gives a substantially better fit to our model than any other locus order; however, the chi-square approximation is not really valid because the expected number of double recombinants in the upper left cell is fewer than 1.

Dan Weeks wrote a very good chapter about different methods for ordering loci (Weeks, 1991), in which he provides a comprehensive overview of the theory and practice of a number of approaches. The user is referred to this source for a detailed analysis of this very important problem in human genetics. For now, we treat only what can be done with the LINKAGE programs. Typically, the analyst is unable to perform the analysis described above, because in real pedigree data, all meioses are not informative and phases are not known for all pairs of markers. The LINKAGE programs can be used to solve this problem. The ILINK program can be used to maximize the likelihood under each possible order by estimating each intermarker recombination fraction jointly. Thus, maximum use is made of all the pedigree

Table 14–2. Representation of the Four Possible Three-locus Recombination Events in a 2 × 2 Table

	Interval 1	
Interval 2	*R*	*NR*
R	W	X
NR	Y	Z

Table 14–3. Representations under Each Possible Locus Order Using a 2×2 Table

	Order ABC		Order ACB		Order BAC	
Interval 2	*R*	*NR*	*R*	*NR*	*R*	*NR*
R	II	III	III	II	I	III
NR	I	IV	I	IV	II	IV

information, including the partially informative meioses. As was mentioned in the previous chapter, however, the general LINKAGE programs are very slow and quickly run out of memory as the number of loci and number of alleles per locus increases. As mentioned in Chapter 13, a special version of LINKAGE, called CLINKAGE, is optimized for likelihood calculations in CEPH-type pedigrees. Using these programs, likelihoods can be computed rapidly for any given marker order and any reasonable number of markers.

14.2 CILINK

For the remainder of this chapter we concentrate on the practical usage of the CILINK program, which is the CEPH-pedigree-specific version of the ILINK program. Consider the case of five CEPH-type pedigrees, each with an identical pedigree structure (as shown in Figure 14–1) with marker locus phenotypes as given in Table 14–5.

Note that in this case, all meioses are fully informative and occur in the same proportions as in Table 14–4. Make a standard LINKAGE format parameter file for this set of pedigrees, with the four allele numbers marker phenotypes as indicated below each individual in file CEPH1.PRE. Then process this file with MAKEPED to produce CEPH1.PED. Call up PREPLINK to create a parameter file (called CEPH1.DAT). You must specify that there are 4 loci, three of them with four equally frequent alleles, and one with eight equally frequent alleles, each locus being of the allele numbers type. Do not worry about the other options, such as locus order, or any of the program-specific parameters, because we use LCP shortly to set this up.

When you finish, call up the LCP program, selecting the *three-generational pedigrees* option (these are the CLINKAGE programs). Choose the CILINK program, *All orders* option, with *No sex difference* in recombination fraction. Then set up the parameter screen as follows:

            Locus Set [] : *1 2 3*
 Recombination Fractions [.1] : *.1 .1*

Note that you need to indicate two recombination fractions here. The program then reorders these three loci in all possible orders and maximizes the

Table 14–4. Sample Data Placed in the Three Possible 2×2 Tables

	Order ABC		Order ACB		Order BAC	
Interval 2	*R*	*NR*	*R*	*NR*	*R*	*NR*
R	3	6	6	3	1	6
NR	1	90	1	90	3	90

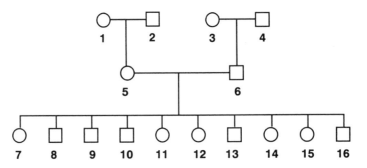

Figure 14–1. Pedigree structure for each of the five CEPH pedigrees in CEPH1.*

likelihood (under the assumption of no interference) for each given order, respectively. Hit ⟨Page Down⟩ to save this analysis setup, then hit ⟨Ctrl-Z⟩ to exit and type *PEDIN* to run the analysis. Note that instead of calling the UNKNOWN program, LCP now calls a program called CFACTOR, which does the CEPH-type pedigree factoring, making these programs so efficient.

When the programs finish running, use the linkage report program (LRP) to examine the output. To do this, type *LRP* at the DOS prompt. The first screen specifies the STREAM file name as *STREAM.OUT*. (Remember this stream file was produced by each of the LINKAGE programs). This name is correct, so hit ⟨Page Down⟩ to continue. At the next screen, select *Three-generation pedigree reports*, and then the *Multi-Point order report* (CILINK) option. Select the *table format*, and request that the report be *output to the screen*. You then see the following information on the screen:

Order	−2LN Like	Odds
.070 .040		
3__1__2	−1.9294E + 02	1.00E+00 <==
.040 .090		
1__2__3	−1.8316E + 02	1.33E + 02
.070 .090		
1__3__2	−1.6602E + 02	7.00E + 05

Just as in our 2 × 2 analysis of this same data set above, note that locus order 3-1-2 (CAB = BAC) is the best. Note that the recombination fraction estimates for each locus order are the same as if they had been estimated from the marginals of the 2 × 2 tables in Table 14–4. The main question here is how to interpret these results. Typically, for a locus order to be conclusive, we must have 1000:1 odds supporting the best order over the second best order, or a $\log_{10}$(likelihood) difference of at least 3 between the top two orders (analogous to the lod score of 3 requirement in a linkage test). In this case, we only have 133:1 odds, as shown in the third column above. To compute the lod scale equivalent, look at the values of −2 ln(Like) shown above. Subtracting the −2 ln(Like) of the best order from each of the others gives us the results shown in Table 14–6 (Lod scale equivalents are computed by dividing

Table 14–5. Genotypes for Each Individual at Four Marker Loci in Five CEPH-type Pedigrees of the Structure Shown in Figure 14–1

Pedigree	Individual	Marker 1	Marker 2	Marker 3	Marker 4
1	1	1 1	1 1	1 1	1 2
1	2	2 2	2 2	2 2	3 4
1	3	3 3	3 3	3 3	5 6
1	4	4 4	4 4	4 4	7 8
1	5	1 2	1 2	1 2	2 3
1	6	3 4	3 4	3 4	6 7
1	7	1 3	1 4	1 3	2 6
1	8	1 4	1 4	1 4	2 7
1	9	1 3	1 3	1 3	2 6
1	10	1 3	1 4	1 3	2 7
1	11	1 3	1 3	1 3	2 6
1	12	2 4	2 4	2 4	3 7
1	13	2 3	2 3	2 3	3 6
1	14	2 4	2 3	2 4	3 7
1	15	2 4	2 4	2 4	3 7
1	16	2 4	2 4	2 4	3 7
2	1	1 1	1 1	1 1	1 2
2	2	2 2	2 2	2 2	3 4
2	3	3 3	3 3	3 3	5 6
2	4	4 4	4 4	4 4	7 8
2	5	1 2	1 2	1 2	2 3
2	6	3 4	3 4	3 4	6 7
2	7	1 3	1 3	1 3	2 6
2	8	2 3	2 3	2 3	3 6
2	9	1 3	1 3	1 3	2 6
2	10	2 3	1 3	1 3	2 6
2	11	1 3	1 3	1 3	2 6
2	12	2 4	2 4	2 4	3 7
2	13	1 4	1 4	1 4	2 7
2	14	2 4	2 4	2 4	3 7
2	15	1 4	1 4	1 4	2 7
2	16	2 4	2 4	2 4	3 7
3	1	1 1	1 1	1 1	1 2
3	2	2 2	2 2	2 2	3 4
3	3	3 3	3 3	3 3	5 6
3	4	4 4	4 4	4 4	7 8
3	5	1 2	1 2	1 2	2 3
3	6	3 4	3 4	3 4	6 7
3	7	1 3	1 3	2 3	2 6
3	8	1 3	1 3	1 3	2 6
3	9	2 4	2 4	2 4	3 7
3	10	1 4	1 4	1 4	2 7
3	11	2 3	2 3	2 3	3 6
3	12	2 4	2 4	1 4	3 7
3	13	1 3	1 3	1 3	2 6
3	14	1 4	1 4	2 4	2 7
3	15	2 3	2 3	2 3	3 6
3	16	2 4	2 4	2 4	3 7
4	1	1 1	1 1	1 1	1 2
4	2	2 2	2 2	2 2	3 4
4	3	3 3	3 3	3 3	5 6
4	4	4 4	4 4	4 4	7 8
4	5	1 2	1 2	1 2	2 3
4	6	3 4	3 4	3 4	6 7
4	7	1 3	1 3	1 3	2 6
4	8	2 3	2 3	2 4	3 6
4	9	1 4	1 4	1 4	2 7
4	10	2 4	2 4	2 4	3 7
4	11	2 3	2 3	2 3	3 6
4	12	1 4	1 4	1 4	2 7
4	13	1 3	1 3	1 3	2 6
4	14	1 4	1 4	1 3	2 7
4	15	1 3	1 3	1 3	2 6
4	16	1 4	1 4	1 4	2 7
5	1	1 1	1 1	1 1	1 2
5	2	2 2	2 2	2 2	3 4
5	3	3 3	3 3	3 3	5 6
5	4	4 4	4 4	4 4	7 8

Table 14–5. (*Continued*)

Pedigree	Individual	Marker 1	Marker 2	Marker 3	Marker 4
5	5	1 2	1 2	1 2	2 3
5	6	3 4	3 4	3 4	6 7
5	7	1 3	1 3	1 3	2 6
5	8	1 3	1 3	1 3	2 6
5	9	1 4	1 4	1 4	2 7
5	10	1 4	1 4	1 3	2 7
5	11	1 4	1 4	1 4	2 7
5	12	1 3	1 3	1 3	2 6
5	13	2 3	2 3	2 3	3 6
5	14	1 3	1 3	1 3	2 6
5	15	1 4	1 4	1 4	2 7
5	16	2 3	2 3	2 3	3 6

the differences in $-2 \ln(\text{Like})$ by $2 \ln(10) \approx 4.6$; odds (likelihood ratio) computed as 10^Z, where Z is the $\log_{10}(\text{Likelihood})$ difference):

Table 14–6. CILINK Analysis of Loci 1, 2, and 3 in Each Possible Order

Order	Δ2 ln(Like)	Lod Scale	Odds
3--1--2	-0-	-0-	1
1--2--3	9.78	2.13	133
1--3--2	26.92	5.85	70,000

In this example, then, we can eliminate order 1-3-2 but cannot distinguish between orders 3-1-2 and 1-2-3 at the level of 1000:1 odds. The final interpretation is that you need to analyze more data to make a *framework map* (a map with best order supported by a likelihood ratio of at least 1000:1 over the next best order), but it seems much more likely that the true order is 3-1-2, though with this small sample size, we have not established that this is the case. The only real solution is to collect more families or type the remainder of the CEPH families for these markers. It is important to realize that this analysis was based on only five CEPH-type families. There are actually many more families than this, so there is certainly better power for locus ordering when the whole panel is typed.

As an exercise to show how much efficiency is gained by using the CILINK program over the ILINK program, repeat the previous analysis using the ILINK program instead of the CILINK program. When you look at the results in Table 14–7, notice that the values of $-2 \ln(\text{Like})$ are very different from those found with CILINK, but that the differences and odds are the same as indicated below, showing that they are equally valid. You cannot compare likelihoods generated with these two programs separately, however, because there are differences due to the factoring algorithms used by CILINK.

Table 14–7. ILINK Analysis of Loci 1, 2, and 3 in Each Possible Order

Order	2 ln(Like)	Δ2 ln(Like)	Lod Scale	Odds
3--1--2	555.66	-0-	-0-	1
1--2--3	565.44	9.78	2.13	133
1--3--2	582.58	26.92	5.85	70,000

□ Exercise 14

Order the set of five loci given in the pre-MAKEPED file shown below. Also, draw out the pedigree structures. Are they all compatible with the CEPH pedigree structural requirements? Enter this file as USEREX14.PRE and process it with MAKEPED to produce USEREX14.PED.

44	1	12	13	1	1 0 0	1 0 1	0 1 1	1 0 0	1 1
44	2	14	15	2	1 0 1	1 1 0	1 0 1	1 0 0	1 0
44	3	1	2	2	0 0 0	1 1 0	1 1 1	1 0 0	1 0
44	4	1	2	2	1 0 0	0 1 1	1 1 1	1 0 0	1 1
44	5	1	2	2	1 0 1	0 1 1	1 1 1	1 0 0	1 1
44	6	1	2	1	1 0 0	0 1 1	1 1 1	1 0 0	1 1
44	7	1	2	1	1 0 1	1 0 1	1 1 1	1 0 0	1 0
44	8	1	2	1	1 0 1	1 0 0	1 1 1	1 0 0	0 0
44	9	1	2	2	1 0 0	0 1 1	1 1 1	1 0 0	1 1
44	10	1	2	2	1 0 1	1 1 0	1 1 1	1 0 0	1 1
44	11	1	2	1	0 0 0	1 0 0	1 1 1	1 0 0	1 0
44	12	0	0	1	1 1 0	0 1 1	0 1 1	1 0 0	0 1
44	13	0	0	2	1 1 0	1 1 0	0 1 1	1 0 0	1 1
44	14	0	0	1	1 0 1	1 0 1	1 0 1	1 0 0	1 1
44	15	0	0	2	1 0 0	0 1 1	1 0 1	1 0 0	1 1
45	1	10	11	1	1 0 0	1 1 0	1 1 1	0 1 1	0 1
45	2	12	13	2	0 1 0	0 1 0	1 0 1	1 0 1	1 1
45	3	1	2	2	1 1 0	1 1 0	1 0 1	0 1 1	1 1
45	4	1	2	1	1 1 0	1 1 0	1 1 1	0 0 1	1 1
45	5	1	2	1	1 1 0	1 1 0	1 0 1	1 1 0	0 1
45	6	1	2	1	1 1 0	0 1 0	1 1 1	0 0 0	1 1
45	7	1	2	2	1 1 0	0 0 0	1 0 1	1 1 0	1 1
45	8	1	2	1	1 1 0	0 1 0	1 1 1	1 0 1	0 1
45	9	1	2	1	1 1 0	1 1 0	1 0 1	1 1 0	0 1
45	10	0	0	1	1 0 0	0 1 0	0 1 1	1 0 1	0 1
45	11	0	0	2	1 0 0	1 1 0	1 1 1	1 1 0	0 1
45	12	0	0	1	0 1 0	0 1 0	1 1 1	1 0 1	1 1
45	13	0	0	2	0 1 0	0 1 0	1 0 1	1 0 0	0 1
46	1	11	12	1	1 1 0	0 0 0	1 1 1	0 1 1	1 1
46	2	13	14	2	1 1 0	1 0 0	1 0 1	1 1 0	0 1
46	3	1	2	1	1 1 0	0 0 0	1 1 1	0 1 1	1 1
46	4	1	2	1	1 1 0	1 1 0	1 1 1	0 1 1	1 1
46	5	1	2	1	1 1 0	0 0 0	1 1 1	0 1 1	1 1
46	6	1	2	1	1 0 0	1 1 0	1 1 1	1 0 1	1 1
46	7	1	2	1	1 1 0	0 0 0	1 1 1	1 0 1	1 1
46	8	1	2	2	0 1 0	0 0 0	1 0 1	1 1 0	0 1
46	9	1	2	2	1 1 0	0 0 0	1 0 1	1 1 0	0 1
46	10	1	2	2	0 1 0	1 0 0	1 0 1	1 1 0	0 1
46	11	0	0	1	0 0 0	0 0 0	1 1 1	0 0 1	1 1
46	12	0	0	2	0 0 0	0 0 0	1 0 1	0 0 0	0 1
46	13	0	0	1	1 1 0	1 0 0	1 1 1	0 1 0	1 1
46	14	0	0	2	1 0 0	1 0 0	1 1 1	0 0 0	0 1
47	1	12	13	1	1 0 0	0 1 0	1 1 1	0 1 0	0 1
47	2	14	15	2	1 0 0	1 1 0	0 1 1	1 1 0	1 1
47	3	1	2	2	1 0 0	0 1 0	0 1 1	1 1 0	0 1
47	4	1	2	1	1 0 0	1 1 0	0 1 1	0 1 0	1 1
47	5	1	2	1	1 0 0	0 1 0	0 1 1	1 1 0	0 1
47	6	1	2	1	1 0 0	1 1 0	0 1 1	1 1 0	1 1
47	7	1	2	2	1 0 0	1 1 0	0 1 1	1 1 0	1 1
47	8	1	2	2	1 0 0	1 1 0	0 1 1	1 1 0	0 1
47	9	1	2	1	1 0 0	0 1 0	1 1 1	0 1 0	1 1
47	10	1	2	1	1 0 0	0 1 0	1 1 1	1 1 0	0 1
47	11	1	2	1	1 0 0	1 1 0	0 1 1	1 1 0	0 1

47	12	0	0	1	1 0 0	0 1 0	1 1 1	0 1 0	1 1
47	13	0	0	2	1 1 0	1 1 0	1 0 1	1 1 0	0 1
47	14	0	0	1	1 0 0	0 1 0	1 1 1	1 0 0	0 1
47	15	0	0	2	1 1 0	1 0 0	1 1 1	0 1 0	1 0
49	1	11	12	1	0 1 0	1 0 0	1 1 1	1 0 0	0 1
49	2	13	14	2	1 1 0	1 1 0	1 1 1	1 1 0	1 1
49	3	1	2	2	1 1 0	1 1 0	0 1 1	1 0 0	1 1
49	4	1	2	1	0 1 0	1 1 0	1 1 1	1 1 0	0 1
49	5	1	2	1	1 1 0	1 1 0	1 1 1	1 0 0	1 1
49	6	1	2	2	1 1 0	1 0 0	1 1 1	1 0 0	1 1
49	7	1	2	2	1 1 0	1 0 0	0 1 1	1 0 0	0 1
49	8	1	2	2	0 1 0	0 0 0	0 1 1	1 0 0	0 1
49	9	1	2	2	0 1 0	0 0 0	1 1 1	1 0 0	0 1
49	10	1	2	1	0 1 0	0 0 0	0 1 1	1 0 0	0 1
49	11	0	0	1	0 1 0	1 1 0	1 1 1	1 1 0	0 1
49	12	0	0	2	1 1 0	1 0 0	1 0 1	1 0 0	0 1
49	13	0	0	1	1 1 0	0 1 0	1 1 1	0 1 0	0 1
49	14	0	0	2	1 0 0	1 0 0	1 1 1	1 1 0	1 1
50	1	10	11	1	1 0 0	0 1 1	1 0 1	0 1 1	0 1
50	2	12	13	2	1 1 0	1 1 0	1 0 1	0 1 1	0 1
50	3	1	2	1	1 0 0	0 1 1	1 0 1	0 1 1	0 1
50	4	1	2	1	1 0 0	0 1 1	1 0 1	0 0 1	0 1
50	5	1	2	2	1 0 0	0 1 1	1 0 1	0 1 0	0 1
50	6	1	2	2	1 1 0	1 1 0	1 0 1	0 1 1	0 1
50	7	1	2	2	1 1 0	1 0 1	1 0 1	0 1 1	0 1
50	8	1	2	2	1 0 0	0 1 1	1 0 1	0 1 1	0 1
50	9	1	2	2	0 0 0	1 0 1	1 0 1	0 1 1	0 1
50	10	0	0	1	1 0 0	1 1 0	1 1 1	0 0 1	0 1
50	11	0	0	2	1 0 0	0 0 0	1 1 1	1 1 0	1 1
50	12	0	0	1	1 0 0	0 1 0	1 0 1	0 1 0	0 1
50	13	0	0	2	0 1 0	1 0 0	1 1 1	0 0 1	0 1
53	1	11	12	1	1 0 1	0 1 0	0 1 1	0 0 0	1 1
53	2	13	14	2	1 0 0	0 0 0	0 1 1	0 1 1	0 1
53	3	1	2	2	1 0 1	0 1 0	0 1 1	0 0 0	0 0
53	4	1	2	2	1 0 1	0 1 0	0 1 1	0 0 0	1 1
53	5	1	2	2	0 0 0	0 1 1	0 1 1	0 0 0	0 1
53	6	1	2	2	1 0 0	0 1 1	0 1 1	1 0 1	0 0
53	7	1	2	1	1 0 0	0 0 0	0 1 1	0 0 0	0 1
53	8	1	2	2	1 0 1	0 1 0	0 1 1	0 0 0	1 1
53	9	1	2	1	1 0 1	0 1 0	0 1 1	1 1 0	1 1
53	10	1	2	2	1 0 1	0 0 0	0 1 1	1 0 1	0 0
53	15	1	2	1	1 0 0	0 0 0	0 1 1	1 0 1	0 1
53	11	0	0	1	0 1 1	0 1 0	1 1 1	0 0 0	0 0
53	12	0	0	2	1 0 0	0 1 1	1 1 1	0 0 0	0 1
53	13	0	0	1	1 0 0	0 0 0	1 1 1	0 1 0	0 1
53	14	0	0	2	1 1 0	0 1 1	0 1 1	0 1 1	1 1
54	1	17	14	1	1 1 0	0 1 1	1 1 1	1 1 0	1 0
54	2	15	16	2	1 0 0	1 0 0	1 1 1	0 1 1	0 1
54	3	1	2	2	1 0 0	1 0 1	1 1 1	0 1 0	1 1
54	4	1	2	2	1 1 0	1 1 0	0 1 1	0 1 1	1 1
54	5	1	2	2	1 1 0	1 1 0	1 1 1	1 0 1	1 1
54	6	1	2	2	1 1 0	1 0 1	1 0 1	1 1 0	1 1
54	7	1	2	2	1 0 0	1 0 1	0 1 1	0 1 0	1 1
54	8	1	2	2	1 0 0	1 0 1	0 1 1	0 1 1	1 1
54	9	1	2	1	1 0 0	0 0 0	1 0 1	1 1 0	1 1
54	10	1	2	1	1 1 0	1 1 0	1 0 1	1 1 0	1 1
54	11	1	2	2	1 1 0	1 1 0	1 1 1	1 1 0	1 1
54	12	1	2	1	1 0 0	1 0 1	1 1 1	0 1 0	1 1
54	13	1	2	1	1 1 0	1 1 0	0 0 0	1 0 1	1 1
54	17	0	0	1	0 0 0	0 0 0	0 0 0	0 0 0	0 0

54	14	0	0	2	1 1 0	1 0 1	1 1 1	1 1 0	1 1
54	15	0	0	1	1 1 0	1 0 1	1 1 1	0 1 1	0 1
54	16	0	0	2	1 1 0	1 1 0	1 0 1	0 1 0	0 1
55	1	15	16	1	1 0 0	0 1 1	1 0 1	0 1 1	0 1
55	2	0	0	2	1 0 0	0 1 0	1 0 1	0 1 1	0 0
55	3	1	2	2	1 0 0	0 1 1	1 0 1	0 1 1	1 1
55	4	1	2	1	1 0 0	0 1 1	1 0 1	0 1 0	1 1
55	5	1	2	1	1 0 0	0 1 1	1 0 1	0 1 1	1 1
55	6	1	2	1	1 0 0	0 1 0	1 0 1	0 1 1	0 1
55	7	1	2	2	1 0 0	0 0 0	1 0 1	0 1 1	0 1
55	8	1	2	1	1 0 0	0 1 1	1 0 1	0 1 1	0 1
55	9	1	2	1	1 0 0	0 1 0	1 0 1	0 1 0	1 1
55	10	1	2	1	1 0 0	0 1 0	1 0 1	0 1 0	0 1
55	11	1	2	1	1 0 0	0 1 1	1 0 1	0 1 1	0 1
55	12	1	2	2	1 0 0	0 1 1	1 0 1	0 1 1	1 1
55	13	1	2	2	1 0 0	0 1 1	1 0 1	0 1 0	1 1
55	14	1	2	1	1 0 0	0 1 1	1 0 1	0 1 0	1 1
55	17	1	2	2	1 0 0	0 1 0	1 0 1	0 1 0	0 1
55	15	0	0	1	1 0 0	0 1 1	1 1 1	1 1 0	0 1
55	16	0	0	2	1 0 0	0 1 0	1 0 1	1 0 1	0 1
56	1	18	13	1	1 0 0	1 0 0	1 0 1	1 1 0	0 1
56	2	12	14	2	1 1 0	1 1 0	1 0 1	1 1 0	1 0
56	3	1	2	1	1 0 0	1 1 0	1 0 1	1 0 0	1 1
56	4	1	2	1	1 1 0	1 1 0	1 0 1	0 1 0	1 1
56	5	1	2	2	1 1 0	1 1 0	1 0 1	0 1 0	1 1
56	6	1	2	2	1 0 0	0 0 0	1 0 1	0 1 0	1 1
56	7	1	2	2	1 1 0	1 1 0	1 0 1	1 1 0	1 1
56	8	1	2	2	1 1 0	0 0 0	1 0 1	0 1 0	1 1
56	9	1	2	1	1 1 0	0 0 0	1 0 1	1 1 0	1 1
56	10	1	2	1	1 1 0	0 0 0	1 0 1	1 1 0	1 1
56	11	1	2	2	1 0 0	1 0 0	1 0 1	1 0 0	1 1
56	15	1	2	2	1 1 0	1 1 0	1 0 1	1 1 0	1 1
56	16	1	2	2	1 1 0	1 1 0	1 0 1	0 1 0	1 1
56	17	1	2	2	1 0 0	1 0 0	1 0 1	1 1 0	1 1
56	18	0	0	1	0 0 0	0 0 0	0 0 0	0 0 0	0 0
56	13	0	0	2	1 0 0	1 0 0	1 1 1	0 1 0	1 1
56	12	0	0	1	0 1 0	1 1 0	1 0 1	1 1 0	1 1
56	14	0	0	2	1 1 0	1 1 0	1 0 1	1 0 0	1 0
57	1	18	15	1	1 1 0	1 1 0	1 0 1	0 1 1	1 0
57	2	19	16	2	0 1 0	1 1 0	1 1 1	0 1 0	0 1
57	3	1	2	2	0 1 0	1 1 0	0 0 0	0 1 1	1 1
57	4	1	2	1	0 1 0	1 0 0	0 0 0	0 1 0	1 1
57	5	1	2	1	0 1 0	1 0 0	0 0 0	0 1 0	1 1
57	6	1	2	2	0 1 0	1 0 0	1 0 1	0 1 1	1 1
57	7	1	2	1	0 1 0	0 1 0	1 0 1	0 1 1	1 1
57	8	1	2	2	0 1 0	1 1 0	1 0 1	0 1 1	1 1
57	9	1	2	1	1 1 0	1 1 0	1 1 1	0 1 0	1 1
57	10	1	2	2	0 0 0	1 1 0	1 0 1	0 1 0	1 1
57	11	1	2	2	0 1 0	1 0 0	1 0 1	0 1 1	1 1
57	12	1	2	1	0 1 0	1 1 0	1 1 1	0 1 0	1 1
57	13	1	2	2	1 1 0	1 1 0	1 1 1	0 1 0	1 1
57	14	1	2	1	0 1 0	1 1 0	1 1 1	0 1 1	1 1
57	17	1	2	2	1 1 0	1 1 0	1 1 1	0 1 0	1 1
57	18	0	0	1	0 0 0	0 0 0	0 0 0	0 0 0	0 0
57	15	0	0	2	1 1 0	1 1 0	1 0 1	1 0 1	1 0
57	19	0	0	1	0 0 0	0 0 0	0 0 0	0 0 0	0 0
57	16	0	0	2	1 1 0	0 1 0	1 0 1	0 1 0	0 1
58	1	11	12	1	0 1 0	1 1 0	0 1 1	0 1 1	0 1
58	2	13	14	2	1 1 0	1 1 0	1 1 1	0 1 0	0 1
58	3	1	2	1	1 1 0	1 1 0	0 1 1	0 1 1	0 1

```
58    4    1    2    1    0 1 0    1 1 0    0 1 1    0 1 1    0 1
58    5    1    2    2    1 1 0    1 1 0    0 1 1    0 1 0    0 1
58    6    1    2    1    0 1 0    1 0 0    0 1 1    0 1 1    0 1
58    7    1    2    1    1 1 0    1 1 0    1 1 1    0 1 1    0 1
58    8    1    2    2    0 1 0    1 0 0    0 1 1    0 1 0    0 1
58    9    1    2    2    0 1 0    1 0 0    1 1 1    0 1 1    0 1
58   10    1    2    1    0 1 0    1 0 0    0 1 1    0 1 0    0 1
58   15    1    2    1    1 1 0    1 1 0    1 1 1    0 1 0    0 1
58   11    0    0    1    1 1 0    0 0 0    0 1 1    0 0 0    1 1
58   12    0    0    2    1 1 0    1 0 0    1 1 1    0 0 0    0 1
58   13    0    0    1    0 0 0    1 1 0    1 1 1    0 1 1    0 1
58   14    0    0    2    1 0 0    0 1 0    1 1 1    0 1 1    1 1
59    1    0    0    1    1 1 0    1 1 0    1 1 1    0 1 0    0 0
59    2    0    0    2    1 1 0    0 1 1    1 0 1    1 1 0    1 1
59    3    1    2    1    0 1 0    0 1 1    1 1 1    0 1 0    1 0
59    4    1    2    2    0 1 0    0 1 1    1 1 1    1 1 0    1 0
59    5    1    2    2    0 0 0    1 0 1    1 1 1    0 1 0    0 1
59    6    1    2    2    1 1 0    0 1 0    1 0 1    1 1 0    1 1
59    7    1    2    2    0 1 0    0 1 0    1 1 1    1 1 0    1 0
59    8    1    2    1    1 1 0    1 1 0    1 0 1    1 1 0    0 0
59    9    1    2    1    1 1 0    1 1 0    1 0 1    0 0 0    1 1
59   10    1    2    1    0 1 0    0 1 0    1 1 1    0 1 0    1 0
59   11    1    2    1    1 1 0    0 1 1    1 1 1    0 1 0    1 0
59   12    1    2    1    1 0 0    1 1 0    1 0 1    0 1 0    0 0
59   13    1    2    1    1 0 0    1 1 0    1 0 1    0 1 0    0 1
59   14    1    2    1    1 0 0    1 1 0    1 0 1    0 1 0    0 1
59   15    1    2    1    1 1 0    0 1 1    1 1 1    0 0 0    1 1
59   16    1    2    1    1 1 0    1 1 0    1 0 1    1 1 0    1 1
59   17    1    2    1    1 1 0    0 1 0    1 0 1    0 1 0    1 1
59   18    1    2    2    1 1 0    0 1 1    1 0 1    1 1 0    1 1
```

The corresponding parameter file is shown below and should be entered as USEREX14.DAT.

```
5 0 0 3
0  0.00000000 0.00000000 0
 1 2 3 4 5

2 3
 0.53571430 0.41785710 0.04642857
3
 1 0 0
 0 1 0
 0 0 1

2 3
 0.34931510 0.54452060 0.10616440
3
 1 0 0
 0 1 0
 0 0 1

2 2
 0.74083770 0.25916230
3
 1 0 1
 0 1 1

2 3
 0.24662160 0.62500000 0.12837840
3
```

```
1 0 0
0 1 0
0 0 1

2 2
 0.33532940 0.66467060
2
 1 0
 0 1

0 0
 0.10000000 0.10000000 0.10000000 0.10000000
0
 1 1 1 1
```

Use CILINK to order these five loci, as was described above. Can you order these five loci conclusively? If not, how many orders cannot be excluded? What conclusions can you draw from this analysis? Can you run this analysis with ILINK?

15.□

CMAP and Adding a New Locus

15.1 Multipoint Lod Scores

You often have some idea of the map of a certain region and desire to add a specific additional marker to this already established map. In such circumstances, it may be beneficial to fix the map of known markers and compute lod scores for each possible location of the new marker. In other words, you move the new marker across the map, computing the likelihood if this new marker was actually located at each possible point along the map. This may be done in one of two ways: (1) the interval lengths of the current map are kept fixed, and only the new locus is moved across the known map (using CMAP); or (2) the new locus is successively placed in each possible interval with reanalysis of each locus order (reestimation of all recombination fractions using CILINK). The second method is in general preferable and was described in Chapter 14. Here, we describe the first method.

Assume that we have a known map of markers with fixed intermarker recombination fractions as shown in Table 15–1.

Now, we have an additional marker to map against this known map. We compute the likelihood for each possible position of the new marker in each interval along the map. The CMAP (and LINKMAP) programs work by placing the new marker in each possible intermarker interval and subdividing each interval into a certain number of equal segments, computing the likelihood at each step. If we divide each interval into two segments, we have likelihoods computed for the positions for the new locus N as shown in Table 15–2.

The program equally divides each interval into two (in this case) segments by dividing the recombination fraction by 2 for the entire interval (i.e.,

Table 15–1. Known Map of Markers 1, 2, and 3

Theta:	0.10 0.10
Locus:	----1----2----3----
Interval:	0 1 2 3

Table 15–2. List of Map Positions for the New Locus (*N*) to Be Analyzed with CMAP against the Fixed Map of Markers 1, 2, and 3

Position	MAP (thetas)
A	*N*-(0.500)-1-(0.100)-2-(0.100)-3
B	*N*-(0.250)-1-(0.100)-2-(0.100)-3
C	*N*-(0.000)-1-(0.100)-2-(0.100)-3
D	1-(0.050)-*N*-(0.056)-2-(0.100)-3
E	1-(0.100)-*N*-(0.000)-2-(0.100)-3
F	1-(0.100)-2-(0.050)-*N*-(0.056)-3
G	1-(0.100)-2-(0.100)-*N*-(0.000)-3
H	1-(0.100)-2-(0.100)-3-(0.250)-*N*
I	1-(0.100)-2-(0.100)-3-(0.500)-*N*

$\theta_{1,2} = 0.100$, so when the new locus is placed in this interval, this recombination fraction is divided by 2 to get $\theta_{1,N} = 0.05$. Note that $\theta_{N,2}$ is not equal to $\theta_{1,N}$ but is computed according to the Haldane mapping function to make the map distance from locus 1 to locus 2 constant in Haldane centiMorgans.

Now that you have the $\log_{10}$ likelihoods computed for each of these points, how can you convert them into lod scores that can be interpreted easily? In this case, our null hypothesis is that the set of markers 1, 2, and 3 are linked to each other at fixed recombination fractions, but that marker *N* is unlinked to the entire map of markers. Thus, we compute multipoint lod scores for map position *D* as $\log_{10}[L(D)/L(A)]$, where *A* and *D* are defined in Table 15–2. Position *A* corresponds to the new marker unlinked to the fixed map of 1-(0.1)-2-(0.1)-3, and thus characterizes our null hypothesis likelihood. Another measure that is often used is the *location score,* which is based on 2 times the natural log likelihood of the same likelihood ratio, $2 \ln[L(D)/L(A)]$. This is often preferred, because it asymptotically follows a chi-square distribution with 1 df. However, it has become traditional to express your results in terms of multipoint lod score for ease of comparison with two-point analyses.

A significant test result is again signified by the magic number of 3, so a multipoint lod score greater than 3 is considered "proof" of linkage to this set of markers. Estimation can also be carried out by this approach analogously to the two-point case, with the most likely location of the new marker being at the point of its maximum likelihood. Be certain to use a 3-unit-of-lod-score support interval for the location of the new marker. Although some investigators have recommended (Conneally et al., 1985) a 1-unit-of-lod-score support interval as acceptable in estimating a two-point recombination fraction, in the multipoint case, the additional problem arises of needing to select one locus order over all other orders at 1000:1 odds. For this reason, a meaningful support interval can only be based on 3-units-of-lod-score ($10^3 = 1000:1$ odds). Even in the two-point case, the 3-unit-of-lod-score support interval may be more appropriate and meaningful, because the hypothesis of $\theta = 0.5$ is only excluded when $Z(\hat{\theta}) - Z(0.5) \geq 3$, which is the same as saying the value $\theta = 0.5$ is outside a 3-unit support interval around the maximum lod score. For these reasons, we advocate the use of the 3-unit-of-lod-score support interval in all situations to avoid logical inconsistencies of the type described above.

15.2 Computing Multipoint Lod Scores with CMAP

Map this new marker with the CMAP program in this family. For now, assume that we actually found a significant result for ordering the first three markers as 3-(0.07)-1-(0.04)-2. Then, use marker 4 as our test locus and compute the multipoint lod scores for this marker at a series of points across the fixed map. To do this, call up the LCP program, entering the appropriate pedigree and parameter file names (CEPH1.*), and specifying the *Three-generational pedigrees* option, and then the *CMAP* program. Choose the *All map intervals* option, and *No sex difference* in recombination fractions. The next screen should be completed as follows:

```
              Test loci [] : 4
        Order of fixed loci [] : 3 1 2
   Recombination fractions [.1] : 0.07 0.04
Number of evaluations in interval [5] : 5
```

The test locus is the new locus (4) for which likelihoods are to be calculated at a series of points across the fixed map of loci (3 1 2), separated by fixed recombination fractions (0.07, 0.04). The last line, for number of evaluations per interval determines the density of the grid of points at which the lod scores will be computed. In this case, each intermarker interval is divided into five equal subintervals, as described above. Please enter this problem and hit ⟨Page Down⟩ to create the batch file. After you run the analysis, call up the LRP program to examine the results. This time, be sure to select the *Location score report (CMAP)* option, instead of the CILINK option you used in the locus-ordering chapter. You should see the results given in Table 15–3.

Note that the first column here is the location score. To compute multipoint lod scores from these location scores, divide each of these location scores by $2 \ln(10) \approx 4.6$. These multipoint lod scores are added to Table 15–3, with their corresponding map locations. In this case, our 3-unit support interval is completely contained within the interval (1, 2), so this locus has been uniquely placed into one interval, and we have significant evidence for this locus order (assuming that the fixed map was correct).

Note that the lod score for map N-(0.000)-3-(0.070)-1-(0.040)-2 was -20.61, whereas the lod score for map 3-(0.000)-N-(0.070)-1-(0.040)-2 was $-\infty$. This happened because sometimes the recombination fractions shown are accurate to only three decimal places. The program divides the recombination fraction into equal segments and computes lod scores for each subdivision of the intervals. However, the division is accurate only to the level of machine precision. When dealing with recombination fractions of 0, the slightest deviation from 0 can have a major effect on the lod score, because only at $\theta = 0$ is the lod score equal to $-\infty$. Therefore, whenever you have two different values for the lod score at $\theta = 0$ from a given marker, and one of them $= -\infty$, the correct value is $-\infty$. In general, when the left-side recombination fraction is 0, it is the more accurate value. Similarly, it is not always the case that the likelihood when the new locus is unlinked to the set of markers on the left side equals that computed with the disease unlinked on the right side. Again, this is due to rounding error, and in every case it is more accurate to use the left-side value. We therefore recommend that you always normalize the lod scores to the likelihood with the new marker unlinked to the set of known loci on the left side of the fixed map.

Table 15–3. Results of CMAP Analysis of the New Locus (4) against the Fixed Map of Loci 1-2-3

Order	Loc. Score	−2 ln Like	Odds		Lod	x
4 = = = = 3 – – – – 1 – – – – 2						
.500 .070 .040	+ 0.0000E + 00	− 1.9294E + 02	7.13E + 28		0.00	− ∞
.400 .070 .040	+ 3.0788E + 01	− 2.2373E + 02	1.47E + 22		6.69	− 0.8047
.300 .070 .040	+ 5.5433E + 01	− 2.4838E + 02	6.54E + 16		12.05	− 0.4581
.200 .070 .040	+ 7.4593E + 01	− 2.6753E + 02	4.52E + 12		16.22	− 0.2554
.100 .070 .040	+ 8.6796E + 01	− 2.7974E + 02	1.01E + 10		18.87	− 0.1116
.000 .070 .040	− 1.1368E + 02	− 7.9266E + 01	3.45E + 53		− 20.61	0
3 = = = = 4 = = = = 1 – – – – 2						
.000 .070 .040		infinity				0
.014 .058 .040	+ 1.0393E + 02	− 2.9687E + 02	1.93E + 06		22.59	0.0142
.028 .044 .040	+ 1.1265E + 02	− 3.0559E + 02	2.46E + 04		24.49	0.0288
.042 .031 .040	+ 1.1696E + 02	− 3.0990E + 02	2.85E + 03		25.43	0.0439
.056 .016 .040	+ 1.1857E + 02	− 3.1151E + 02	1.27E + 03		25.78	0.0594
3 – – – – 1 = = = = 4 = = = = 2						
.070 .000 .040		infinity				0.0754
.070 .008 .033	+ 1.3115E + 02	− 3.2409E + 02	2.37E + 00		28.51	0.0835
.070 .016 .025	+ 1.3281E + 02	− 3.2575E + 02	1.03E + 00		28.87	0.0917
.070 .024 .017	+ 1.3287E + 02	− 3.2581E + 02	1.00E + 00	⟨ = =	28.88	0.1000
.070 .032 .009	+ 1.3134E + 02	− 3.2429E + 02	2.15E + 00		28.55	0.1085
.070 .040 .000		infinity				0.1171
3 – – – – 1 – – – – 2 = = = = 4						
.070 .040 .000		infinity				0.1171
.070 .040 .100	+ 1.0877E + 02	− 3.0171E + 02	1.71E + 05		23.65	0.2287
.070 .040 .200	+ 8.8456E + 01	− 2.8140E + 02	4.41E + 09		19.23	0.3725
.070 .040 .300	+ 6.3906E + 01	− 2.5685E + 02	9.46E + 14		13.86	0.5752
.070 .040 .400	+ 3.4843E + 01	− 2.2778E + 02	1.94E + 21		7.57	0.9218
.070 .040 .500	+ 0.0000E + 00	− 1.9294E + 02	7.13E + 28		0.00	∞

15.3 Map Distance

It is always useful to be able to represent the multipoint lod scores in graphical format. To do this, you need to express each putative location of the new marker in terms of its map location in Morgans. For arguments' sake, we typically take the location of the leftmost marker to be at map position 0. All other map distances can be computed by the Haldane mapping function. The Haldane mapping function must, in principle, be used here, because the likelihood computations are all performed assuming absence of interference (although some researchers often erroneously use the Kosambi mapping function to give the illusion of a shorter map). For example, in interval 0 (to the left of marker 3), the map distances of each point from marker 3 can be computed by converting the recombination fractions $\theta_{N,3}$ to map distance by the relationship

$$x_{Hald}(\theta) = -\frac{1}{2}\ln(1-2\theta)$$

where x_{Hald} is the distance in Haldane morgans corresponding to recombination fraction θ. In this case, because these recombination fractions are to the left of locus 3 since we are standardizing locus 3 to be map position 0, we prefix them with a minus sign, without loss of generality. Map positions between loci 3 and 1 can be computed similarly, by converting $\theta_{3,N}$ to map distance by the same formula. However, after you get to the right of locus 1, things get more complicated. You no longer are given recombination fractions $\theta_{3,N}$, but instead have $\theta_{3,1}$ and $\theta_{1,N}$. At this point convert $\theta_{3,1}$ to map distance and $\theta_{1,N}$ to map distance and add them together. Similarly, for points to the right of marker 2, you have $\theta_{3,1}$, $\theta_{1,2}$, and $\theta_{2,N}$. Convert each of these to map distance using the above formula and sum the map distances together. For example, for map position 3-(0.07)-1-(0.04)-2-(0.20)-N, the corresponding map position (distance from locus 3) is $x_{Hald}(0.07) + x_{Hald}(0.04) + x_{Hald}(0.20) = 0.0754 + 0.0417 + 0.2554 = 0.3725$. These θ to x conversions can be performed with linkage utility program MAPFUN. To do this, call up the MAPFUN program. The program prompts you with the following:

```
Calculate Map distance from given theta [M, or MS for summing ts]
    or Theta from given map distance [T]? (-1 exits)
```

In this situation we want to compute map distances from given θ's, so select option M. You are then asked:

```
Enter theta [+ mapping parameters] (-1 exits)
```

Enter the appropriate value of θ, for example 0.07 ($= \theta_{3,1}$). Do not worry about other mapping parameters. These have to do with other mapping functions, which we do not need to discuss now. The program gives you the following results:

```
Theta   xHALD    xKOS     xCaFal    xRAO    xFELS  xSTURT  xBINOM
                           param=>   0.350   0.000   2.000   4.000
0.0700  0.0754  0.0705     0.0700  0.0701  0.0705  0.0751  0.0740
```

The only map distance you need is the Haldane map distance. The other mapping functions are obtained from various models of interference (cf. Chapter 19). In general, if you compute multipoint lod scores with the LINKAGE or CLINKAGE programs, the programs base the likelihood calculations on the assumption of no interference, so the only valid and meaningful conversion is from θ to x_{Hald}. Two-point θ's can be converted validly by any map function you choose to assume, because no multilocus gamete probabilities are involved therein. So, for our purposes, all the other output can safely be ignored. Our result is $x_{Hald} = 0.0754$. Now enter -1 twice to exit the program. Note that the reverse transformation ($x \to \theta$) can also be performed by this program for a variety of mapping functions. The map distances for the example with CMAP are given in Table 15–3. A graphical display of the multipoint lod score curve is then possible by plotting $Z(x)$ versus x, as shown in Figure 15–1.

☐ Exercise 15

As an exercise, use CMAP to map locus 4 against the second-best locus order determined with CILINK, 1-(0.04)-2-(0.09)-3, for the data in files CEPH1.*. Can the locus 4 be uniquely assigned to one of these map intervals by the 3-unit support interval criterion? Compute map distances and multipoint lod scores across this other map.

Go back and run CILINK on all four loci together. Note that this would be impossible with regular ILINK, just as this whole chapter's exercises would've been impossible with regular LINKMAP on a PC. Is one order preferred significantly above all others? Is there anything interesting about the

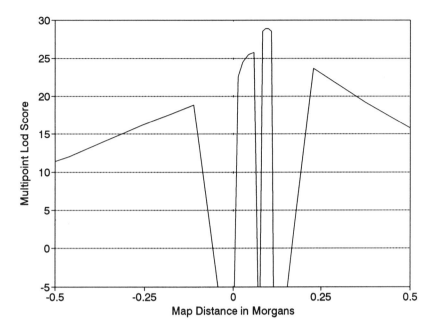

Figure 15-1. Graph of multipoint lod scores from Table 15-3

two best orders? Does the addition of this new marker locus help us at all in ordering loci 1, 2, and 3? Why or why not?

Go back to the data set from Exercise 14 and use CILINK to make a map of loci 1, 2, and 3. Then, fixing this map, go back and add locus 4. Check and see if these results are compatible with four-point CILINK results. Then add locus 5 to the same map of loci 1, 2, and 3. Compute all multipoint lod scores and their corresponding map locations as detailed in this chapter. Are the results compatible with the CILINK results from the previous chapter? What differences, if any, are there in the results and the significance levels of our test for locus order and why?

16.

Mapping a Disease Locus against a Fixed Map of Markers

16.1 Multipoint Testing and Estimating Linkage with Diseases

There are two phases of any genetic linkage analysis: the testing phase and the estimation phase. To prevent logical inconsistencies, you must have a significant test result before proceeding to the estimation step. In the testing phase, there is no great advantage to using multipoint analysis when analyzing highly polymorphic markers. The maximum multipoint lod score possible is equal to the maximum possible two-point lod score when all meioses are informative in both cases. A benefit is obtained in the testing phase only when multipoint analysis allows us to increase the percentage of meioses informative for at least one marker and the disease. In general, however, when there are questions about the model parameters or diagnostic criteria, as is common in complex disorders, it is advisable to rely on some kind of two-point analysis for the testing phase of any linkage analysis. Not only is two-point analysis more robust in testing situations, but it also can be done at a much lower cost in computer time. Because the mode of inheritance of complex traits is typically unknown and the analysis model presumably is different from the true model, estimates of θ tend to be inflated (Risch, 1990). In multipoint analysis, this inflation tends to "drive" the trait outside of a map even though the trait locus may be in the middle of the map of markers (Risch, 1990a). Complex traits will be discussed in more detail in Part III.

The greatest utility of multilocus analysis comes in estimating the location of your linked disease gene, provided that the mode of inheritance is well known. As we saw in the previous few chapters, multipoint analysis can be a very powerful tool for ordering loci along a chromosome. The simplest way of doing this is by selecting the location for a new gene so as to minimize the number of double (and to a lesser extent, single) recombinants. We saw how the CILINK and CMAP programs can be used to localize a new marker relative to other nearby markers. However, when the new locus to be mapped is a disease gene, the situation becomes somewhat different. No longer do we have the advantage of a 1:1 correspondence between phenotype and genotype because now we deal with this additional variable of penetrance. Because more complicated penetrance models are required for disease mapping than for marker mapping, we can no longer take advantage of the rapid and efficient algorithm used by the CLINKAGE programs. Instead, we must rely on the general LINKAGE programs, which are much more restrictive in terms of the number of loci that can be used and the maximum number of permissible alleles at each locus. The fundamental concepts and usage of ILINK and LINKMAP are the same as those you have already seen for CILINK and CMAP, but computing efficiency is lower and the generality higher.

16.2 Disease Gene Mapping

Create pedigree and parameter files (MULTDIS1.*) for the two pedigrees shown in Figure 16–1 (with marker locus phenotypes indicated in Table 16–1).

The disease is assumed to be a fully penetrant dominant disorder, with gene frequency of 0.0001, and each of the eight markers is assumed to have two equally frequent codominant alleles.

Now that we have the pedigree and parameter files prepared, we must decide on a course of action for this analysis. Before going any further with a multipoint analysis, it is wise to perform two-point analysis with the disease versus each of the markers to see if there is any two-point evidence to support a linkage to this region. We want to use the LCP program to prepare a batch file that performs two-point analyses with the disease versus each of the markers. To do this, invoke LCP and specify the appropriate parameter file and pedigree file. Then, select the *MLINK* program, with the *specific evaluations*

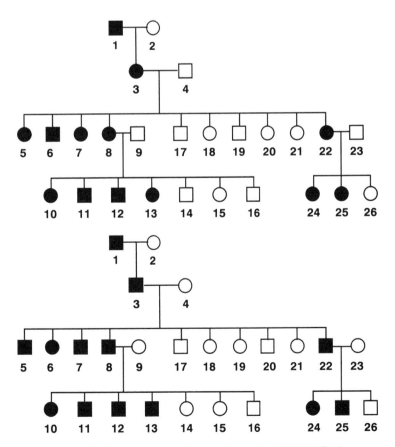

Figure 16–1. Pedigree structures for pedigrees in MULTDIS1.*

Table 16–1. Marker Locus Phenotypes for the Pedigree in Figure 16–1

Pedigree	Individual	M1	M2	M3	M4	M5	M6	M7	M8
1	1	2 2	2 2	2 2	2 2	2 2	2 2	2 2	2 2
1	2	1 1	1 1	1 1	1 1	1 1	1 1	1 1	1 1
1	3	1 2	1 2	1 2	1 2	1 2	1 2	1 2	1 2
1	4	1 1	1 1	1 1	1 1	1 1	1 1	1 1	1 1
1	5	1 2	1 2	1 1	1 2	1 2	1 1	1 2	1 1
1	6	1 1	1 2	1 2	1 1	1 2	1 2	1 1	1 2
1	7	1 2	1 2	1 2	1 1	1 2	1 2	1 2	1 2
1	8	1 2	1 2	1 2	1 2	1 2	1 2	1 2	1 2
1	9	1 2	1 2	1 2	1 2	1 2	1 2	1 2	1 2
1	10	1 2	2 2	1 2	1 2	2 2	1 2	2 2	2 2
1	11	1 1	1 2	1 2	2 1	1 2	1 2	1 2	2 2
1	12	1 1	2 1	1 2	1 1	2 2	1 2	1 1	2 2
1	13	1 2	1 2	1 1	2 2	1 2	1 2	1 2	1 1
1	14	1 1	2 1	1 1	1 1	2 1	1 2	1 1	1 1
1	15	1 2	1 1	1 1	2 2	1 1	1 1	2 2	1 1
1	16	1 2	2 1	1 1	1 2	2 1	1 2	1 2	1 1
1	17	1 2	1 1	1 1	1 2	1 1	1 1	1 2	1 1
1	18	1 1	1 1	1 1	1 1	1 1	1 2	1 1	1 2
1	19	1 1	1 1	1 1	1 1	1 1	1 1	1 1	1 1
1	20	1 2	1 1	1 1	1 2	1 1	1 2	1 2	1 1
1	21	1 2	1 1	1 1	1 1	1 1	1 1	1 2	1 1
1	22	1 2	1 2	1 2	1 2	1 2	1 2	1 2	1 2
1	23	1 2	1 2	1 2	1 2	1 2	1 2	1 2	1 2
1	24	1 1	2 2	2 2	1 1	2 2	2 2	2 2	2 2
1	25	1 2	1 2	1 2	1 2	1 2	1 1	1 2	1 1
1	26	1 2	1 2	1 1	1 2	1 1	1 1	1 2	1 1
2	1	2 2	2 2	2 2	2 2	2 2	2 2	2 2	2 2
2	2	1 1	1 1	1 1	1 1	1 1	1 1	1 1	1 1
2	3	1 2	1 2	1 2	1 2	1 2	1 2	1 2	1 2
2	4	1 1	1 1	1 1	1 1	1 1	1 1	1 1	1 1
2	5	1 2	1 2	1 1	1 2	1 2	1 1	1 2	1 1
2	6	1 2	1 2	1 2	1 2	1 2	1 2	1 2	1 2
2	7	1 2	1 2	1 2	1 2	1 2	1 2	1 2	1 2
2	8	1 2	1 2	1 2	1 2	1 2	1 2	1 2	1 2
2	9	1 1	1 1	1 1	1 1	1 1	1 1	1 1	1 1
2	10	1 2	1 2	1 2	1 2	1 2	1 2	1 2	1 2
2	11	1 1	1 2	1 2	1 1	1 2	1 2	1 2	1 2
2	12	1 1	1 1	1 2	1 1	1 2	1 2	1 1	1 2
2	13	1 2	1 2	1 2	1 2	1 2	1 2	1 2	1 2
2	14	1 1	1 1	1 1	1 1	1 1	1 2	1 1	1 1
2	15	1 2	1 1	1 1	1 2	1 1	1 1	1 2	1 1
2	16	1 1	1 1	1 1	1 1	1 1	1 1	1 1	1 1
2	17	1 1	1 1	1 1	1 1	1 1	1 1	1 1	1 1
2	18	1 1	1 1	1 1	1 1	1 1	1 1	1 1	1 1
2	19	1 1	1 1	1 1	1 1	1 1	1 1	1 1	1 1
2	20	1 2	1 1	1 1	1 2	1 1	1 1	1 2	1 1
2	21	1 2	1 1	1 1	1 1	1 1	1 1	1 2	1 1
2	22	1 2	1 2	1 2	1 2	1 2	1 2	1 2	1 2
2	23	1 2	1 2	1 2	1 2	1 2	1 2	1 2	1 2
2	24	2 2	2 2	2 2	2 2	2 2	2 2	2 2	2 2
2	25	1 2	1 2	1 2	1 2	1 2	1 1	1 2	1 1
2	26	1 1	1 1	1 1	1 1	1 1	1 1	1 1	1 1

and *No sex difference* options. Enter the appropriate analyses to be done as follows: First, to analyze locus 1 (disease) versus locus 2, enter the following options:

```
           Locus Order [ ] : 1 2
Recombination Fractions [.1] : 0
    Recombination varied [1] : 1
        Increment value [.1] : .1
             Stop value [.5] : .5
```

followed by ⟨Page Down⟩. To analyze the disease versus locus 3, repeat the process, except instead of entering locus order [ ] : 1 2, enter 1 3. Normally, you continue doing this until you have selected the disease to be analyzed versus each of the loci, but in the interest of time, only go up to disease versus 4. At this point, press ⟨Ctrl-Z⟩ to exit from LCP and write the batch file. To perform these analyses, you type *PEDIN* to invoke your newly created batch file PEDIN.BAT. To produce similar results use the ILINK program, which iteratively finds the maximum likelihood estimate of the recombination fraction. Try this analysis again with ILINK to verify that your results are consistent; note that ILINK results give you an estimate, and MLINK gives you a sense of the shape of the likelihood curve. To do this, again invoke the LCP program, select parameter and pedigree files as before, and then select the *ILINK* program, with the *Specific orders* and *No sex difference* options. Then enter your problems. The following example is as shown above for the comparison of markers 1 and 2:

```
Locus Order [ ] : 1 2
Recombination Fractions [.1] : 0.1
```

Then hit ⟨Page Down⟩ and enter the next comparison, 1 versus 3. Normally, you continue in this manner until all possible two-point comparisons involving the disease locus (i.e., 1 vs. 2, . . . , 1 vs. 9) have been specified, but again, to save time, analyze only the disease versus the first three loci (2, 3, and 4). Note that sometimes ILINK gives an estimate of $\hat{\theta} > 0.50$. This is an artifact of the method the program uses to maximize the likelihood. All such estimates can be thought of as being equal to 0.5 because that is the maximum meaningful value for a recombination fraction. Lod scores at $\theta > 0.5$ may serve as a check of data consistency; if $Z(\hat{\theta} > \frac{1}{2})$ is large (> 2, say), the data may contain errors and should be checked. Table 16–2 is a table of two-point intermarker recombination fractions that should coincide with those estimates you obtained, though there may be some minor differences.

The most tightly linked marker appears to be locus 6. For this locus, please perform an MLINK analysis in steps of 0.01 to find the upper bound for the 3-unit-of-lod-score support interval. In this case, the support interval covers the interval [0, 0.19), because the lod score at 0 is 10.225, and the lod score first falls below 7.225 ($= 10.225 - 3$) at $\theta = 0.19$, where $Z(0.19) = 7.12$. So, we can see that in the two-point analysis, we have a support interval for the location of our disease gene covering

$$-\frac{1}{2} \ln[1 - 2(0.19)] = 0.239 \text{ M} = 23.9 \text{ cM}$$

Furthermore, the support interval can extend on either side (proximal or distal) of our marker, so the support interval is actually twice this long or 47.8 cM. Now, we should use multipoint analysis to determine its effect on the length of our support interval and the accuracy with which we can map our disease gene.

Assume we have a fixed map of our markers from the CEPH pedigrees as follows: 5-2-8-3-6-4-9-7, with intermarker θ's as follows: 0.075, 0.075, 0.225,

Table 16–2. ILINK Estimates of Two-point θ, and $Z(\hat{\theta})$ for Each Marker Locus versus Disease

	2	3	4	5	6	7	8	9
$\hat{\theta}$:	0.363	0.031	0.085	0.324	0.000	0.206	0.295	0.150
$Z(\hat{\theta})$:	0.540	7.700	6.090	0.940	10.225	2.727	1.290	4.698

0.075, 0.075, 0.075, 0.075. We must now find the location of our disease gene along this map of markers. To do this, we must use the LINKMAP program and move the disease locus through each of the intervals along our fixed map of loci, as was done in the CMAP example. We are unable to analyze all the loci jointly in a nine-point analysis with the general pedigrees version of LINKMAP because of memory constraints. To circumvent this problem, we use the technique of sliding our group of four loci down the map and analyzing the disease only in the middle interval (i.e., with two flanking markers on each side) of each set of markers. We first analyze the disease against markers 5, 2, 8, and 3, allowing the disease locus to move over the region from the left of locus 5 up to locus 8. At that point we switch to looking at the set of loci 2-8-3-6, when we move the disease in the middle interval of this set of loci, 8-3. We proceed like this until we have covered the entire length of our map, as shown in Table 16–3.

In this way, we can compute multipoint lod scores across the map, using the nearest markers to each interval in which the disease is placed. Although these lod scores are not the same as those obtained from a putative nine-point analysis, this type of analysis would be impossible on a PC with the LINKAGE programs. After computing all the multipoint lod scores across this map of markers, we find our estimated map position for the disease and a multipoint 3-unit-of-lod-score support interval for the map position, as before.

To perform these multipoint analyses, invoke LCP and this time choose the *LINKMAP* program. Because we are going to analyze the disease in each interval with a different set of markers, we need to specify the *Specific intervals* option, with *No sex difference*. Now, for our first few analyses we use the set of markers 5, 2, 8, and 3. Normally we only use a specific set of markers to analyze the disease in the middle interval, but in this case, we have no markers farther out so we can get the best results from these four markers. Our test locus is the disease. This means that the disease moves throughout whatever interval we specify on the fixed map of loci 5-2-8-3. For the entry of recombination fractions, we must input the KNOWN, FIXED recombination fractions between each of the loci. In this case, they are 0.075 between 5 and 2, 0.075 between 2 and 8, and 0.225 between 8 and 3. The test interval must be specified next. It is imperative to have one evaluation for each set of markers with the disease fixed at $\theta = 0.50$ to the left of the leftmost marker. This value of the log likelihood at this point must be subtracted from the log likelihoods at all points analyzed with this specific marker set to calculate multipoint lod scores and location scores. To do this we specify *test interval = 0*, meaning to the left of the fixed map, and we request *1* evaluation, so it only does calculations at $\theta = 0.5$, and possibly also at $\theta = 0$ from the leftmost marker. Otherwise, test interval refers to the intermarker interval you want the disease (test locus) to move through. In our example, test interval 1 causes the disease to be moved between markers 5 and 2, interval 2 refers to that

Table 16–3. Demonstration of Strategy for Picking Which Markers to Use in a Multipoint LINKMAP Analysis of Disease (=) versus a Map of Eight Markers, when Only Five-point Analysis Is Possible

```
= = = =5= = = =2= = = =8– – – –3
        2– – – –8= = = =3– – – –6
                8– – – –3= = = =6– – – –4
                        3– – – –6= = = =4– – – –9
                                6– – – –4= = = =9= = = =7= = = =
```

between 2 and 8, and so forth. Note that the largest value possible is interval 4, meaning to the right of the rightmost (fourth) locus. You may specify any number of points at which the likelihood should be calculated, but in general 5 is sufficient, unless you want a finer map, in which case you can raise it. For our purposes, we use five evaluations per interval. In other words, to analyze the disease to the left of our map enter the following:

```
              Test loci [ ] : 1
      Order of fixed loci [ ] : 5 2 8 3
Recombination fractions [.1] : 0.075 0.075 0.225
          Test interval [0] : 0
    Number of evaluations [5] : 5
```

To analyze the disease between 5 and 2, change the test interval to 1. Furthermore, to analyze the disease between loci 2 and 8, change the test interval to 2. Note that in this case we didn't have to specify separately an analysis to the left of the map of markers with one evaluation to get the value of the log likelihood at $\theta = 0.5$, because that is calculated anyway when the disease has moved through all points to the left of our map of loci. However, in the next interval, between 8 and 3, we need to change our set of marker loci to 2, 8, 3, and 6. In this case we need to do a separate entry to calculate the value at $\theta = 0.5$ to the left of this new set of markers as follows:

```
              Test loci [ ] : 1
      Order of fixed loci [ ] : 2 8 3 6
Recombination fractions [.1] : 0.075 0.225 0.075
          Test interval [0] : 0
    Number of evaluations [5] : 1
```

to get the value at $\theta = 0.5$, and then

```
              Test loci [ ] : 1
      Order of fixed loci [ ] : 2 8 3 6
Recombination fractions [.1] : 0.075 0.225 0.075
          Test interval [0] : 2
    Number of evaluations [5] : 5
```

to move the disease between loci 8 and 3. Also note that as we changed the loci in the analysis we also had to enter the correct recombination fractions for each interval, because this is crucial to the analysis. Continue this process until you have prepared a batch file that runs the disease over every point on the map using this sliding window type of method. We want you to calculate the location scores and lod scores across the map, using the output from LRP to help you if you wish. Everything is essentially the same as for the analysis of CMAP output in the previous chapter and is presented in Table 16–4, and the multipoint lod scores are illustrated graphically in Figure 16–2. The calculation of location scores is left as an exercise.

In this example, we see that our maximum multipoint lod score is 9.011, which is actually lower than that achieved in the two-point analysis with marker 6, though the MLE of the disease location is still at marker 6. In this analysis, the 3-unit-of-lod-score support interval encompasses only those regions with lod scores greater than 6.011, which in this example extends within the region between markers 3 and 4 and slightly to the right of marker 3, where a lod score of 6.518 was achieved at 0.07 to the right of marker 3. In this case, our support interval is disjoint, covering a range of 14.52 cM between the markers 3 and 4 and up to 7.58 cM to the right of marker 3. Although the region is disjoint, it has an absolute length less than the entire 22.1 cM range.

Remember that in the two-point example, the support interval of 47.8 cM is more than twice this length. If we had more tightly linked markers in our map, the properties would be different, and we could potentially isolate the location of our disease gene even further.

Table 16–4. Results of LINKMAP Analysis with Disease against the Fixed Map of Eight Markers

Intermarker Thetas	ln(like)	log(like)	Map Distance from Locus 5	Location Scores	Lod Scores
LOCI: 1 5 2 8 3					
0.5 0.075 0.075 0.225	−192.690	−83.684	−∞	0	0
0.4 0.075 0.075 0.225	−190.952	−82.929	−0.80471		0.755
0.3 0.075 0.075 0.225	−190.572	−82.764	−0.45814		0.920
0.2 0.075 0.075 0.225	−191.961	−83.367	−0.25541		0.317
0.1 0.075 0.075 0.225	−196.877	−85.502	−0.11157		−1.819
0 0.075 0.075 0.225	−∞	−∞	0	−∞	−∞
LOCI: 5 1 2 8 3					
0.015 0.062 0.075 0.225	−236.121	−102.545	0.015229		−18.862
0.03 0.048 0.075 0.225	−231.712	−100.631	0.030937		−16.947
0.045 0.033 0.075 0.225	−231.877	−100.702	0.047155		−17.018
0.06 0.017 0.075 0.225	−236.789	−102.836	0.063916		−19.152
0.075 0 0.075 0.225	−∞	−∞	0.081259	−∞	−∞
LOCI: 5 2 1 8 3					
0.075 0 0.075 0.225	−∞	−∞	0.081259	−∞	−∞
0.075 0.015 0.062 0.225	−237.803	−103.276	0.096489		−19.592
0.075 0.03 0.048 0.225	−231.880	−100.704	0.112197		−17.020
0.075 0.045 0.033 0.225	−230.579	−100.139	0.128414		−16.455
0.075 0.06 0.017 0.225	−233.556	−101.432	0.145176		−17.748
0.075 0.075 0 0.225	−∞	−∞	0.162518	−∞	−∞
LOCI: 1 2 8 3 6					
0.500 0.075 0.225 0.075	−185.8052	−80.694			
LOCI: 2 8 1 3 6					
0.075 0 0.225 0.075	−∞	−∞	0.162518	−∞	−∞
0.075 0.045 0.198 0.075	−184.419	−80.092	0.209674		0.602
0.075 0.09 0.165 0.075	−177.598	−77.130	0.261744		3.564
0.075 0.135 0.123 0.075	−173.590	−75.389	0.319874		5.305
0.075 0.18 0.07 0.075	−170.796	−74.176	0.385662		6.518
0.075 0.225 0 0.075	−∞	−∞	0.461437	−∞	−∞
LOCI: 1 8 3 6 4					
0.500 0.225 0.075 0.075	−183.599	−79.735			
LOCI: 8 3 1 6 4					
0.225 0 0.075 0.075	−∞	−∞	0.461437	−∞	−∞
0.225 0.015 0.062 0.075	−165.297	−71.787	0.476667		7.948
0.225 0.03 0.048 0.075	−164.244	−71.330	0.492375		8.405
0.225 0.045 0.033 0.075	−163.575	−71.039	0.508592		8.696
0.225 0.06 0.017 0.075	−163.117	−70.840	0.525354		8.895
0.225 0.075 0 0.075	−162.850	−70.724	0.542696		9.011
LOCI 1 3 6 4 9					
0.500 0.075 0.075 0.075	−176.860	−76.809			
LOCI: 3 6 1 4 9					
0.075 0 0.075 0.075	−156.197	−67.835	0.5427		8.974
0.075 0.015 0.062 0.075	−156.679	−68.044	0.5579		8.765

Table 16–4. (*Continued*)

Intermarker Thetas	ln(like)	log(like)	Map Distance from Locus 5	Location Scores	Lod Scores
0.075 0.03 0.048 0.075	− 157.363	− 68.342	0.5736		8.467
0.075 0.045 0.033 0.075	− 158.403	− 68.793	0.5899		8.016
0.075 0.06 0.017 0.075	− 160.302	− 69.618	0.6066		7.191
0.075 0.075 0 0.075	− ∞	− ∞	0.6240	− ∞	− ∞

LOCI 1 6 4 9 7

0.500 0.075 0.075 0.075	− 178.324	− 77.445			

LOCI: 6 4 1 9 7

0.075 0 0.075 0.075	− ∞	− ∞	0.623956	− ∞	− ∞
0.075 0.015 0.062 0.075	− 173.943	− 75.542	0.639185		1.903
0.075 0.03 0.048 0.075	− 173.317	− 75.270	0.654894		2.174
0.075 0.045 0.033 0.075	− 174.253	− 75.677	0.671111		1.768
0.075 0.06 0.017 0.075	− 177.254	− 76.980	0.687873		0.465
0.075 0.075 0 0.075	− ∞	− ∞	0.705215	− ∞	− ∞

LOCI: 6 4 9 1 7

0.075 0.075 0 0.075	− ∞	− ∞	0.705215	− ∞	− ∞
0.075 0.075 0.015 0.062	− 191.679	− 83.245	0.720445		− 5.800
0.075 0.075 0.03 0.048	− 189.469	− 82.285	0.736153		− 4.840
0.075 0.075 0.045 0.033	− 189.804	− 82.430	0.752371		− 4.986
0.075 0.075 0.06 0.017	− 192.860	− 83.757	0.769132		− 6.313
0.075 0.075 0.075 0	− ∞	− ∞	0.786475	− ∞	− ∞

LOCI: 6 4 9 7 1

0.075 0.075 0.075 0	− ∞	− ∞	0.786475	− ∞	− ∞
0.075 0.075 0.075 0.1	− 172.369	− 74.858	0.898047		2.586
0.075 0.075 0.075 0.2	− 170.619	− 74.099	1.041888		3.346
0.075 0.075 0.075 0.3	− 171.654	− 74.548	1.244620		2.897
0.075 0.075 0.075 0.4	− 174.283	− 75.690	1.591194		1.755

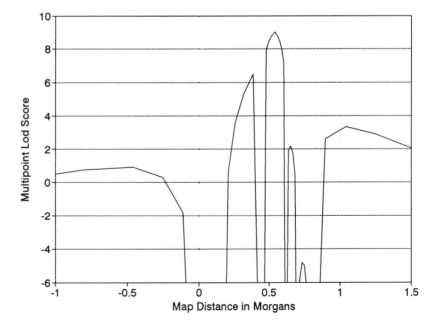

Figure 16–2. Graph of multipoint lod scores from Table 16–4

☐ **Exercise 16**

Assume for the moment that the map was actually the following:

5-(0.02)-2-(0.02)-8-(0.04)-3-(0.01)-6-(0.01)-4-(0.02)-9-(0.03)-7

Now, rerun the LINKMAP analysis. In this case, what is the effect on the maximum lod score, and the 3-unit-of-lod-score support interval? How long is the support interval now, and how many intervals are covered? This points out the importance of having an accurate map of your markers before doing the LINKMAP analysis, because the results are highly dependent on the initial map distance estimates, in terms of the length of the 3-unit-of-lod-score support intervals, and sometimes the lod score values themselves. Remember that irrespective of the specific map of markers, the two-point support interval is still 47.8 cM long for this example, so if this were the true map of markers, multipoint analysis would have reduced the length of our support interval to a small fraction of its original length.

17 □

Exclusion Mapping

In this chapter, we introduce the concept of exclusion mapping. Issues surrounding the usage of negative test results are considered, including the relative power of two-point and multipoint methods for excluding chromosomal regions, and various pitfalls in the interpretation of negative linkage test results. Two methods of exclusion mapping are in general use. The first is based on the log likelihood of a trait versus a marker or map of markers; the second employs Bayesian arguments (prior–posterior probability of map position) and has been employed for two-point analysis in a program called EXCLUDE (Edwards, 1987). Here, only the likelihood-based approach is illustrated.

17.1 Using Negative Test Results

In linkage analysis, the interest is primarily in localizing putative disease genes relative to well-characterized marker loci. As we have discussed thus far, the focus of such analysis is obtaining a positive test result for linkage (lod score > 3) and then trying to fine map the precise chromosomal location of the disease gene, as a prelude to isolating the genetic effect by molecular methods. However, with any given marker, the probability of finding a positive test result is quite low, because the human genome is very large and most randomly selected markers are not linked to the putative disease gene. Further, even if the selected marker is linked to the disease gene, there is no guarantee of a positive test result in any finite pedigree sample. In light of this, we need some way to accommodate negative test results as well so as to eliminate various chromosomal regions from consideration. In doing this, we concentrate the remainder of our genomic search without repeating redundant work, in areas where the gene most likely is not. One way of doing this is *exclusion mapping*.

The methodology of exclusion mapping is quite different from that of the test-and-estimate approach to positive "inclusion" mapping. Obviously, if the test statistic being applied is

$$Z_{max} = \log_{10} \frac{L(\hat{\theta})}{L\left(\theta = \frac{1}{2}\right)}$$

$Z_{max} \geq 0$ always. It is important to remember that the likelihood ratio test is a test of the hypothesis of no linkage, such that in the absence of a significant test result, you fail to reject H_0, meaning that there is no significant evidence for linkage. However, this does not mean that you accept H_0 and have proved by the failure to achieve a significant positive test result that there is no linkage. It is quite another thing to prove the absence of linkage—a problem that can be statistically very complicated.

Morton has proposed (1955) that the test of linkage be treated as a sequential likelihood ratio test (LRT) of a simple hypothesis, $\theta = \theta_1$. He proposed that new families continue to be sampled until either the criterion $Z(\theta_1) > 3$ is fulfilled, in which case you would reject the hypothesis of no linkage, or until $Z(\theta_1) < -2$, in which case you would reject the hypothesis of linkage. As long as $-2 < Z(\theta_1) < 3$, no conclusions can be made. As described by Chotai (1984), this concept was extended to the general case such that the positive test is considered significant whenever $Z_{max} > 3$; and the negative test is considered significant on $\{\theta \mid Z(\theta) < -2\}$, and the disease gene is said to be excluded from this region of the genome, where the lod scores fall below -2. The same criteria are routinely accepted for multipoint lod scores as well, though the theory is less well characterized in this case.

17.2 Two-point Exclusion Mapping

Consider an example of exclusion mapping to see how it can be applied in practice. Go back to the data set from the previous chapter (files MULTDIS1.*) and compute lod scores for the disease versus marker 2 with MLINK, starting from $\theta = 0$, in steps of 0.01 up to $\theta = 0.5$. Then, examine the output using the LRP program. In this two-point analysis, there is clearly no significant positive test result, so we cannot estimate the location of the putative disease gene. However, examining the lod scores, you see that on the interval $[0, 0.13]$, $Z(\theta) < -2$, so the disease gene can be excluded from being in this region. This exclusion covers a range of 13% recombination on either side of marker 2, which is a total genetic distance of 30.1 cM excluded.

Now, repeat the analysis using marker 9 and the disease. In this case, there is a positive test result for linkage between these two loci, with $Z_{max} = 4.698$ at $\theta = 0.15$. However, we also note that $Z(\theta = 0) = -\infty$, so we also have a negative test result with the same marker. These two results can be reconciled if you go back to the original formulation of the sequential test as a test of each simple hypothesis, $\theta = \theta_1$. Thus, the hypothesis $\theta = 0$ is rejected in favor of the hypothesis $\theta = 0.15$. The conclusion is that there is linkage between the disease and marker 9, but that $\theta > 0$. In this case, the 3-unit-of-lod-score support interval for the estimate of θ is $\theta \in (0.02, 0.43)$, since $Z(\theta) > 1.698 \ (= 4.698 - 3)$ at all values of $\{\theta \mid 0.02 < \theta < 0.43\}$. In general, exclusion mapping is most useful when there is no positive test result, because a positive test result allows us to develop a support interval for the location of the disease gene. Further exclusion information is not of use in this situation, because the gene was already localized to some degree and now fine mapping can begin.

17.3 Multipoint Exclusion Mapping

Exclusion mapping is also routinely performed using multipoint analysis based on the same criteria. In general, a much greater exclusion map can be obtained using multipoint analysis than using two-point analysis, because under certain incorrect locus orders, obligate double recombinants can be quite prevalent, greatly lowering the multipoint lod score. Let us go back to the example from the previous chapter and look at the multipoint lod scores we generated in that analysis. If you look at all points with lod scores lower than -2, you see that the regions from map positions [0, 0.162518] and [0.720445, 0.786475] can be excluded. Furthermore, the disease gene is mapped to the region (0.3856, 0.6066) by the 3-unit-of-lod-score support criterion. Hence, we have the ability to exclude regions of the genome that are only 12 cM away from the region to which the disease was mapped, with such region covering a 6 cM range. The total exclusion region in this analysis is 22 cM in an analysis with a positive lod score of 12. This is impossible with two-point analysis in this pedigree set. We saw that a 35-cM region can be excluded with one two-point analysis, but when the two-point result contained a positive test result, the maximum exclusion was extremely small (<1 cM). In fact, the two-point analysis with which the lod score of 10 was obtained allows for the exclusion of none of the genome. When there is no linkage, multipoint analysis can generally provide a much more complete exclusion map than two-point analysis.

17.4 Model Errors and Exclusion Mapping

It has been shown that using an incorrect model for the disease does not in general lead to an increased false-positive rate (Clerget-Darpoux et al., 1986), although maximizing the lod score over models does (Weeks et al., 1990a). In other words, you are not more likely to obtain spurious lod scores of 3 in the absence of linkage at a higher rate under the wrong model than using the correct model. If there is linkage, however, there is lower power to detect it when the model parameters are incorrectly specified. Furthermore, the estimates of the recombination fraction are typically inflated.

Contrary to the lack of false positives, the false-negative rate can be astronomical when an analysis is performed under an incorrect model. It is very simple to design cases in which the disease can be "excluded" from its true location by the $Z(\theta) < -2$ criterion, when the analysis is done under an incorrect model. For this reason, when doing a linkage analysis with a complex disease for which the model is not accurately known, it is not wise to use exclusion analysis because the exclusion results obtained apply only to that specific model. You can only say that a given region was excluded if the analysis model is correct. Thus, we do not advocate any kind of exclusion analysis when the model is not known with a high degree of accuracy. There is of course an additional problem with exclusion mapping when there is the possibility of genetic heterogeneity, or diagnostic instability (see Part III). If there is linkage in only 20% of families, then summing the lod scores across families can easily lead to spurious exclusions. Similarly, if there is a significant rate of diagnostic uncertainty or instability, then it is again easy to induce false recombinants, leading to mistaken exclusion of the true disease map location.

☐ **Exercise 17**

Consider again the disease pedigrees from Chapter 16 (Files MULTDIS1.*). This time, however, repeat the analysis using an incorrect model, assuming the disease to be autosomal recessive with 80% penetrance.

Next analyze the disease under the fully penetrant dominant model with the assumption that all unaffected persons are actually unaffected with only 75% certainty (see Chapter 10). How does altering the model change your conclusions from the linkage analysis, including both positive and negative results?

18 □

Sex Difference in Recombination Rates: Multipoint Case

In this chapter you learn how to treat sex difference in recombination rates. You estimate them in CILINK and then use them in LINKMAP to help refine your estimates of gene location.

Gametes are produced in males and females by the extremely different processes of spermatogenesis and oogenesis. As a by-product of the different processes involved, the recombination rates in the two sexes are known to be quite different. In fact, with the exception of the telomeres, males tend to exhibit much lower rates of recombination than females. The precise biological reason for this is not important to the linkage analyst but rather it is the quantification of the effect that is of greatest concern. If male and female recombination rates are really so different, then this fact should be used in the linkage analysis to glean maximal information from the data at hand. Much finer recombination estimates can be obtained and higher power can be gained in multipoint analyses by using this information. The LINKAGE programs are equipped to estimate sex-specific recombination rates in ILINK and CILINK, and to utilize this information for fine mapping in LINKMAP and CMAP, as you will see below.

18.1 Estimating Sex-specific Recombination Rates

Estimating sex-specific rates of recombination in the ILINK or CILINK program is simple. To illustrate, reconsider the data set from Chapter 14. Call up the LCP program to analyze the appropriate pedigree and parameter files (CEPH1.*). Then select the following options in order: *Three-generation pedigrees, CILINK, All Orders,* and *Varying sex difference.* The *varying sex difference* option means that separate male and female recombination fractions should be estimated for each interval. Now, set up the analysis exactly as you had done for the previous exercise, as follows:

```
                 Locus set [ ] : 1 2 3
    Male recombination fractions [.1] : .1 .1
  Female recombination fractions [.1] : .1 .1
```

Then, hit ⟨Page Down⟩ to save the analysis and ⟨Ctrl-Z⟩ to exit the program. Run the analysis by typing *PEDIN* at the DOS prompt and then examine the results in the LRP program, exactly as you did before. You should find the following results:

Order	−2 LN Like	Odds
.060 .060 3 − − − −1 − − − −2 .080 .020	−1.9418E+02	1.00E+00 <= =
.060 .120 1 − − − −2 − − − −3 .020 .060	−1.8537E+02	8.21E+01
.060 .119 1 − − − −3 − − − −2 .080 .060	−1.6730E+02	6.90E+05

In this analysis, there was even less significance than when the sex-difference in recombination rates was not allowed for.

18.2 Constant Female-to-male Map Distance Ratio

Also, you should notice that in each case, the estimates for the male recombination fractions are presented on top, and the estimates for the female recombination fractions are on the bottom. Note that under order 3-1-2 in interval 1, the female recombination rate is higher than the male rate, whereas in interval 2 the male rate is higher than the female rate. The same applies to order 1-3-2. This is highly unlikely in reality because the region is so small that the difference in recombination rates might reasonably be expected to be somewhat comparable. The programs allow you to fix such a restriction in the form of a constant ratio of female-to-male map distance. This means that $x_{Hald}(\theta_f)/x_{Hald}(\theta_m) = R$, where R is held constant over the entire set of markers to be analyzed together. Now, instead of independently estimating four recombination fractions (two male and two female) for each locus order, only three free parameters are estimated jointly: two male θ's, and the constant female-to-male map distance ratio. In this way, the number of free parameters can be reduced, and the restriction (that sex difference in recombination is held constant over the region under consideration) is allowed for, which is a reasonable thing to believe over a short map length. Furthermore, in this way, you are using more data to estimate the constant ratio of recombination rates, making the estimated sex difference more precise. To do this, repeat the analysis above, only choose the *Constant sex difference* rather than the *Varying sex difference* option in LCP. Then, set up the following screen:

```
                Locus set [ ] : 1 2 3
Male recombination fractions [.1] : .1 .1
Female-to-male distance ratio [1] : 1
```

Then, perform the analysis and read the output into LRP. You should see the following results:

Order	−2 LN Like	Odds
.076 .044 3 − − − −1 − − − −2 .064 .036	−1.9304E+02	1.00E+00 <==
.056 .124 1 − − − −2 − − − −3 .024 .056	−1.8529E+02	4.81E+01
.079 .101 1 − − − −3 − − − −2 .061 .079	−1.6630E+02	6.42E+05

So, we see that allowing for a constant sex difference in recombination rates reduces our power to order these three loci even further. Looking at the estimated recombination rates, the value of the constant sex ratio is not at all clear. Let us compute the value of this ratio for the order 3-1-2. In interval 1, we have $\theta_m = 0.076$ and $\theta_f = 0.064$. Converting these into map distances using the Haldane mapping function (which in this case is mandatory because the distance ratio is set to a constant in the program under this mapping function only!), we have

$$x_m = -0.5 \ln(1 - 2(0.076)) = 0.0824$$

$$x_f = -0.5 \ln(1 - 2(0.064)) = 0.0685$$

From this, we can compute

$$R = \frac{x_f}{x_m} = \frac{0.0685}{0.0824} = 0.831$$

Similarly, for interval 2, we have

$$R = \frac{x(0.036)}{x(0.044)} = \frac{0.0374}{0.0461} = 0.0811$$

Likewise, in the outer interval

$$x_m(3,2) = 0.0824 + 0.0461 = 0.1285$$

$$x_f(3,2) = 0.0685 + 0.0374 = 0.1059$$

$$R = \frac{x_f}{x_m} = \frac{0.1059}{0.1285} = 0.824$$

These values are all very close to each other, and given the degree of rounding error present in these estimated θ's and map distance conversions, they can be considered to be equal. In fact, a theoretical formulation of the female-to-male map distance can be written in one equation as

$$R = \frac{\ln(1 - 2\theta_f)}{\ln(1 - 2\theta_m)}.$$

Substituting our values, for interval 1 we get

$$\frac{\ln[1 - 2(0.064)]}{\ln[1 - 2(0.076)]} = 0.831$$

as above. Because we know that all these estimates of the ratio of female-to-male map distance are approximate (subject to rounding error), let us use LRP to determine what value of R was really estimated by the program. To do this, call up LRP as before, only this time, select the Full format option. You should see the following screen for the analysis of constant sex ratio:

```
        Initial Male Recomb. : 0.076 0.044
                Locus Order : 03 — — — — —01 — — — — —02
      Female Recombination : 0.064 0.036
         Constant Sex Ratio : 0.824

      Generalized LOD Score : +4.191800E+01



                       Data : Valid
                  Data Type : Autosomal



    Maximum −2 LN Likelihood : −1.930400E+02
                        PTG : −6.665120E−05
        Number of Iterations : 8
        Likelihood Validity : Valid
      Gemini Exit Condition : Specified tolerance on normalized
                              gradient met.
     Iterated Parameter List :            1          1          1
       Final Parameter Values : +7.624180E−02 +4.373910E−02
                               +8.240760E−01
       Final Gradient Values : +0.000000E+00 +4.419420E−01
                               +0.000000E+00
```

This tells us that the estimated constant sex ratio was 0.824. Let us determine the female recombination fraction from the estimates of male recombination fraction and sex ratio. To do this (for interval 1), we need first to convert the male recombination fraction to map distance, according to

$$x_m = -0.5\ln[1 - 2(0.076)] = 0.0824$$

Then, we know that $R = \frac{x_f}{x_m}$; so

$$x_f = Rx_m = (0.824)(0.0824) = 0.0679$$

Converting this back to recombination fraction, you get $\theta_f = 0.5$ $(1 - e^{-2(0.0679)}) = 0.0635$. To three decimal places, this estimate is 0.064, exactly what was given by the CILINK program. To see how the rounding error caused all the deviations we observed in calculating the ratio for each interval do the same calculations for the second interval. You should again get results corresponding to those in the CILINK output file. Internally, the program estimates two parameters: the male recombination fractions, and the female-to-male map distance ratio (Haldane). From these values, it computes the corresponding female recombination fractions at the end. Hence, when we replicated this procedure exactly, the estimates presented in CILINK's output file are completely consistent.

Now, we need to look at our data again to see if we had significant evidence in favor of either model for sex difference in recombination. Consider the fixed order 3-1-2, and look at the values of $-2 \ln$ (Like) under each of these three models of sex difference in recombination rate. You should obtain the results summarized in Table 18–1 in your analysis.

The difference in $-2 \ln$(Like) can be thought of as a chi-square statistic with the number of degrees of freedom equal to the difference in degrees of freedom between the models being compared. In this study, therefore, a test

Table 18–1. Results of Analysis of Sex Difference in Recombination Rates with CILINK under Locus Order 3-1-2

Model	df	−2 ln Like	Δ(−2 ln Like)
Varying sex difference:	4	−194.18	0.00
Constant sex difference:	3	−193.04	1.14
No sex difference:	2	−192.94	1.24

of constant sex difference versus no sex difference has $(3 - 2 =)$ 1, df and the value of the statistic is $[-192.94 - (-193.04)] = 0.10$. This is clearly insignificant. Likewise, if we want to test varying sex difference against no sex difference, the statistic has $(4 - 2 =)$ 2 df and has a value of $[-192.94 - (-194.18)] = 1.24$, which is again insignificant. The exact p-value, as computed with the CHIPROB program is 0.537944, which is completely insignificant, so you cannot reject the null hypothesis of no sex difference in this sample.

Repeat the analysis above using all four loci in this data set. At the end, you should have the results shown in Table 18–2.

In this case, it is clear that the hypothesis of constant sex difference is not significantly better than that of no sex difference ($\chi^2_{(1)} = 0.10$), whereas that of varying sex difference is somewhat more supported ($\chi^2_{(3)} = 2.97$), but the p-value is still only 0.396277, so no significant evidence exists for sex difference in recombination rates in this pedigree set. It is interesting to examine more closely the results of the analysis with varying sex difference. The estimated recombination rates in this analysis are:

```
 .060 .020 .040
3----1----4----2
 .080 .021 .001
```

Computing the female-to-male map distance ratios for each intermarker region, we find $R_1 = 1.35$, $R_2 = 1.044$, $R_3 = 0.016$. In fact, the estimated recombination rate between loci 4 and 2 should have been 0, making this ratio 0, which shows that in this family set every recombination event between markers 4 and 2 occurred in males. If you remember, this family had 100 informative meioses: 50 in females, and 50 in males. Only four meioses showed a recombination between loci 4 and 2, and all of them seem to have occurred in males. Because this rate is so small anyway, it is not extremely rare to observe no recombinants by chance in a given sex. For this reason, it is often safer to estimate a constant sex ratio of map distances to prevent having frequent estimates of $\theta = 0$ in one sex, with a somewhat larger estimate in the other. If a recombination occurred in one sex between two markers, the recombination fraction must be greater than 0 in the other sex as well, because there is obviously some genetic distance between the markers.

Table 18–2. Results of Analysis of Sex Difference in Recombination Rates with CILINK Using All Four Loci Jointly

Model	df	−2 ln Like	Δ(−2 ln Like)
Varying sex difference:	6	−328.91	0.00
Constant sex difference:	4	−326.04	2.87
No sex difference:	3	−325.94	2.97

18.3 Using Sex Difference in General Pedigree Data

We now want to see how information about sex difference in recombination rates can be used in general pedigree data. Reconsider the autosomal dominant disease from Chapter 16 in two new pedigrees, structurally and phenotypically (at the trait locus) identical to those in Figure 16–1, with different marker locus genotypes as indicated in Table 18–3. Assume the same markers have been typed here as well (make files MULTDIS2.* - Note that

Table 18–3. Genotypes for Pedigrees with Structure as Shown in Figure 16–1, to Be Entered in Files MULTDIS2.*

Pedigree	Individual	M1	M2	M3	M4	M5	M6	M7	M8
1	1	2 2	2 2	2 2	2 2	2 2	2 2	2 2	2 2
1	2	1 1	1 1	1 1	1 1	1 1	1 1	1 1	1 1
1	3	1 2	1 2	1 2	1 2	1 2	1 2	1 2	1 2
1	4	1 1	1 1	1 1	1 1	1 1	1 1	1 1	1 1
1	5	1 2	1 2	1 1	1 2	1 2	1 1	1 2	1 1
1	6	1 1	1 2	1 2	1 1	1 2	1 2	1 1	1 2
1	7	1 2	1 2	1 2	1 1	1 2	1 2	1 2	1 2
1	8	1 2	1 2	1 2	1 2	1 2	1 2	1 2	1 2
1	9	1 1	1 1	1 1	1 1	1 1	1 1	1 1	1 1
1	10	1 2	1 2	1 2	1 2	1 2	1 2	1 2	1 2
1	11	1 1	1 2	1 2	1 1	1 2	1 2	1 2	1 2
1	12	1 1	1 1	1 2	1 1	1 2	1 2	1 1	1 2
1	13	1 2	1 2	1 1	1 2	1 2	1 1	1 2	1 1
1	14	1 1	1 1	1 1	1 1	1 1	1 2	1 1	1 1
1	15	1 2	1 1	1 1	1 2	1 1	1 1	1 2	1 1
1	16	1 2	1 1	1 1	1 2	1 1	1 1	1 2	1 1
1	17	1 2	1 1	1 1	1 2	1 1	1 1	1 2	1 1
1	18	1 1	1 1	1 1	1 1	1 1	1 2	1 1	1 2
1	19	1 1	1 1	1 1	1 1	1 1	1 1	1 1	1 1
1	20	1 2	1 1	1 1	1 2	1 1	1 2	1 2	1 1
1	21	1 2	1 1	1 1	1 1	1 1	1 1	1 2	1 1
1	22	1 2	1 2	1 2	1 2	1 2	1 2	1 2	1 2
1	23	1 1	1 1	1 1	1 1	1 1	1 1	1 1	1 1
1	24	1 1	1 2	1 2	1 1	1 2	1 2	1 2	1 2
1	25	1 2	1 2	1 2	1 2	1 2	1 1	1 2	1 1
1	26	1 2	1 2	1 1	1 2	1 1	1 1	1 2	1 1
2	1	2 2	2 2	2 2	2 2	2 2	2 2	2 2	2 2
2	2	1 1	1 1	1 1	1 1	1 1	1 1	1 1	1 1
2	3	1 2	1 2	1 2	1 2	1 2	1 2	1 2	1 2
2	4	1 1	1 1	1 1	1 1	1 1	1 1	1 1	1 1
2	5	1 2	1 2	1 1	1 2	1 2	1 1	1 2	1 1
2	6	1 2	1 2	1 2	1 2	1 2	1 2	1 2	1 2
2	7	1 2	1 2	1 2	1 2	1 2	1 2	1 2	1 2
2	8	1 2	1 2	1 2	1 2	1 2	1 2	1 2	1 2
2	9	1 1	1 1	1 1	1 1	1 1	1 1	1 1	1 1
2	10	1 2	1 2	1 2	1 2	1 2	1 2	1 2	1 2
2	11	1 1	1 2	1 2	1 1	1 2	1 2	1 2	1 2
2	12	1 1	1 1	1 2	1 1	1 2	1 2	1 1	1 2
2	13	1 2	1 2	1 2	1 2	1 2	1 2	1 2	1 2
2	14	1 1	1 1	1 1	1 1	1 1	1 2	1 1	1 1
2	15	1 2	1 1	1 1	1 2	1 1	1 1	1 2	1 1
2	16	1 1	1 1	1 1	1 1	1 1	1 1	1 1	1 1
2	17	1 1	1 1	1 1	1 1	1 1	1 1	1 1	1 1
2	18	1 1	1 1	1 1	1 1	1 1	1 1	1 1	1 1
2	19	1 1	1 1	1 1	1 1	1 1	1 1	1 1	1 1
2	20	1 2	1 1	1 1	1 2	1 1	1 1	1 2	1 1
2	21	1 2	1 1	1 1	1 1	1 1	1 1	1 2	1 1
2	22	1 2	1 2	1 2	1 2	1 2	1 2	1 2	1 2
2	23	1 1	1 1	1 1	1 1	1 1	1 1	1 1	1 1
2	24	1 2	1 2	1 2	1 2	1 2	1 2	1 2	1 2
2	25	1 2	1 2	1 2	1 2	1 2	1 1	1 2	1 1
2	26	1 1	1 1	1 1	1 1	1 1	1 1	1 1	1 1

Table 18–4. Results (Incorrect) from First Attempt at Analysis of Loci 4, 9, and 7 on Pedigrees from MULTDIS2.*

Model	df	− 2 ln Like	Δ(− 2 ln Like)
Varying sex difference:	4	181.90	0.00
Constant sex difference:	3	181.90	0.00
No sex difference:	2	181.25	− 0.75

MULTDIS2.DAT should be identical to MULTDIS1.DAT because the markers and trait locus have the same parameters as before).

Ignoring the disease, for the moment test whether there is a significant sex difference in recombination rates in these families. Consider only locus order 4-9-7, which we already know is the true order of these loci. Ideally, we want to check for sex differences in recombination rates using the CEPH pedigrees, but in this case it is not possible. Therefore, we must use the general pedigree version of ILINK and a correspondingly reduced set of loci, in this case, three. Now, analyze these three loci in ILINK, using the *Specific order,* and each of the following options in turn: *No sex difference, Constant sex difference,* and *Varying sex difference.* Use starting values of *0.1* for all recombination fractions, and *1* for the female-to-male map distance ratio. When you finish running the analysis, examine the results in LRP, which yields the results shown in Table 18–4.

Note that you have achieved an impossible result, in which the hypothesis of no sex difference has a higher likelihood than varying or constant sex difference, even though no sex difference is a nested hypothesis. This should tell you something is wrong. The other thing that should alert you that an error occurred is that the final estimates of the recombination fractions and female-to-male distance ratios are all the same as the starting values, meaning the program didn't do any maximization at all. ILINK has the peculiar property of not always converging, depending on the initial values given to it. Whenever running this program, it is always advisable to examine the conditions under which the program finished the maximization of the likelihood. To examine the exiting conditions, call up the LRP program again, only this time select the option for *Full format* rather than *Table format.* The results there should contain the following message:

```
Likelihood Validity : Not completely converged (**)
Gemini Exit Condition : Excessive cancellation in gradient
```

This means that the likelihood was not successfully maximized in this analysis and that you should attempt the analysis again with different starting values. Call up LCP and set up another run with the following starting values:

Table 18–5. Correct Results from Analysis of Loci 4, 9, and 7 on Pedigrees from MULTDIS2.*

Model	df	− 2 ln Like	Δ(− 2 ln Like)
Varying sex difference:	4	180.52	0.00
Constant sex difference:	3	180.52	0.00
No sex difference:	2	181.25	0.63

Table 18–6. Analysis of Loci 3, 6, 4, 9, 7 from Pedigrees in MULTDIS2.*

Model	df	− 2 ln Like	Δ(− 2 ln Like)
Varying sex difference:	8	277.8569	0.0000
Constant sex difference:	5	277.8570	0.0001
No sex difference:	4	279.3242	1.4671

```
No sex difference:

                    Locus order [ ] : 4 9 7
      Recombination fractions [.1] : 0.2 0.2

Constant sex difference:

                    Locus order [ ] : 4 9 7
    Male recombination fractions [.1] : 0.2 0.2
      Female/Male distance ratio [1] : 2

Varying sex difference:

                    Locus order [ ] : 4 9 7
    Male recombination fractions [.1] : 0.2 0.2
  Female recombination fractions [.1] : 0.05 0.05
```

Then, run the analysis and examine the output in LRP. This time, first check the exit conditions and likelihood validity with the Full format option. This time the message should say

```
  Likelihood validity : Valid
Gemini exit condition : Specified tolerance on normalized
                        gradient met
```

This should be the case for each sex difference option. Examining the likelihoods you should see the results given in Table 18–5.

None of these comparisons is significant. So, for the purposes of testing on this set of data, nothing is significant at all. However, there is always the option of using more loci together. On the PC it should be possible to analyze five loci together. So, try looking jointly at loci 3-6-4-9-7. When this analysis is finished, the results should look like those given in Table 18–6.

So, in this case, our test for constant sex difference versus no sex difference is again insignificant, but it has a *p*-value of only 0.2257, as opposed to the three-locus case, in which the *p*-value was 0.4273. It turns out that if you can use all the loci jointly, the statistic becomes marginally significant, with an estimated ratio of female-to-male map distance of about 2.113:1.

18.4 Using Sex Difference in Recombination Fraction in LINKMAP

To take advantage of the sex differences in recombination fraction using the LINKMAP program is simple. Analyze loci 3, 6, and 4 versus the disease, moving the disease across the entire length of the map, with five evaluations per interval. The map of this region was 3-(0.075)-6-(0.075)-4, under no sex difference; 3-(0.05)-6-(0.05)-4, with a ratio of female-to-male map distance of 2.113, and male thetas indicated for constant sex difference; 3-(0.05/0.10)-6-(0.05/0.10)-4, in format (θ_m/θ_f), under varying sex difference. Let us reanalyze the data with LINKMAP now. First, call up LCP and select the *LINKMAP* program, *All intervals* option, followed by *No sex difference*. Set up the next screen as:

```
              Test loci [ ] : 1
        Order of fixed loci [ ] : 3 6 4
     Recombination fractions [.1] : 0.075 0.075
Number of evaluations in interval [5] : 5
```

Then, do the same thing with the *Constant sex difference* option, setting up the screen as follows:

```
              Test loci [ ] : 1
        Order of fixed loci [ ] : 3 6 4
   Male recombination fractions [.1] : 0.05 0.05
       Female/Male distance ratio [1] : 2.113
Number of evaluations in interval [5] : 5
```

Finally, set up a third analysis with *Varying sex difference,* as follows:

```
              Test loci [ ] : 1
        Order of fixed loci [ ] : 3 6 4
   Male recombination fractions [.1] : 0.05 0.05
 Female recombination fractions [.1] : 0.10 0.10
Number of evaluations in interval [5] : 5
```

Run these analyses. When you finish, you should obtain the results given in Table 18–7.

In this example, the two situations—constant sex difference, and varying sex difference—give identical results, because the recombination fractions are the same under both models in this case. However, you can see that there is a slight difference between the magnitude of some of the lod scores in the analyses with sex difference and those without, though in general, the differences are minimal. In general applications, however, always use the best supported model. If there is significant evidence for sex difference in recombi-

Table 18–7. LINKMAP Results with and without Allowing for Sex Difference in Recombination Rates. Disease versus Loci 3, 6, and 4.

Thetas			Sex-Averaged Map Distance (in morgans)	No Sex Difference		Sex Ratio = 2.113	
				Location Scores	Lod Scores	Location Scores	Lod Scores
0.5	0.075	0.075		0	0	0	0
0.4	0.075	0.075	−0.80471	12.15294	2.638971	7.527224	1.634513
0.3	0.075	0.075	−0.45814	21.83398	4.741182	15.99249	3.472719
0.2	0.075	0.075	−0.25541	29.28252	6.358606	24.89760	5.406436
0.1	0.075	0.075	−0.11157	33.83958	7.348158	32.66120	7.092278
0	0.075	0.075	0	−4.0E+20	−8.7E+19	−4.0E+20	−8.7E+19
0.015	0.062	0.075	0.015229	45.33776	9.844952	45.46628	9.872858
0.03	0.048	0.075	0.030934	49.54470	10.75847	49.63480	10.77804
0.045	0.033	0.075	0.047157	52.06690	11.30616	52.12358	11.31847
0.06	0.017	0.075	0.063916	53.92788	11.71027	53.95502	11.71616
0.075	0	0.075	0.081257	55.45176	12.04117	55.45176	12.04117
0.075	0.015	0.062	0.096486	54.13072	11.75431	54.08710	11.74484
0.075	0.03	0.048	0.112193	52.46032	11.39159	52.37892	11.37391
0.075	0.045	0.033	0.128414	50.12484	10.88445	50.01056	10.85963
0.075	0.06	0.017	0.145174	46.10902	10.01242	45.96564	9.981292
0.075	0.075	0	0.162518	−4.0E+20	−8.7E+19	−4.0E+20	−8.7E+19
0.075	0.075	0.1	0.274090	33.83958	7.348158	32.66120	7.092278
0.075	0.075	0.2	0.417931	29.28252	6.358606	24.89760	5.406435
0.075	0.075	0.3	0.620664	21.83398	4.741181	15.99249	3.472719
0.075	0.075	0.4	0.967237	12.15293	2.638971	7.527224	1.634513

nation fractions, then use this information when doing a LINKMAP analysis, because it allows for a more accurate likelihood analysis. In any of the situations discussed thus far, the inclusion of sex-specific recombination rates is simple and straightforward, so we do not go into specific details about how to include it in each possible application. Unless stated otherwise, all analyses to be discussed using the LINKAGE programs can be adapted for sex-specific recombination rates with a minimum of additional effort.

□ Exercise 18

Go back to the set of CEPH pedigrees from Exercise 14 (files USEREX14.*). Reanalyze the data allowing for sex difference in recombination under both the constant and varying sex difference options, using all five loci jointly.

Then, repeat the LINKMAP–ILINK analyses of sex difference in recombination fraction with our disease, using the data in the pedigrees from Chapter 16 (MULTDIS1.*). Is there strong evidence for sex difference in recombination fraction with loci 3-6-4-9-7? Which hypothesis is supported: constant or varying sex difference? What happens if you combine the pedigrees in the two disease data sets with the dominant disease (MULTDIS1.* and MULTDIS2.*) and analyze them together? Is there more evidence for sex difference in recombination? Is there anything interesting about these two data sets?

19.

Introduction to Interference

In this chapter, the concept of genetic interference is introduced. Although there is currently no overwhelming support for any specific model of interference in humans, it is believed to be present. Clearly, if an accurate model for positive interference were available, it would greatly increase the power of multipoint linkage analysis. In this chapter, we introduce how to allow for interference in three-point analysis with the ILINK program and briefly discuss preliminary versions of the CLINKAGE programs that allow for interference according to certain models.

19.1 What Is Interference?

Interference is the phenomenon whereby crossovers do not occur independently along a chromosome, and the presence of a crossover at any given location affects the probability of finding another crossover in a nearby chromosomal region. It is a well-known phenomenon in many species, such as mice, and *Drosophila*. Typically, such interference is positive, meaning that a crossover at one location decreases the probability of another crossover in a nearby region, perhaps due to a stearic hindrance or other biochemical reaction. Researchers often postulate that positive interference exists in humans, though it has not yet been demonstrated by rigorous statistical examination (Sturt, 1976). The presence and characterization of such interference may be of utility in linkage mapping. Presently, the LINKAGE programs perform multipoint likelihood calculations that assume the absence of interference. If positive interference is present in humans, double recombinants in a small region are then accorded too large a probability of occurrence, so allowing for it in the analysis could allow potentially for somewhat increased power in locus ordering and for further accuracy in fine scale linkage mapping. The first problems, however, are to prove its existence and to develop a quantification of the phenomenon.

19.2 Three-point Analysis of Interference

The simplest and most straightforward manner of solving the problem is based on three-point analysis, as described in Ott (1991). Assume three colinear markers, A-B-C, and then estimate θ_{AB}, θ_{BC}, and θ_{AC}, without restricting that there be no interference. The likelihood could then be reparametrized, as shown in Table 19–1.

The ILINK program has an option to analyze three-point data according to the above parametrization. Basically, the program estimates the probabilities α, β, and γ, with $\delta = 1 - \alpha - \beta - \gamma$. From these estimates, it determines the estimates of the three recombination fractions, $\theta_{AB} = \alpha + \gamma$; $\theta_{BC} = \alpha + \beta$; $\theta_{AC} = \beta + \gamma$, as should be clear from Table 19–1 (Remember from Chapter 14 that the recombination events in two intervals uniquely determine the third interval's recombination status in a three-point analysis). A more common and meaningful parametrization of this analysis is to express the results as estimates of θ_{AB}, θ_{BC}, and c, the coefficient of coincidence, which is a measure of the type and strength of interference.

Interference can be quantified in three-point analysis by the coefficient of coincidence

$$c = \frac{\theta_{AB} + \theta_{BC} - \theta_{AC}}{2\theta_{AB}\theta_{BC}}$$

This quantity c can be interpreted as follows: if $c = 0$, then there is complete positive interference, meaning that a recombination in interval A-B makes it impossible for a second recombination to occur in interval B-C; if $c = 1$, there is no interference (and the Haldane mapping function applies), because then the recombination fractions are independent; if $0 < c < 1$, there is some positive interference, and presence of a recombination decreases the probability of further recombination to some degree in that immediate area; and if $c > 1$, there is negative interference, meaning that one crossover increases the probability of a second crossover in adjacent chromosomal regions. We are thus dealing with the three parameters, θ_{AB}, θ_{BC}, and c, and can perform a likelihood ratio test of the absence of interference, as

$$2 \ln \frac{L(\theta_{AB},\theta_{BC},\hat{c})}{L(\theta_{AB},\theta_{BC},c=1)} \sim \chi^2_{(1)}$$

where the θ's should be estimated separately in numerator and denominator.

Consider the set of pedigrees from Exercise 14 and use the LSP program to extract loci 3, 1, and 2 from the pedigree and parameter files you created in that chapter (USEREX14.*), in a form readable by ILINK, to estimate the recombination fractions θ_{31}, θ_{12}, and θ_{32}, allowing for the presence of interfer-

Table 19–1. Reparametrization of Probabilities of Each Meiosis Type Allowing for Interference, Where $\delta = 1 - \alpha - \beta - \gamma$

Interval B-C	Interval A-B		Total
	Recombinant	*Nonrecombinant*	
Recombinant	α	β	θ_{BC}
Nonrecombinant	γ	δ	$1 - \theta_{BC}$
Total	θ_{AB}	$1 - \theta_{AB}$	

ence. To do so, proceed as follows. First, call up the LSP program by typing LSP at the DOS prompt. Then, respond to its queries as follows:

```
Command                          [ILINK] : ILINK
Pedigree File                [PEDIN.DAT] : USEREX14.PED
Parameter File              [DATAIN.DAT] : USEREX14.DAT
Number of Loci                       [] : 3
Locus Order                          [] : 3 1 2
Interference                        [0] : 1 (To allow interference)
Sex Difference                      [0] : 0 (No sex difference)
Male Recombination Fractions [0.1] : 0.1 0.1 0.1
```

The LSP program then constructs new pedigree and parameter files for this analysis, with only the three specified loci in the new files. This program is called by the PEDIN.BAT files created in LCP in the performance of every linkage analysis done with LCP. However, as in this case, you can see where the LSP program can be a useful tool on its own, to prepare files for such analyses as this one. Your LSP-created parameter file (*DATAFILE.DAT*) and pedigree file (*PEDFILE.DAT*) are ready to be analyzed directly by the UN-KNOWN and ILINK programs (you *cannot use* LCP at this point because the files are named *PEDFILE.DAT* and *DATAFILE.DAT!*). The *DATA-FILE.DAT* file should resemble the following:

```
3 0 0 3
0 0.00000000 0.00000000 0
 3 1 2

2 3
 0.53571430 0.41785710 0.04642857
3
 1 0 0
 0 1 0
 0 0 1

2 3
 0.34931510 0.54452060 0.10616440
3
 1 0 0
 0 1 0
 0 0 1

2 2
 0.74083770 0.25916230
3
 1 0 1
 0 1 1

0 1
 0.10000000 0.10000000 0.10000000
0
 1 1 1
```

The important features of this data file relative to the interference option are indicated on the last four lines. The fourth line from the bottom, *0 1,* has a 0 for *no sex difference,* and a *1* for *allow for interference.* The third line from the bottom contains starting values for the *three* recombination fractions. The second line from the bottom contains a *0,* because we do not wish to estimate other parameters for any of the loci, and the last line contains three *1*'s to tell the program to estimate all three recombination fractions in the manner described above. To use the files created by LSP to test and estimate interference, please call up the *UNKNOWN* program followed by the *ILINK* program. Then, look at the FINAL.DAT file in your word processor. The file should look like the following:

```
CHROMOSOME ORDER OF LOCI :
  3  1  2
************************************************************
P VALUES:
 0.194 0.120 0.077
THETAS:
 0.270 0.197 0.314
************************************************************
-2 LN(LIKE)  =  8.787537241097E+002
OTTS GENERALIZED LOD SCORE  =  5.573634329867E+000
NUMBER OF ITERATIONS  =      6
NUMBER OF FUNCTION EVALUATIONS  =      33
PTG  =  -4.659531440578E-005
************************************************************
************************************************************
```

In this file, you are provided with estimates of *P-VALUES* and *THETAS*. First, the *THETAS* are the estimates of θ_{31}, θ_{12}, and θ_{32}, respectively. The *P-VALUES* are not *p*-values in the statistical sense. They are merely the estimates of the parameters γ, β, and α from Table 19–1 and can be used to recreate the recombination fraction estimates as described above. The other important value to compute in this case is *c*, the coefficient of coincidence. Using the formula given above, for this example

$$c = \frac{0.270 + 0.197 - 0.314}{2(.270)(.197)} = 1.44$$

indicating that in this example the estimated interference is negative because $1.44 > 1$. The next thing to consider is testing whether or not the evidence for interference is significant. Sometimes, only those values of $\hat{c} \leq 1$ are tested against $c = 1$ (one-sided test). On the other hand, significant evidence for negative interference might be indicative of errors in marker typing in your pedigree data, or it might provide evidence for gene conversion at the middle locus. If you wanted to test for any deviation from $c = 1$, you would proceed as follows. The likelihood ratio test is of the form

$$-2 \ln\left[\frac{L(\hat{\theta}_{AB}, \hat{\theta}_{BC}, c = 1)}{L(\hat{\theta}_{AB}, \hat{\theta}_{BC}, \hat{c})}\right] \approx \chi^2_{(1)}$$

The value of $-2 \ln L(\hat{\theta}_{AB}, \hat{\theta}_{BC}, \hat{c})$ is 878.75 from the FINAL.DAT file above. The value of $-2 \ln L(\hat{\theta}_{AB}, \hat{\theta}_{BC}, c = 1)$ can be found by running ILINK on this locus order without allowing for interference. Perform this analysis, and you find that $-2 \ln L(\hat{\theta}_{AB}, \hat{\theta}_{BC}, c = 1) = 878.94$, making our likelihood ratio statistic = $878.94 - 878.75 = 0.19$, for a highly nonsignificant *p*-value of 0.66. Hence, there is no evidence for interference in this sample. Ott et al. (1994) examined a large number of such triples of loci in the CEPH chromosome consortium data and never found any significant evidence for interference in that data set with this approach.

19.3 Sex-specific Interference Analysis

It has also been shown that when there is a sex difference in recombination rates, it must be allowed for to test interference validly, as follows. The sex-pooled coefficient of coincidence c_T is biased upward in general when there really is a sex difference in recombination fractions. If we assume complete interference, $c = 0$ in both males and females, then they showed that c_T is asymptotically unbiased, but when interference is absent in both males and females separately

$$c_T = 1 + \frac{(\theta_{f1} - \theta_{m1})(\theta_{f2} - \theta_{m2})}{(\theta_{f1} + \theta_{m1})(\theta_{f2} + \theta_{m2})}$$

and therefore c_T is asymptotically biased, and inconsistent (as opposed to the consistent result when $c = 0$). Further, asymptotically

$$L(\hat{\theta}_1, \hat{\theta}_2, c = 1) < L(\hat{\theta}_1, \hat{\theta}_2, c = \hat{c}_T (\neq 1))$$

so

$$\frac{L(\hat{\theta}_1, \hat{\theta}_2, \hat{c}_T)}{L(\hat{\theta}_1, \hat{\theta}_2, c = 1)} \to \infty$$

as $n \to \infty$, and the chi-square test fails.

In general, c_T is always greater than the sex-specific coefficients of coincidence. For example, if you estimate $c_T = 1$, you know that $c_T > c_m$ (likewise for c_f). So when you estimate no interference from sex-pooled data, and there is a sex difference in recombination fraction, this implies there is positive interference in each sex separately.

Because there is usually significant evidence for sex differences in the recombination fraction, it is imperative to allow for sex difference in the recombination fractions (and coefficient of coincidence) in your ILINK estimation and testing for the presence of interference in your data. Reconsider the data set used above, loci 3-1-2 in USEREX14.*. And let us use LSP to extract these loci and prepare the files for the interference analysis under the various sex difference options. Repeat everything exactly as before, only now when you are prompted with *Sex Difference* [0]:, enter a *1* to specify a constant sex difference in recombination. Then, analyze the data with ILINK as described before. The FINAL.DAT file should resemble the following:

```
CHROMOSOME ORDER OF LOCI :
   3   1   2
****************************************************
P VALUES:
 0.171 0.087 0.000
FEMALE:
 0.304 0.164 0.095
THETAS:
 0.171 0.087 0.258
FEMALE:
 0.399 0.259 0.469
CONSTANT FEMALE/MALE DIST RATIO :
3.821
****************************************************
-2 LN(LIKE)  = 8.730176055538E+002
OTTS GENERALIZED LOD SCORE = 6.819214051328E+000
NUMBER OF ITERATIONS  =    14
NUMBER OF FUNCTION EVALUATIONS  =     88
PTG = -6.854390155713E-004
****************************************************
****************************************************
```

In this situation, the estimated coefficient of coincidence is

$$c_m = \frac{0.171 + 0.087 - 0.258}{2(0.171)(0.087)} = 0$$

indicating complete positive interference in males, and

$$c_f = \frac{0.399 + 0.259 - 0.469}{2(0.399)(0.259)} = 0.914$$

indicating very slight positive interference in females, assuming a constant sex ratio of 3.821. However, it is probably more appropriate to assume a varying sex ratio, because the sex ratio forces some constraints on the sex-specific coefficients of coincidence, so analyze the data with *Sex difference [0]:* set to *2* in LSP. Then, reanalyzing the data should yield the following FINAL.DAT file:

```
CHROMOSOME ORDER OF LOCI :
  3  1  2
**********************************************************
P VALUES:
 0.146 0.107 0.000
FEMALE:
 0.348 0.115 0.130
THETAS:
 0.146 0.107 0.252
FEMALE:
 0.479 0.245 0.463
FEMALE/MALE DIST RATIO :
 9.161 2.802 3.701
**********************************************************
-2 LN(LIKE) = 8.726082665176E+002
OTTS GENERALIZED LOD SCORE = 6.908100708333E+000
NUMBER OF ITERATIONS =     14
NUMBER OF FUNCTION EVALUATIONS =      117
PTG = -7.623469083546E-004
**********************************************************
**********************************************************
```

In this example, the value of

$$c_m = 0.146 + 0.107 - \frac{0.252}{2(0.146)(0.107)} = 0.03$$

and

$$c_f = 0.479 + 0.245 - \frac{0.463}{2(0.479)(0.245)} = 1.11$$

Again, there is almost complete positive interference in males and slightly negative interference in females. We still must test the hypothesis of interference under each of these models, as before. So, we need to use ILINK to compute the -2 ln(Like) for this locus order under the two sex difference options. The results of this analysis should show that for *Constant sex difference,* -2 ln(Like) = 873.45, and for *Varying sex difference,* -2 ln(Like) = 873.15. Therefore, subtracting the values obtained with interference, our chi-square statistic for *Constant sex difference* = 873.45 − 873.02 = 0.43 ($p = 0.51$); *Varying sex difference* = 873.15 − 872.61 = 0.54 ($p = 0.46$). Thus, when sex difference in recombination fraction is properly allowed for we still have no significant evidence for interference in this data set.

In this chapter, the concept of interference was introduced on a basic level, and testing and estimating interference from three-point data was explained using the ILINK program of the LINKAGE package. To date, no conclusive evidence of interference has been found in man using this approach. This can be due to either a lack of interference in humans or simply that our sample sizes are too small to detect what interference may exist. Ott (1991) determined that for Kosambi level interference, with three equally spaced markers ($\theta = 0.15$) and fully informative phase-known data, 847 meioses are required to reject the null hypothesis of no interference at the 0.05 level with 80% power. With this in mind, it is not surprising that the results of the small analyses done in this chapter proved nonsignificant, whether or not interference is actually present. There are more sophisticated methods currently under development by Weeks and colleagues (1991) and Ott et al (1994) to handle more than three loci at a time in a test for interference in humans. Their preliminary results suggest that the Sturt mapping function (Sturt, 1976) may be the best fitting model for interference in humans, and they have potentially significant evidence for interference of this nature in one six-point analysis. Further investigation is necessary, however, to prove that interference exists as a general phenomenon in human genetics. They are developing a modified version of the CILINK program, called CINTMAX (Weeks et al., 1991), which is capable of analyzing CEPH pedigree data under a variety of possible models of interference. This technique may become useful in gene mapping in the future.

☐ Exercise 19

Consider the data from MULTDIS2.*. Is there any evidence of interference in this data set? Ott (1991) reported that the optimum intermarker spacing to detect interference is approximately $\theta = 0.15 - 0.20$, assuming phase-known data (which we have in this data set for the most part). Choose all ordered triples of loci with $0.125 \leq \theta \leq 0.225$ (to allow us to have more possible triples to consider that are nearly optimal) for both adjacent θ's, assuming the sex-averaged map.

5-(0.075)-2-(0.075)- 8-(0.225)-3-(0.075)-6-(0.075)-4-(0.075)-9-(0.075)-7

Then, test for the presence of interference on each such triple of loci, and report the value of the appropriate χ^2 statistic and the coefficient of coincidence. Repeat this analysis under *no sex difference, constant sex difference,* and *varying sex difference,* providing the values of c_m and c_f separately, where applicable. What are your conclusions about interference in this data set?

20.

Solutions to the Exercises in Part II

☐ Exercise 14

The output from your CILINK analysis should resemble the results shown in Table 20–1. In order to order the loci conclusively, the best order must be at least 1000 times more likely than the second-best order. In this case, you can see that the first four orders are all about equally well supported, and none of them can be excluded. Still, the remaining 56 possible orders can be excluded, because they are more than 1000 times less likely than the best order. Looking closely at the set of orders that cannot be excluded, notice that they all involve three basic groupings as follows: (3, 4) - (5, 1) - 2. Each order in the set of possible orders represents a simple inversion of the order of loci within one of the groups. All possible orders involving mere flips of 3 and 4 or 5 and 1 are approximately equally supported. Hence, the only firm conclusion is that the order is (3, 4)-(5, 1)-2 with odds of over 1000:1. Notice that LCP presents the user with an option *Inversions of adjacent loci*. This option allows the user to see if flipping any pair of loci increases the likelihood significantly, or if all inversions of adjacent loci are still excluded from being possible orders. It is possible to run this analysis with ILINK instead of CILINK only if your computer has the capacity to compile the program with the constant *maxneed* set to 782, and *maxhap* = 108 (See Appendix B for more information about program constants). This is not possible in the Turbo PASCAL version of LINKAGE.

☐ Exercise 15

The results of the CMAP analysis are presented in Table 20–2, including multipoint lod scores and map distance from marker 1. In this analysis, it is impossible to localize new locus 4 to any one map interval, because the 3-unit support interval extends throughout the region between loci 1 and 3, and therefore cannot be uniquely placed with the required odds of 1000:1.

If you attempt to order the four loci with CILINK, the results should be similar to those in Table 20–3. In this case, the odds for order were relatively quite good. Order 3-1-4-2 is the best order (consistent with our CMAP results

Table 20–1. Solutions to Exercise 14 (Files USEREX14.*). Orders Followed by * Are within 3 Lod Units of the Best Order and Cannot Be Excluded

Locus Order	Intermarker θ's	−2 ln Like	Odds
3----4----5----1----2	.049 .251 .049 .207	−1.0395E+02	1.00E+00*
4----3----5----1----2	.058 .234 .049 .207	−1.0380E+02	1.08E+00*
3----4----1----5----2	.052 .239 .036 .231	−1.0339E+02	1.33E+00*
4----3----1----5----2	.056 .224 .035 .231	−1.0292E+02	1.68E+00*
5----1----2----3----4	.049 .199 .350 .060	−8.9534E+01	1.35E+03
5----1----2----4----3	.049 .200 .365 .050	−8.8096E+01	2.78E+03
5----1----4----3----2	.046 .215 .055 .348	−8.7737E+01	3.32E+03
1----5----2----3----4	.036 .212 .347 .061	−8.7002E+01	4.80E+03
5----1----3----4----2	.045 .202 .051 .361	−8.5734E+01	9.05E+03
1----5----2----4----3	.036 .213 .363 .051	−8.5543E+01	9.95E+03
1----5----4----3----2	.044 .229 .054 .352	−8.4005E+01	2.15E+04
1----5----3----4----2	.045 .215 .051 .365	−8.2188E+01	5.33E+04
4----1----5----3----2	.221 .044 .122 .247	−8.0629E+01	1.16E+05
4----5----3----1----2	.204 .041 .140 .211	−7.9706E+01	1.84E+05
4----1----5----2----3	.249 .035 .214 .258	−7.7912E+01	4.52E+05
4----5----1----2----3	.264 .047 .200 .263	−7.7315E+01	6.09E+05
5----3----4----1----2	.207 .051 .240 .212	−7.7158E+01	6.59E+05
5----4----3----1----2	.226 .052 .227 .212	−7.6256E+01	1.03E+06
3----4----1----2----5	.049 .252 .188 .248	−7.4951E+01	1.99E+06
4----3----1----2----5	.060 .237 .187 .248	−7.4873E+01	2.06E+06
1----2----5----3----4	.182 .268 .231 .0581	7.2637E+01	6.32E+06
1----2----5----4----3	.182 .268 .255 .049	−7.1152E+01	1.33E+07
3----5----1----2----4	.166 .055 .190 .375	−7.0649E+01	1.71E+07
3----5----1----4----2	.135 .051 .193 .342	−7.0533E+01	1.81E+07
4----1----3----5----2	.213 .103 .044 .269	−6.8821E+01	4.26E+07
3----5----4----1----2	.064 .177 .229 .209	−6.7046E+01	1.03E+08
1----4----3----5----2	.204 .051 .201 .294	−6.4836E+01	3.12E+08
1----2----3----4----5	.197 .369 .053 .241	−6.4442E+01	3.80E+08
1----2----4----3----5	.197 .385 .053 .222	−6.3806E+01	5.22E+08
3----1----5----2----4	.225 .034 .211 .375	−6.2956E+01	7.99E+08
1----3----4----5----2	.194 .048 .223 .296	−6.2816E+01	8.57E+08
3----1----5----4----2	.185 .040 .209 .345	−6.2414E+01	1.05E+09
1----2----3----5----4	.186 .287 .065 .213	−6.1752E+01	1.46E+09
5----1----4----2----3	.044 .212 .317 .254	−6.0779E+01	2.37E+09
1----3----5----4----2	.125 .036 .183 .359	−5.9809E+01	3.85E+09
1----5----3----2----4	.048 .142 .216 .357	−5.9713E+01	4.04E+09
5----3----1----4----2	.051 .116 .189 .348	−5.8925E+01	6.00E+09
5----1----3----2----4	.046 .169 .199 .348	−5.7962E+01	9.71E+09
1----5----4----2----3	.042 .229 .320 .253	−5.6793E+01	1.74E+10
5----3----1----2----4	.056 .145 .194 .376	−5.6600E+01	1.92E+10
1----4----3----2----5	.213 .054 .333 .281	−5.4754E+01	4.83E+10
1----4----5----3----2	.196 .175 .069 .304	−5.3920E+01	7.32E+10
4----1----2----5----3	.271 .184 .259 .113	−5.3479E+01	9.13E+10
1----2----4----5----3	.198 .380 .196 .0651	5.3306E+01	9.96E+10
4----1----2----3----5	.270 .186 .263 .101	−5.2910E+01	1.21E+11
1----3----4----2----5	.202 .051 .345 .283	−5.2858E+01	1.25E+11
5----4----1----3----2	.221 .196 .150 .245	−4.7971E+01	1.43E+12
5----4----1----2----3	.228 .234 .201 .265	−4.7799E+01	1.56E+12
3----1----2----5----4	.221 .171 .246 .279	−4.7184E+01	2.13E+12
4----5----1----3----2	.100 .100 .100 .100	−4.6881E+01	2.47E+12
1----3----5----2----4	.119 .043 .246 .362	−4.6853E+01	2.51E+12
4----1----3----2----5	.224 .141 .218 .256	−4.5488E+01	4.96E+12
3----1----4----5----2	.171 .174 .209 .285	−4.3895E+01	1.10E+13
3----1----2----4----5	.220 .185 .363 .261	−3.7472E+01	2.73E+14
1----4----5----2----3	.197 .209 .258 .251	−3.6318E+01	4.86E+14
1----3----2----5----4	.175 .195 .246 .269	−3.6267E+01	4.99E+14
3----1----4----2----5	.170 .187 .327 .281	−3.4021E+01	1.53E+15
1----4----2----3----5	.218 .321 .275 .111	−3.2839E+01	2.77E+15
1----4----2----5----3	.218 .323 .283 .102	−3.2614E+01	3.10E+15
1----3----2----4----5	.181 .203 .335 .261	−2.9718E+01	1.32E+16

Table 20–2. Results of CMAP Analysis of CEPH1.*; Assuming Locus Order 1-(0.04)-2-(0.09)-3; Adding New Locus 4 to This Map

Locus Order	Loc Score	−2 ln Like	Odds		Lod Score	Map Distance
4 = = = = 1 − − − − 2 − − − − 3						
.500 .040 .090	+ 0.0000E + 00	− 1.8316E + 02	7.13E + 28		0.00	− ∞
.400 .040 .090	+ 3.4842E + 01	− 2.1800E + 02	1.94E + 21		7.57	− 0.805
.300 .040 .090	+ 6.3905E + 01	− 2.4707E + 02	9.46E + 14		13.88	− 0.458
.200 .040 .090	+ 8.8455E + 01	− 2.7162E + 02	4.42E + 09		19.21	− 0.255
.100 .040 .090	+ 1.0877E + 02	− 2.9193E + 02	1.71E + 05		23.62	− 0.112
.000 .040 .090	+ 6.6542E + 01	− 2.4970E + 02	2.53E + 14		14.45	0
1 = = = = 4 = = = = 2 − − − − 3						
.000 .040 .090	− ∞	∞	∞		− ∞	0
.008 .033 .090	+ 1.3115E + 02	− 3.1431E + 02	2.37E + 00		28.48	0.008
.016 .025 .090	+ 1.3281E + 02	− 3.1597E + 02	1.03E + 00		28.84	0.016
.024 .017 .090	+ 1.3287E + 02	− 3.1604E + 02	1.00E + 00	⟨ = =	28.85	0.025
.032 .009 .090	+ 1.3134E + 02	− 3.1451E + 02	2.15E + 00		28.52	0.033
.040 .000 .090	− ∞	∞	∞		− ∞	0.042
1 − − − − 2 = = = = 4 = = = = 3						
.040 .000 .090	− ∞	∞	∞		− ∞	0.042
.040 .018 .075	+ 1.2875E + 02	− 3.1191E + 02	7.87E + 00		27.96	0.060
.040 .036 .058	+ 1.2769E + 02	− 3.1085E + 02	1.34E + 01		27.72	0.079
.040 .054 .040	+ 1.2398E + 02	− 3.0714E + 02	8.53E + 01		26.92	0.099
.040 .072 .021	+ 1.1595E + 02	− 2.9911E + 02	4.73E + 03		25.18	0.120
.040 .090 .000	− ∞	∞	∞		− ∞	0.141
1 − − − − 2 − − − − 3 = = = = 4						
.040 .090 .000	− ∞	∞	∞		− ∞	0.141
.040 .090 .100	+ 8.6796E + 01	− 2.6996E + 02	1.01E + 10		18.85	0.253
.040 .090 .200	+ 7.4592E + 01	− 2.5775E + 02	4.52E + 12		16.20	0.396
.040 .090 .300	+ 5.5432E + 01	− 2.3859E + 02	6.54E + 16		12.04	0.599
.040 .090 .400	+ 3.0787E + 01	− 2.1395E + 02	1.47E + 22		6.69	0.946
.040 .090 .500	+ 0.0000E + 00	− 1.8316E + 02	7.13E + 28		0.00	∞

of Chapter 15), but the second-best order is only 133 times less likely, so it cannot be excluded. That order is 1-4-2-3. All other orders can be excluded, leaving us with a definitive locus order of 1-4-2, with 3 either proximal to 1 or distal to 2. Again, however, we are left with no additional power to order loci 1, 2, and 3. The odds for ordering are identical, at 133:1 in favor of 3-1-2. However, we were able conclusively to order loci 1-4-2 relative to each other. You may verify with a three-point CILINK run that this order would still have been uniquely determined without including locus 3 in the analysis. Because all markers are typed, phase-known, and fully informative in these families, the addition of further markers does not help in ordering the original loci. The

Table 20–3. CILINK Results for Files CEPH1.*; Loci 1, 2, 3, and 4

Locus Order	Thetas	−2 ln Like	Odds
3----1----4----2	.070 .020 .020	− 3.2594E + 02	1.00E + 00 ⟨ = =
1----4----2----3	.020 .020 .089	− 3.1616E + 02	1.33E + 02
1----2----4----3	.040 .020 .070	− 3.1196E + 02	1.09E + 03
3----1----2----4	.070 .040 .020	− 3.1196E + 02	1.09E + 03
3----4----1----2	.070 .020 .040	− 3.1196E + 02	1.09E + 03
4----1----2----3	.020 .040 .090	− 3.0218E + 02	1.44E + 05
1----3----4----2	.070 .070 .020	− 2.9482E + 02	5.73E + 06
4----1----3----2	.020 .070 .090	− 2.8505E + 02	7.61E + 08
1----4----3----2	.020 .070 .090	− 2.8505E + 02	7.61E + 08
1----3----2----4	.070 .090 .020	− 2.8505E + 02	7.61E + 08
4----3----1----2	.070 .070 .040	− 2.8084E + 02	6.22E + 09
1----2----3----4	.048 .093 .078	− 2.7081E + 02	9.37E + 11

Table 20–4. CILINK Results for Files USEREX14.*; Loci 1, 2, and 3

Locus Order	Thetas	− 2 ln Like	Odds
1----2----3	.197 .294	− 2.4795E + 01	1.00E + 00 ⟨ = =
3----1----2	.249 .191	− 2.4725E + 01	1.04E + 00
1----3----2	.187 .226	− 1.5197E + 01	1.21E + 02

only situation in which the addition of further markers can help is when some markers are phase-unknown in some meioses, or markers are informative in some meioses but not in others. In this case, neither situation obtained, and thus no net change in odds for ordering was possible.

For the data in files USEREX14.*, the results from the CILINK analysis of loci 1, 2, and 3 are given in Table 20–4. In this case, using only the three loci, it is impossible to exclude any of the possible locus orders at the 1000:1 level. So, let us add in locus 4 to the analysis, and see if it helps us order loci 1, 2, and 3. In this case, for the four loci jointly, the CILINK results are shown in Table 20–5. When all four loci are analyzed together, we see that the best four-locus order has 3-1-2 within it. The best order with 1-2-3 in it has odds of 145:1 against it, and the best order with 1-3-2 in it has odds of 2220:1, and can thus be excluded. In contrast to the situation in files CEPH1.*, this example has a great deal more uncertainty in it, and therefore, we improve our locus ordering ability by adding an additional locus as a sort of nuisance parameter. There is still no conclusive ordering of the three loci, so we should analyze all five together, which we did in Chapter 14. The best order had 3-1-2 in it, the best order with order 1-2-3 in it had odds of 1350:1 against it, and the best five-locus order with 1-3-2 in it had odds of 3320:1 against it. Thus, we can establish the order 3-1-2 with the required 1000:1 odds criterion only by adding in the additional loci 4 and 5. Now, we need to compute the intermarker recombination fractions for this locus order from the five-point ordering estimates

$$3\text{-}(0.049)\text{-}4\text{-}(0.251)\text{-}5\text{-}(0.049)\text{-}1\text{-}(0.207)\text{-}2$$

We need to find the recombination between loci 3 and 1 under this scenario. To do this, call up the MAPFUN program, which was introduced in Chapter 15, and select the MS (summing θ's) option. Then, enter successively the values of $\theta_{3,4} = 0.049$, $\theta_{4,5} = 0.251$, and $\theta_{5,1} = 0.049$. The program then gives the result that $\theta_{3,1} = 0.2974$, assuming the Haldane mapping function. This could also have been done by hand by converting all the recombination fractions

Table 20–5. CILINK Results for Files USEREX14.*; Loci 1, 2, 3, and 4

Locus Order	Thetas	− 2 ln Like	Odds
3----4----1----2	.049 .254 .210	− 6.2575E + 01	1.00E + 00 ⟨ = =
4----3----1----2	.059 .239 .209	− 6.2475E + 01	1.05E + 00
1----2----3----4	.199 .379 .058	− 5.2629E + 01	1.45E + 02
1----2----4----3	.199 .400 .051	− 5.1394E + 01	2.68E + 02
1----4----3----2	.217 .053 .351	− 4.7168E + 01	2.22E + 03
1----3----4----2	.206 .051 .365	− 4.5381E + 01	5.42E + 03
4----1----2----3	.272 .197 .266	− 3.5169E + 01	8.94E + 05
4----1----3----2	.223 .147 .244	− 3.4711E + 01	1.12E + 06
3----1----2----4	.225 .188 .391	− 2.7989E + 01	3.24E + 07
3----1----4----2	.170 .191 .347	− 2.6190E + 01	7.96E + 07
1----3----2----4	.183 .206 .356	− 2.0028E + 01	1.73E + 09
1----4----2----3	.221 .321 .253	− 1.8631E + 01	3.49E + 09

into map distance by using the Haldane function $x = -\frac{1}{2}\ln(1 - 2\theta)$, adding the three map distances together, and then converting the total map distance back into a recombination fraction by the relation $\theta = \frac{1}{2}(1 - e^{-2x})$. The result should come out the same, $\theta \approx 0.297$. Now, you can do the CMAP analysis requested with locus order 3-(0.297)-1-(0.207)-2. Try adding locus 4 and 5 to this constant map of markers with the CMAP program as an exercise in general, because we used them to order the loci 3-1-2, we wouldn't bother with CMAP analysis at this point, but do it anyway as an exercise with CMAP. The results are shown in Table 20–6 for locus 4 and in Table 20–7 for locus 5. The CMAP results for locus 4 are somewhat interesting. The entire region between loci 1 and 2 is excluded by the $Z(x) < -2$ criterion, as is much of the region to the right of locus 2. The maximum lod score of 8.27 occurs between loci 3 and 1, very close to locus 3, but the 3-unit support interval extends for about 25 cM on either side of locus 3, giving us no power to place locus 4 uniquely in an interval of this map. It is interesting to note that when the disease is unlinked to the map of markers ($\theta = 0.500$) on the right-hand side, the lod score is not 0, but 0.14. This is because there is often some rounding error in that direction, and the recombination fraction at which that lod score was computed was not exactly 0.500, but slightly smaller. This phenomenon is similar to that observed when 4-(0.000)-3-(0.297)-1-(0.207)-2 has a lod score of -4.18, and 3-(0.000)-4-(0.297)-1-(0.207)-2 has a lod score of $-\infty$, even though they are ostensibly the same point. This is, as well, due to the fact that the first lod score is computed at $\theta > 0.000$, and the value of θ we see in the output is rounded to three decimal places. For this reason, we always use the value with $\theta = 0.500$ to the left as our normalizing value in computing lod or location scores. The analysis with locus 5 allows for no exclusion region but does show evidence for linkage, with a maximum lod score of 8.42 between loci 3 and 1, very close to locus 1, with the 3-unit support interval extending between loci 3 and 2, again not allowing us to order the locus with the required 1000:1 odds.

If we look back at our four-point CILINK analysis with loci 1, 2, 3, and 4, we see that the order 3-4-1-2 was the best order, 4-3-1-2 had odds of 1.05:1 against it (here as well, it was within the support interval), 3-1-2-4 had odds of 32,400,000:1 against it, and 3-1-4-2 had odds of 79,600,000:1 against it. This is compatible with the exclusion results we obtained in the CMAP analysis. Because the recombination fractions were estimated separately in each order with CILINK, the odds are naturally somewhat better than with CMAP, which gave odds against the same orders of 3.08:1, 49,500,000:1, and 1,010,000,000,000,000:1, respectively. In general, unless the map is known with a high degree of certainty, it is more conservative and reliable to use CILINK rather than CMAP for such ordering problems. Similar results are found if you run CILINK to order loci 1, 2, 3, and 5 and compare those results with the output from CMAP.

□ Exercise 16

Results from the LINKMAP analysis are given in Table 20–8 and shown graphically in Figure 20–1. First compare this graph with Figure 16–2 under the alternative locus order. How much can you tell about the analysis from the picture alone? In this analysis, our maximum lod score is reduced to only 7.16 from 9.011 in the example from Chapter 16. Furthermore, our 3-unit support interval is also reduced to only 3.5 cM on the interval (0.066, 0.101). So, you can see that having a finer marker map can help you to narrow the support

Table 20–6. CMAP Results of Locus 4 versus Map 3-(0.297)-1-(0.207)-2

Locus Order/θ's	Location Score	−2 ln Like	Odds		Lod Score	Map Distance
4 = = = =3 − − − −1 − − − −2						
.500 .297 .207	+0.0000E+00	−2.4286E+01	1.88E+08		0.00	−∞
.400 .297 .207	+9.9910E+00	−3.4277E+01	1.27E+06		2.17	−0.805
.300 .297 .207	+2.0518E+01	−4.4804E+01	6.58E+03		4.46	−0.458
.200 .297 .207	+2.9457E+01	−5.3743E+01	7.54E+01		6.40	−0.255
.100 .297 .207	+3.5852E+01	−6.0137E+01	3.08E+00		7.79	−0.112
.000 .297 .207	−1.9271E+01	−5.0145E+00	2.87E+12		−4.18	0.000
3 = = = =4 = = = =1 − − − −2						
.000 .297 .207	−∞	∞	∞		−∞	0.000
.059 .270 .207	+3.8103E+01	−6.2388E+01	1.00E+00	⟨ = =	8.27	0.063
.119 .234 .207	+3.5723E+01	−6.0008E+01	3.29E+00		7.76	0.136
.178 .185 .207	+2.9975E+01	−5.4261E+01	5.82E+01		6.51	0.220
.238 .113 .207	+1.6710E+01	−4.0996E+01	4.42E+04		3.63	0.323
3 − − − −1 = = = =4 = = = =2						
.297 .000 .207	−∞	∞	∞		−∞	0.450
.297 .041 .181	−3.8826E+01	+1.4540E+01	5.07E+16		−8.43	0.493
.297 .083 .149	−3.0996E+01	+6.7104E+00	1.01E+15		−6.73	0.541
.297 .124 .110	−3.7932E+01	+1.3646E+01	3.24E+16		−8.24	0.593
.297 .166 .062	−6.4530E+01	+4.0244E+01	1.93E+22		−14.01	0.652
.297 .207 .000	−∞	∞	∞		−∞	0.718
3 − − − −1 − − − −2 = = = =4						
.297 .207 .000	−∞	∞	∞		−∞	0.718
.297 .207 .100	−4.4800E+01	+2.0514E+01	1.00E+18		−9.72	0.830
.297 .207 .200	−1.2589E+01	−1.1697E+01	1.02E+11		−2.73	0.973
.297 .207 .300	−3.5960E−01	−2.3926E+01	2.25E+08		−0.08	1.176
.297 .207 .400	+2.6670E+00	−2.6953E+01	4.95E+07		0.58	1.523
.297 .207 .500	+6.6360E−01	−2.4949E+01	1.35E+08		0.14	∞

Table 20–7. CMAP Results of Locus 5 versus Map 3-(0.297)-1-(0.207)-2

Locus Order/θ's	Location Score	−2 ln Like	Odds		Lod Score	Map Distance
5 = = = =3 − − − −1 − − − −2						
.500 .297 .207	+0.0000E+00	−2.4285E+01	2.65E+08		0.00	−∞
.400 .297 .207	+6.0046E+00	−3.0290E+01	1.32E+07		1.30	−0.805
.300 .297 .207	+1.2257E+01	−3.6542E+01	5.78E+05		2.66	−0.458
.200 .297 .207	+1.7746E+01	−4.2032E+01	3.71E+04		3.85	−0.255
.100 .297 .207	+2.1638E+01	−4.5923E+01	5.31E+03		4.70	−0.112
.000 .297 .207	−3.5068E+01	+1.0782E+01	1.09E+16		−0.76	0.000
3 = = = =5 = = = =1 − − − −2						
.000 .297 .207	−∞	∞	∞		−∞	0.000
.059 .270 .207	+2.8783E+01	−5.3069E+01	1.49E+02		6.25	0.063
.119 .234 .207	+3.2422E+01	−5.6707E+01	2.42E+01		7.04	0.136
.178 .185 .207	+3.5563E+01	−5.9849E+01	5.02E+00		7.72	0.220
.238 .113 .207	+3.8791E+01	−6.3077E+01	1.00E+00	⟨ = =	8.42	0.323
3 − − − −1 = = = =5 = = = =2						
.297 .000 .207	−∞	∞	∞		−∞	0.450
.297 .041 .181	+3.2667E+01	−5.6953E+01	2.14E+01		7.09	0.493
.297 .083 .149	+2.8794E+01	−5.3080E+01	1.48E+02		6.25	0.541
.297 .124 .110	+2.0955E+01	−4.5241E+01	7.47E+03		4.55	0.593
.297 .166 .062	+4.9642E+00	−2.9250E+01	2.22E+07		1.08	0.652
.297 .207 .000	−∞	∞	∞		−∞	0.718
3 − − − −1 − − − −2 = = = =5						
.297 .207 .000	−∞	∞	∞		−∞	0.718
.297 .207 .100	−5.1220E−01	−2.3773E+01	3.42E+08		−0.11	0.830
.297 .207 .200	+9.7451E+00	−3.4031E+01	2.03E+06		2.12	0.973
.297 .207 .300	+1.0337E+01	−3.4623E+01	1.51E+06		2.24	1.176
.297 .207 .400	+6.2507E+00	−3.0536E+01	1.16E+07		1.36	1.523
.297 .207 .500	+1.0000E−04	−2.4286E+01	2.65E+08		0.00	∞

Table 20–8. LINKMAP Results: Files MULTDIS1.*

Locus Order/θ's	Location Score	− 2 ln Like	Lod Score	Map Distance
1 = = = = 5 – – – – 2 – – – – 8 – – – – 3				
.500 .020 .020 .040	+ 0.0000E + 00	+ 4.2881E + 02	0.00	− ∞
.400 .020 .020 .040	+ 3.4775E + 00	+ 4.2533E + 02	0.76	− 0.805
.300 .020 .020 .040	+ 4.2394E + 00	+ 4.2457E + 02	0.92	− 0.458
.200 .020 .020 .040	+ 1.4615E + 00	+ 4.2735E + 02	0.32	− 0.255
.100 .020 .020 .040	− 8.3698E + 00	+ 4.3718E + 02	− 1.81	− 0.112
5 = = = = 1 = = = = 2 – – – – 8 – – – – 3				
.000 .020 .020 .040	− ∞	∞	− ∞	0.000
.004 .016 .020 .040	− 1.3563E + 02	+ 5.6444E + 02	− 2.94	0.004
.008 .012 .020 .040	− 1.2733E + 02	+ 5.5614E + 02	− 2.76	0.008
.012 .008 .020 .040	− 1.2822E + 02	+ 5.5703E + 02	− 2.78	0.012
.016 .004 .020 .040	− 1.3865E + 02	+ 5.6746E + 02	− 3.01	0.016
.020 .000 .020 .040	− ∞	∞	− ∞	0.020
5 – – – – 2 = = = = 1 = = = = 8 – – – – 3				
.020 .000 .020 .040	− ∞	∞	− ∞	0.020
.020 .004 .016 .040	− 1.3883E + 02	+ 5.6763E + 02	− 3.01	0.024
.020 .008 .012 .040	− 1.2746E + 02	+ 5.5627E + 02	− 2.77	0.028
.020 .012 .008 .040	− 1.2539E + 02	+ 5.5420E + 02	− 2.72	0.032
.020 .016 .004 .040	− 1.3193E + 02	+ 5.6074E + 02	− 2.86	0.037
.020 .020 .000 .040	− ∞	∞	− ∞	0.041
1 = = = = 2 – – – – 8 – – – – 3 – – – – 6				
.500 .020 .040 .010	+ 0.0000E + 00	+ 4.0999E + 02		
2 – – – – 8 = = = = 1 = = = = 3 – – – – 6				
.020 .000 .040 .010	− ∞	∞	− ∞	0.041
.020 .008 .033 .010	− 6.1661E − 01	+ 4.1061E + 02	− 0.13	0.049
.020 .016 .025 .010	+ 1.2609E + 01	+ 3.9738E + 02	2.74	0.057
.020 .024 .017 .010	+ 1.9822E + 01	+ 3.9017E + 02	4.30	0.066
.020 .032 .009 .010	+ 2.4068E + 01	+ 3.8592E + 02	5.23	0.074
.020 .040 .000 .010	− ∞	∞	− ∞	0.083
1 = = = = 8 – – – – 3 – – – – 6 – – – – 4				
.500 .040 .010 .010	+ 0.0000E + 00	+ 4.0455E + 02		
8 – – – – 3 = = = = 1 = = = = 6 – – – – 4				
.040 .000 .010 .010	− ∞	∞	− ∞	0.083
.040 .002 .008 .010	+ 2.8807E + 01	+ 3.7574E + 02	6.26	0.085
.040 .004 .006 .010	+ 3.0757E + 01	+ 3.7379E + 02	6.68	0.087
.040 .006 .004 .010	+ 3.1931E + 01	+ 3.7262E + 02	6.93	0.089
.040 .008 .002 .010	+ 3.2653E + 01	+ 3.7190E + 02	7.09	0.091
.040 .010 .000 .010	+ 3.2952E + 01	+ 3.7160E + 02	7.16	0.093
1 = = = = 3 – – – – 6 – – – – 4 – – – – 9				
.500 .010 .010 .020	+ 0.0000E + 00	+ 3.7942E + 02		
3 – – – – 6 = = = = 1 = = = = 4 – – – – 9				
.010 .000 .010 .020	+ 3.2911E + 01	+ 3.4651E + 02	7.15	0.093
.010 .002 .008 .020	+ 3.1948E + 01	+ 3.4747E + 02	6.94	0.095
.010 .004 .006 .020	+ 3.0542E + 01	+ 3.4888E + 02	6.63	0.097
.010 .006 .004 .020	+ 2.8388E + 01	+ 3.5103E + 02	6.16	0.099
.010 .008 .002 .020	+ 2.4478E + 01	+ 3.5494E + 02	5.32	0.101
.010 .010 .000 .020	− ∞	∞	− ∞	0.103
1 = = = = 6 – – – – 4 – – – – 9 – – – – 7				
.500 .010 .020 .030	+ 0.0000E + 00	+ 3.7765E + 02		
6 – – – – 4 = = = = 1 = = = = 9 – – – – 7				
.010 .000 .020 .030	− ∞	∞	− ∞	0.103
.010 .004 .016 .030	− 7.4645E + 00	+ 3.8511E + 02	− 1.62	0.107
.010 .008 .012 .030	− 6.3847E + 00	+ 3.8403E + 02	− 1.38	0.111
.010 .012 .008 .030	− 8.4791E + 00	+ 3.8613E + 02	− 1.84	0.115
.010 .016 .004 .030	− 1.4758E + 01	+ 3.9241E + 02	− 3.20	0.119
.010 .020 .000 .030	− ∞	∞	− ∞	0.124

Table 20–8. (*Continued*)

Locus Order/θ's	Location Score	−2 ln Like	Lod Score	Map Distance
6 − − − −4 − − − −9 = = = =1 = = = =7				
.010 .020 .000 .030	−∞	∞	−∞	0.124
.010 .020 .006 .024	−4.9452E+01	+4.2710E+02	−10.74	0.130
.010 .020 .012 .018	−4.5242E+01	+4.2289E+02	−9.82	0.136
.010 .020 .018 .012	−4.6160E+01	+4.2381E+02	−10.02	0.142
.010 .020 .024 .006	−5.2556E+01	+4.3021E+02	−11.41	0.149
6 − − − −4 − − − −9 − − − −7 = = = =1				
.010 .020 .030 .000	−∞	∞	−∞	0.155
.010 .020 .030 .100	+1.1874E+01	+3.6578E+02	2.58	0.267
.010 .020 .030 .200	+1.5418E+01	+3.6223E+02	3.35	0.410
.010 .020 .030 .300	+1.3358E+01	+3.6429E+02	2.90	0.613
.010 .020 .030 .400	+8.0961E+00	+3.6955E+02	1.76	0.960

interval for the location of your putative disease gene. In general, it is true that the finer the grid of markers analyzed against a disease, the smaller the support interval is in expectation, almost independent of marker heterozygosity (Terwilliger et al., 1992).

☐ **Exercise 17**

The results of the analysis under the assumption of a recessive disease with 80% penetrance are presented in Table 20–9 and shown graphically in Figure 20–2 for purposes of visual comparison with Figure 16–2. In this analysis, the maximum lod score was obtained at the same location as in the dominant model, only the maximum lod score was only 0.38 under this model. Similarly, there was much less exclusion power. Fortunately, in this case, due to the low

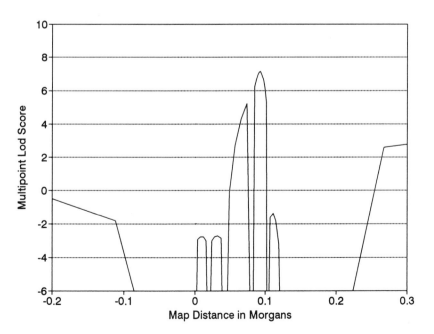

Figure 20–1. Graph of multipoint lod scores from Table 20–8

Table 20–9. Analysis of MULTDIS1.PED under Autosomal Recessive Model with 80% Penetrance

Locus Order/θ's	Location Score	−2 ln Like	Lod Score	Map Distance
1 = = = =5 − − − −2 − − − −8 − − − −3				
.500 .075 .075 .225	+0.0000E+00	+5.6631E+02	0.00	−∞
.400 .075 .075 .225	−6.4885E−02	+5.6637E+02	−0.01	−0.80471
.300 .075 .075 .225	−2.9353E−01	+5.6660E+02	−0.06	−0.45814
.200 .075 .075 .225	−8.1105E−01	+5.6712E+02	−0.18	−0.25541
.100 .075 .075 .225	−2.0020E+00	+5.6831E+02	−0.43	−0.11157
5 = = = =1 = = = =2 − − − −8 − − − −3				
.000 .075 .075 .225	−2.3051E+01	+5.8936E+02	−5.01	0.000000
.015 .062 .075 .225	−3.0653E+00	+5.6937E+02	−0.67	0.015229
.030 .048 .075 .225	−1.5937E+00	+5.6790E+02	−0.34	0.030937
.045 .033 .075 .225	−7.4906E−01	+5.6706E+02	−0.16	0.047155
.060 .017 .075 .225	−1.9528E−01	+5.6650E+02	−0.04	0.063916
.075 .000 .075 .225	+1.6389E−01	+5.6614E+02	0.04	0.081259
5 − − − −2 = = = =1 = = = =8 − − − −3				
.075 .000 .075 .225	+1.6389E−01	+5.6614E+02	0.04	0.081259
.075 .015 .062 .225	−1.4129E−01	+5.6645E+02	−0.03	0.096489
.075 .030 .048 .225	−6.2496E−01	+5.6693E+02	−0.14	0.112197
.075 .045 .033 .225	−1.3942E+00	+5.6770E+02	−0.30	0.128414
.075 .060 .017 .225	−2.7949E+00	+5.6910E+02	−0.61	0.145176
.075 .075 .000 .225	−2.3051E+01	+5.8936E+02	−5.01	0.162518
1 = = = =2 − − − −8 − − − −3 − − − −6				
.500 .075 .225 .075	+0.0000E+00	+5.5254E+02		
2 − − − −8 = = = =1 = = = =3 − − − −6				
.075 .000 .225 .075	−2.3129E+01	+5.7567E+02	−5.02	0.162518
.075 .045 .198 .075	−2.5648E+00	+5.5510E+02	−0.56	0.209674
.075 .090 .165 .075	−8.5232E−01	+5.5339E+02	−0.19	0.261744
.075 .135 .123 .075	+2.4066E−01	+5.5230E+02	0.05	0.319874
.075 .180 .070 .075	+1.0938E+00	+5.5144E+02	0.23	0.385662
1 = = = =8 − − − −3 − − − −6 − − − −4				
.500 .225 .075 .075	+0.0000E+00	+5.4812E+02		
8 − − − −3 = = = =1 = = = =6 − − − −4				
.225 .000 .075 .075	−2.2855E−01	+5.4835E+02	−0.05	0.461437
.225 .015 .062 .075	+1.8114E−01	+5.4794E+02	0.04	0.476667
.225 .030 .048 .075	+5.5754E−01	+5.4757E+02	0.12	0.492375
.225 .045 .033 .075	+9.0693E−01	+5.4722E+02	0.20	0.508592
.225 .060 .017 .075	+1.2339E+00	+5.4689E+02	0.27	0.525354
.225 .075 .000 .075	+1.5421E+00	+5.4658E+02	0.33	0.542696
1 = = = =3 − − − −6 − − − −4 − − − −9				
.500 .075 .075 .075	+0.0000E+00	+5.3465E+02		
3 − − − −6 = = = =1 = = = =4 − − − −9				
.075 .000 .075 .075	+1.7344E+00	+5.3291E+02	0.38	0.5427
.075 .015 .062 .075	+1.4036E+00	+5.3324E+02	0.30	0.5579
.075 .030 .048 .075	+9.9157E−01	+5.3366E+02	0.22	0.5736
.075 .045 .033 .075	+4.5373E−01	+5.3419E+02	0.10	0.5899
.075 .060 .017 .075	−3.0710E−01	+5.3496E+02	−0.07	0.6066
.075 .075 .000 .075	−1.5850E+00	+5.3623E+02	−0.34	0.6240
1 = = = =6 − − − −4 − − − −9 − − − −7				
.500 .075 .075 .075	+0.0000E+00	+5.3758E+02		
6 − − − −4 = = = =1 = = = =9 − − − −7				
.075 .000 .075 .075	−1.5850E+00	+5.3916E+02	−0.34	0.623956
.075 .015 .062 .075	−2.8257E+00	+5.4040E+02	−0.61	0.639185
.075 .030 .048 .075	−3.5801E+00	+5.4116E+02	−0.78	0.654894
.075 .045 .033 .075	−4.6283E+00	+5.4220E+02	−1.01	0.671111
.075 .060 .017 .075	−7.4094E+00	+5.4499E+02	−1.61	0.687873
.075 .075 .000 .075	−6.8973E+01	+6.0655E+02	−14.98	0.705215

Table 20–9. (*Continued*)

Locus Order/θ's	Location Score	−2 ln Like	Lod Score	Map Distance
6 − − − −4 − − − −9= = = =1 = = = =7				
.075 .075 .000 .075	−6.8973E+01	+6.0655E+02	−14.98	0.705215
.075 .075 .015 .062	−2.7083E+01	+5.6466E+02	−5.88	0.720445
.075 .075 .030 .048	−2.4572E+01	+5.6215E+02	−5.34	0.736153
.075 .075 .045 .033	−2.4399E+01	+5.6198E+02	−5.30	0.752371
.075 .075 .060 .017	−2.6332E+01	+5.6391E+02	−5.72	0.769132
.075 .075 .075 .000	−5.1009E+01	+5.8859E+02	−11.08	0.786475
6 − − − −4 − − − −9 − − − −7= = = =1				
.075 .075 .075 .000	−5.1009E+01	+5.8859E+02	−11.08	0.786475
.075 .075 .075 .100	−4.9218E+00	+5.4250E+02	−1.06	0.898047
.075 .075 .075 .200	−1.8085E+00	+5.3938E+02	−0.39	1.041888
.075 .075 .075 .300	−5.6751E−01	+5.3814E+02	−0.12	1.244620
.075 .075 .075 .400	−1.0589E−01	+5.3768E+02	−0.02	1.591194

penetrance for the disease, much ambiguity remained about the genotypes for the unaffected individuals. Moreover, the analysis was using almost exactly the meioses that could not be used in the dominant analysis, because now all affected individuals were considered to be homozygous, so all the information about linkage comes from the heterozygous (at the disease locus) mothers. In light of this, it is clear that the maximum lod score occurred at the same $\hat{\theta}$ primarily by chance and not through a meaningful correlation in the data between the dominant and recessive analyses, in these pedigrees.

When the uncertainty of diagnosis is entered for the *unaffected* individuals in this pedigree, it is necessary to allow for an additional liability class, (because *affected* individuals are still affected with 100% certainty). So, we must go back into the parameter file and add an additional liability class for

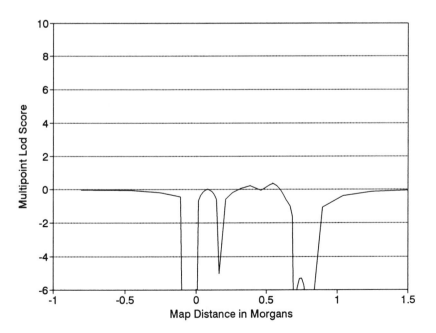

Figure 20–2. Graph of multipoint lod scores from Table 20–9

the unaffected individuals. Remember from Chapter 10 that to allow for uncertainty of diagnosis, then the new penetrances should be computed as

$$(p)P(\text{affected} \mid \text{genotype}) + (1 - p)P(\text{unaffected} \mid \text{genotype})$$

where in this case, p = the probability that the person really is affected. Thus, in our situation, with a 75% chance that the people are unaffected, we have a 25% chance that they are affected, so $p = 0.25$. Then our penetrances should be $f(+/+) = 0.25(0) + 0.75(1) = 0.75$; $f(D/+) = f(+/+) = 0.25(1) + 0.75(0) = 0.25$. Thus, our two liability classes are as follows:

GENOTYPE	$+/+$	$D/+$	D/D
Affecteds	0	1	1
Unaffecteds	0.75	0.25	0.25

Unaffected individuals in the pedigree file then have affection status phenotype 2 2, and affected persons have phenotype 2 1. The resulting LINKMAP output is shown in Table 20–10, and illustrated graphically in Figure 20–3. The maximum lod score in this example is only 6.77, with a support interval covering the range (0.3199, 0.6066), for a 28.67-cM support interval. The exclusion regions are fairly similar to those obtained with 100% diagnostic certainty, though the magnitude of the lod scores is much smaller (i.e., the values are much *less* negative in this example), implying that many of the "obligate" recombination events occurred in unaffected individuals.

☐ Exercise 18

The top 20 orders found with CILINK are presented in Table 20–11 under the assumption of constant sex difference and in Table 20–12 under the assumption of varying sex difference. The same four orders are always the top four, under any of the three sex difference models. To test the significance of the evidence for sex difference in recombination, again consider the three hypotheses given the top ranked order, as outlined in Table 20–13. From this table, we see that the test of H_1 versus H_0 has a chi-square value of 7.32 with (5-4) = 1 df, with a corresponding p-value of 0.008. The test of H_2 versus H_1, however has a chi-square value of 2.63 with (8-5) = 3 df, for a p-value of only 0.45, which is not at all significant. In light of this analysis, our best conclusion is that there is a constant sex difference, with a female-to-male map distance ratio of 2.573. It is interesting to note that some of the map distance ratios are enormous under the varying sex difference option. Usually this occurs when $\theta_m = 0.001$, meaning that no recombinants were seen in this data set in males, even though many recombinants were seen in females. This phenomenon can lead to estimates of the map distance ratio as high as 641.752 in the small sample in Table 20–12.

In the files MULTDIS1.* the evidence for sex difference in recombination is outlined in Table 20–14. As you can see, there is very little evidence for sex difference in recombination, with completely nonsignificant chi-square test results. However, notice the estimated constant sex ratio for this set of loci. The ratio in this example was estimated to be 0.599, meaning that there were higher rates of recombination in males than females by almost 2:1. If you remember back in the original analysis with the data set in MULTDIS2.*, the

Table 20–10. Analysis of MULTDIS1.* with LINKMAP, Assuming 75% Certainty of Diagnosis of Unaffected Individuals

Locus Order/θ's	Location Score	−2 ln Like	Lod Score	Map Distance
1 = = = =5 − − − −2 − − − −8 − − − −3				
.500 .075 .075 .225	+0.0000E+00	+3.8998E+02	0.00	−∞
.400 .075 .075 .225	+2.7396E+00	+3.8724E+02	0.59	−0.80471
.300 .075 .075 .225	+3.7225E+00	+3.8626E+02	0.81	−0.45814
.200 .075 .075 .225	+2.4881E+00	+3.8749E+02	0.54	−0.25541
.100 .075 .075 .225	−2.8903E+00	+3.9287E+02	−0.63	−0.11157
5 = = = =1 = = = =2 − − − −8 − − − −3				
.000 .075 .075 .225	−2.4547E+01	+4.1453E+02	−5.33	0.000000
.015 .062 .075 .225	−2.4432E+01	+4.1441E+02	−5.31	0.015229
.030 .048 .075 .225	−2.4383E+01	+4.1436E+02	−5.29	0.030937
.045 .033 .075 .225	−2.4731E+01	+4.1471E+02	−5.37	0.047155
.060 .017 .075 .225	−2.5559E+01	+4.1554E+02	−5.55	0.063916
.075 .000 .075 .225	−2.6670E+01	+4.1665E+02	−5.79	0.081259
5 − − − −2 = = = =1 = = = =8 − − − −3				
.075 .000 .075 .225	−2.6670E+01	+4.1665E+02	−5.79	0.081259
.075 .015 .062 .225	−1.9969E+01	+4.0995E+02	−4.33	0.096489
.075 .030 .048 .225	−1.7256E+01	+4.0724E+02	−3.75	0.112197
.075 .045 .033 .225	−1.5866E+01	+4.0585E+02	−3.45	0.128414
.075 .060 .017 .225	−1.5848E+01	+4.0583E+02	−3.44	0.145176
.075 .075 .000 .225	−2.4010E+01	+4.1399E+02	−5.21	0.162518
1 = = = =2 − − − −8 − − − −3 − − − −6				
.500 .075 .225 .075	+0.0000E+00	+3.7621E+02		
2 − − − −8 = = = =1 = = = =3 − − − −6				
.075 .000 .225 .075	−2.3982E+01	+4.0019E+02	−5.21	0.162518
.075 .045 .198 .075	+7.7635E+00	+3.6845E+02	1.69	0.209674
.075 .090 .165 .075	+1.4509E+01	+3.6170E+02	3.15	0.261744
.075 .135 .123 .075	+1.9169E+01	+3.5704E+02	4.16	0.319874
.075 .180 .070 .075	+2.2689E+01	+3.5352E+02	4.93	0.385662
1 = = = =8 − − − −3 − − − −6 − − − −4				
.500 .225 .075 .075	+0.0000E+00	+3.7180E+02		
8 − − − −3 = = = =1 = = = =6 − − − −4				
.225 .000 .075 .075	+6.2405E+00	+3.6556E+02	1.36	0.461437
.225 .015 .062 .075	+2.6736E+01	+3.4506E+02	5.81	0.476667
.225 .030 .048 .075	+2.8731E+01	+3.4307E+02	6.24	0.492375
.225 .045 .033 .075	+2.9977E+01	+3.4182E+02	6.51	0.508592
.225 .060 .017 .075	+3.0818E+01	+3.4098E+02	6.69	0.525354
.225 .075 .000 .075	+3.1299E+01	+3.4050E+02	6.80	0.542696
1 = = = =3 − − − −6 − − − −4 − − − −9				
.500 .075 .075 .075	+0.0000E+00	+3.5832E+02		
3 − − − −6 = = = =1 = = = =4 − − − −9				
.075 .000 .075 .075	+3.1178E+01	+3.2714E+02	6.77	0.5427
.075 .015 .062 .075	+3.0155E+01	+3.2817E+02	6.55	0.5579
.075 .030 .048 .075	+2.8738E+01	+3.2958E+02	6.24	0.5736
.075 .045 .033 .075	+2.6620E+01	+3.3170E+02	5.78	0.5899
.075 .060 .017 .075	+2.2791E+01	+3.3553E+02	4.95	0.6066
.075 .075 .000 .075	−1.7001E+01	+3.7532E+02	−3.69	0.6240
1 = = = =6 − − − −4 − − − −9 − − − −7				
.500 .075 .075 .075	+0.0000E+00	+3.6125E+02		
6 − − − −4 = = = =1 = = = =9 − − − −7				
.075 .000 .075 .075	−1.7001E+01	+3.7825E+02	−3.69	0.623956
.075 .015 .062 .075	−1.1794E+00	+3.6243E+02	−2.56	0.639185
.075 .030 .048 .075	+1.6468E−01	+3.6108E+02	0.04	0.654894
.075 .045 .033 .075	−1.3096E+00	+3.6256E+02	−0.28	0.671111
.075 .060 .017 .075	−6.2153E+00	+3.6746E+02	−1.34	0.687873
.075 .075 .000 .075	−2.2096E+01	+3.8335E+02	−4.79	0.705215

Table 20–10. (*Continued*)

Locus Order/θ's	Location Score	−2 ln Like	Lod Score	Map Distance
6 − − − −4 − − − −9 = = = =1 = = = =7				
.075 .075 .000 .075	−2.2096E+01	+3.8335E+02	−4.79	0.705215
.075 .075 .015 .062	−1.9667E+01	+3.8092E+02	−4.27	0.720445
.075 .075 .030 .048	−1.8273E+01	+3.7952E+02	−3.97	0.736153
.075 .075 .045 .033	−1.8599E+01	+3.7985E+02	−4.04	0.752371
.075 .075 .060 .017	−2.0947E+01	+3.8220E+02	−4.55	0.769132
.075 .075 .075 .000	−2.5225E+01	+3.8647E+02	−5.48	0.786475
6 − − − −4 − − − −9 − − − −7 = = = =1				
.075 .075 .075 .000	−2.5225E+01	+3.8647E+02	−5.48	0.786475
.075 .075 .075 .100	+1.0971E+01	+3.5028E+02	2.38	0.898047
.075 .075 .075 .200	+1.2544E+01	+3.4871E+02	2.72	1.041888
.075 .075 .075 .300	+1.0447E+01	+3.5080E+02	2.27	1.244620
.075 .075 .075 .400	+6.1823E+00	+3.5507E+02	1.34	1.591194

estimated sex ratio was 2.113, meaning that in that data set, females showed twice the recombination rate of males. In light of this information, it is not surprising that when the two data sets are combined, the estimated map distance ratio was only 1.23, implying that there is a negligible sex difference. This is caused by the two data sets canceling each other, in terms of recombination sex differences. It is therefore also not surprising that the combined data sets provided a much less significant test than either of the two data sets separately, as shown in Table 20–15.

☐ **Exercise 19**

In this exercise, the only triples of loci meeting the criterion that $0.125 \leq \theta_{AB}$, $\theta_{BC} \leq 0.225$ are 5-(0.139)-8-(0.225)-3, 8-(0.225)-3-(0.139)-4, and 3-(0.139)-4-

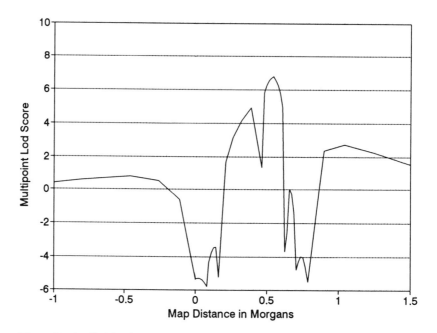

Figure 20–3. Graph of multipoint lod scores from Table 20–10.

Table 20–11. Top Twenty Orders of Loci in USEREX14.*: Constant Sex Difference

Locus Order	Male Thetas	X_f/X_m	-2 ln Like	Odds
3----4----5----1----2	.033 .173 .031 .131	2.573	$-1.1127E+02$	$1.00E+00$
4----3----5----1----2	.034 .165 .031 .132	2.497	$-1.1075E+02$	$1.29E+00$
3----4----1----5----2	.035 .162 .021 .156	2.459	$-1.0981E+02$	$2.07E+00$
4----3----1----5----2	.035 .154 .022 .158	2.391	$-1.0916E+02$	$2.87E+00$
5----1----2----3----4	.022 .091 .269 .029	3.983	$-9.8521E+01$	$5.85E+02$
5----1----2----4----3	.022 .092 .274 .026	3.900	$-9.7107E+01$	$1.19E+03$
1----5----2----3----4	.014 .099 .266 .028	4.388	$-9.5537E+01$	$2.60E+03$
1----5----2----4----3	.015 .103 .271 .026	4.043	$-9.4139E+01$	$5.24E+03$
5----1----4----3----2	.022 .123 .032 .290	3.175	$-9.3867E+01$	$6.00E+03$
1----5----4----3----2	.022 .118 .028 .291	3.918	$-9.1877E+01$	$1.62E+04$
5----1----3----4----2	.023 .118 .027 .295	3.020	$-9.1621E+01$	$1.84E+04$
1----5----3----4----2	.022 .114 .023 .295	3.803	$-8.9630E+01$	$4.99E+04$
5----3----4----1----2	.112 .027 .163 .118	3.109	$-8.7881E+01$	$1.20E+05$
5----4----3----1----2	.118 .029 .156 .114	3.265	$-8.7735E+01$	$1.29E+05$
4----5----3----1----2	.126 .029 .101 .140	2.436	$-8.6845E+01$	$2.01E+05$
3----4----1----2----5	.028 .172 .097 .143	3.491	$-8.6645E+01$	$2.22E+05$
4----3----1----2----5	.030 .165 .095 .142	3.537	$-8.6459E+01$	$2.44E+05$
1----2----5----3----4	.083 .175 .132 .026	3.986	$-8.4785E+01$	$5.63E+05$
1----2----5----4----3	.081 .177 .132 .026	4.165	$-8.3896E+01$	$8.77E+05$
4----5----1----2----3	.179 .030 .125 .228	2.597	$-8.3733E+01$	$9.52E+05$

Table 20–12. Top Twenty Orders of Loci in USEREX14.*: Varying Sex Difference

Locus Order	Male Thetas	Female-to-Male Map Distance Ratios				-2 ln Like	Odds
3----4----5----1----2	.001 .173 .001 .181	248.051	2.448	141.771	1.514	$-1.1390E+02$	$1.00E+00$
3----4----1----5----2	.001 .161 .001 .152	309.807	2.236	135.184	2.563	$-1.1224E+02$	$2.29E+00$
4----3----1----5----2	.001 .202 .001 .154	171.897	1.463	98.958	2.494	$-1.1134E+02$	$3.60E+00$
4----3----5----1----2	.001 .208 .001 .167	324.302	2.979	383.886	2.369	$-1.0749E+02$	$2.47E+01$
5----1----2----3----4	.001 .128 .262 .001	133.534	2.720	3.728	445.905	$-9.9185E+01$	$1.57E+03$
1----5----2----3----4	.001 .111 .283 .001	106.745	3.648	2.355	236.959	$-9.6968E+01$	$4.76E+03$
5----1----4----3----2	.001 .132 .001 .291	161.494	2.272	360.817	1.344	$-9.5964E+01$	$7.86E+03$
1----5----2----4----3	.001 .101 .285 .001	105.075	4.047	2.460	244.922	$-9.5814E+01$	$8.47E+03$
5----1----2----4----3	.001 .113 .355 .001	190.615	4.265	16.182	252.037	$-9.5347E+01$	$1.07E+04$
5----1----3----4----2	.001 .144 .001 .322	134.152	2.026	167.749	1.757	$-9.4186E+01$	$1.91E+04$
5----3----4----1----2	.047 .001 .166 .161	10.334	197.781	2.448	1.857	$-9.1709E+01$	$6.60E+04$
5----4----3----1----2	.046 .001 .166 .161	11.813	193.495	2.368	1.842	$-9.1464E+01$	$7.46E+04$
4----5----3----1----2	.001 .037 .131 .188	638.115	1.656	1.722	1.446	$-9.1238E+01$	$8.35E+04$
3----4----1----2----5	.001 .193 .106 .069	259.719	1.956	2.806	10.297	$-9.0782E+01$	$1.05E+05$
1----5----3----4----2	.001 .194 .001 .312	170.584	1.773	218.382	2.397	$-9.0130E+01$	$1.45E+05$
4----3----1----2----5	.001 .204 .105 .075	195.450	1.881	3.010	11.845	$-9.0002E+01$	$1.55E+05$
3----5----4----1----2	.029 .001 .169 .132	6.854	523.242	2.084	2.399	$-8.8610E+01$	$3.11E+05$
1----5----4----3----2	.001 .088 .001 .394	130.390	8.277	641.752	12.875	$-8.6367E+01$	$9.54E+05$
1----2----5----3----4	.074 .145 .187 .001	4.668	5.108	2.309	195.065	$-8.5768E+01$	$1.29E+06$
1----2----5----4----3	.088 .177 .161 .001	4.362	3.951	2.977	243.203	$-8.4972E+01$	$1.92E+06$

Table 20–13. Likelihoods of Order 3-4-5-1-2 under Various Sex Difference Models

Model	df	-2 ln(Like)	$\Delta -2$ ln(Like)
H_2 Varying Sex Difference	8	-113.90	0.00
H_1 Constant Sex Difference	5	-111.27	2.63
H_0 No Sex Difference	4	-103.95	9.95

Table 20–14. Likelihoods of Order 3-6-4-9-7 under Various Sex Difference Models: Files MULTDIS1.*

Model	df	-2 ln(Like)	$\Delta -2$ ln(Like)
H_2 Varying Sex Difference	8	309.76	0.00
H_1 Constant Sex Difference	5	310.34	0.58
H_0 No Sex Difference	4	310.83	1.07

Table 20–15. Likelihoods of Order 3-6-4-9-7 under Various Sex Difference Models: Files MULTDIS1.* and MULTDIS2.* Together

Model	df	$-2\ln(\text{Like})$	$\Delta -2\ln(\text{Like})$
H_2 Varying Sex Difference	8	590.60	0.00
H_1 Constant Sex Difference	5	590.61	0.01
H_0 No Sex Difference	4	590.82	0.22

(0.139)-7. The results of the analyses of these triples of loci are presented in Table 20–16, with the values of c_m, c_f, and $-2\ln(\text{Likelihood})$ given for each analysis (θ's not shown). Does the great disparity in the estimates of c_m and c_f under the assumption of constant sex difference make sense to you? The reason is quite simple. You see, the *constant sex difference* option forces the recombination fractions in males and females to fit the constant map distance ratio criterion, which assumes the Haldane mapping function. Because the Haldane mapping function is incompatible with interference, you mix apples and oranges when doing such an analysis, and the analysis simply doesn't make any sense. The analysis with loci 8-3-4 points it out quite nicely, because although c_m is essentially 0 (to fit the constant map distance criterion), the female θ's are computed such that $\theta_f = 0.60$, when the *variable sex difference* and *constant sex difference* options both yielded an estimate of $c_m = c_f = 0$. Clearly, it is impossible for this to hold under the constant sex difference option unless the sex ratio was 1. Prove this to yourself as an exercise. To demonstrate further the poor fit of the *constant sex difference* model to the interference analysis, take a look at the likelihood ratio χ^2 values shown in Table 20–16. Notice that with the exception of the first triple of loci (for which no evidence of interference was found), the *constant sex difference* option performed the worst of all, due to its internal incompatibility. In the set of loci 8-3-4, we have our strongest evidence for interference, with a *p*-value of 0.05 for the test. This is pretty convincing evidence, given the small data set we had to work with and the fact that our estimated coefficients of coincidence were all 0 under the *Varying sex difference* model. Because we already established that this data set shows sex difference in recombination rates and that the *Constant sex difference* option is invalid for interference calculations in ILINK, the only valid test to consider is the *Varying sex difference* test. So, we conclude that there is some evidence for positive interference in this data set, although not very powerful evidence. Because we looked at three separate samples, we need to correct for multiple testing. Because the one triple

Table 20–16. Interference Analysis of Loci in MULTDIS2.* with ILINK

Loci	Sex Difference	c_m	c_f	$-2\ln L(c=1)$	$-2\ln L(c=\hat{c})$	χ^2	*p*-value
5-8-3	None	1.48	1.48	215.10	214.66	0.44	0.50
	Constant	2.32	1.31	213.00	212.15	0.85	0.36
	Varying	3.33	0.83	212.99	211.35	1.64	0.20
8-3-4	None	0.00	0.00	215.10	211.75	3.35	0.07
	Constant	0.03	0.60	213.00	211.16	1.84	0.17
	Varying	0.00	0.00	212.99	209.04	3.95	0.05
3-4-7	None	0.00	0.00	206.26	204.14	2.12	0.15
	Constant	0.00	0.58	204.67	203.41	1.26	0.26
	Varying	0.00	0.00	204.67	202.20	2.47	0.12

of loci that gave a significant test result was only marginally significant, after applying a correction for the three tests we carried out, this value is no longer significant, but combined with the reasonably powerful test result from locus order 3-4-7 and the fact that it also yielded estimates of $\hat{c} = 0$, we can safely say that there is suggestive evidence of positive interference in this data set, but not conclusively so.

PART III

Advanced Topics
in Linkage Analysis

21.

Mutation Rates and the LINKAGE Programs

In this chapter, we introduce the concept of mutation and the way in which it is used in the LINKAGE programs. We explain why it is sometimes obligatory to use this option, especially when analyzing sex-linked recessive lethal diseases.

21.1 Mutations

It is often possible for a child to inherit an allele from a parent, which is not found in that parent. In other words, it is sometimes seen that a *1/1* father and a *2/2* mother might have a child with genotype *2/2*. Clearly, this is inconsistent with normal mendelian laws as introduced in Chapter 1. However, the process of *mutation* can cause one parental allele to mutate or change into a different allele, and this mutant allele can then be transmitted to the offspring. Other mechanisms can lead to this situation (as discussed in Ott, 1991, p. 256 and Malcolm et al., 1990), but in LINKAGE the only such phenomenon that can be directly dealt with is mutation. Many biochemical explanations can be given for the existence of such genetic mutations, and they are the primary source of the genetic variability and genetic diseases that exist. It is often essential to allow for the occurrence of mutations in performing a linkage analysis. If the mutation rate is not allowed for, a situation like the one described above causes the LINKAGE programs to complain about a genetic inconsistency in the data. However, if we perform the linkage analysis assuming some fixed rate of mutation, then the mendelian inconsistency could be explained away as a newly mutated allele.

Frequently, when performing a linkage analysis with certain genetic diseases, we might want to assume a certain rate of mutation creating new disease alleles, and when analyzing a sex-linked recessive disease that is lethal, it is mandatory to allow for a certain fixed mutation rate, as you will see below.

21.2 Allowing for Mutation Rates in LINKAGE

In general, we define separate mutation rates to and from each different allele at a locus. For example, if we have a locus with two alleles, separate mutation rates $\mu_{1\to 2}$ and $\mu_{2\to 1}$, for the two possible types of mutation. In general, these are not likely to be equal. Further, it is likely the case that there are different rates of mutation in males and females, because the processes of spermatogenesis and oogenesis are very different.

In the LINKAGE programs, however, the use of mutation rates is extremely limited. The restriction is so severe that only one locus (of any locus type) is allowed to have mutations, and one constant rate is permitted for males and another for females. Furthermore, the mutation can only be specified unidirectionally from any allele to the last (i.e. highest numbered) allele. For this reason, an affection status locus is usually set up with the disease allele as allele *2*, so mutation can be allowed to the disease allele but not from disease to normal. Typically, the disease allele frequency is so small that any such back-mutation occurs at a negligible frequency.

This option is used primarily when considering disease loci, with mutation occurring from the normal allele to the disease allele at the disease locus. This is the purpose for which this option was originated, and it remains a restriction in the applicability of LINKAGE with highly mutable loci.

Let us return to the phase-known example from Chapter 5 Figure 5–1. In this pedigree, we now assume that there is a mutation rate μ, where μ is the probability that any normal allele mutates to a disease allele in one meiosis. Read the parameter file from that example into PREPLINK, and select option *(d) Mutation*. The screen looks like the following:

```
************************************************
(a) MUTATION LOCUS            :  0
(b) MUTATION RATE MALES       :  0.00000E+00
(c) MUTATION RATE FEMALES     :  0.00000E+00
(d) MUTATION                  :  N
(e) RETURN TO MAIN MENU
************************************************
enter letter to modify values
```

At this point, select option (a) and respond to the questions as follows:

```
ENTER NEW MUTATION LOCUS
1              (The disease locus)
ENTER NEW MUTATION RATE MALES
.000001    (Here you enter whatever the value is for μ)
ENTER NEW MUTATION RATE FEMALES
.000001    (If we assume equal rates in males and females, enter μ)
```

Then, write this data file, and rerun the analysis of the pedigree in question, varying values for the mutation rate to visualize its effect on the analysis. The results should resemble those given in Table 21–1.

In this example, it is clear that allowing for mutation has little effect on the likelihood, implying that there are most likely no new mutations in this pedigree. This makes sense in light of the pedigree structure and phenotypes. Let us look at this analytically to confirm that this is so.

We know that the disease locus genotype of *father* is $D/+$, and that *mother* is $+/+$. Because of the low gene frequency, we can assume that *fgrandma* has genotype $D/+$, and we know that *fgrandpa* has genotype $+/+$. Because of the mutation rate, however, *father* could have gotten the D

Table 21–1. Effects of Mutation Rate on the MLE of θ, and the Corresponding Lod Score on a Phase-known Pedigree

μ	$\hat{\theta}$	$Z(\hat{\theta})$
$<10^{-5}$	0.798	0.4185
10^{-4}	0.798	0.4183
10^{-3}	0.799	0.4168
10^{-2}	0.797	0.4015
10^{-1}	0.775	0.2746
0.5	0.655	0.0456

allele from either parent because a mutation could have occurred coming from *fgrandma*. Hence, there are two possible phases for *father*. We must look at the likelihood of *father* having received genotype $D/+$, given the D allele came from *fgrandma*, compared with the likelihood given the D allele came from *fgrandpa*. The likelihood of *father* receiving the D allele from *fgrandma* and the $+$ allele from *fgrandpa* is

$$\left[\left(\frac{1}{2}\right) + \left(\frac{1}{2}\right)\mu\right][1 - \mu] = \left(\frac{1}{2}\right)(1 - \mu)(1 + \mu)$$

and the likelihood of his receiving the $+$ allele from *fgrandma* and the D allele from *fgrandpa* is $\mu(1 - \mu)/2$. Thus, the probability that *father* received the D allele from *fgrandpa* is

$$\frac{\left(\frac{1}{2}\right)(1 - \mu)\mu}{\left(\frac{1}{2}\right)(1 - \mu)(1 + 2\mu)} = \frac{\mu}{1 + 2\mu}$$

Clearly, for $\mu = 0$, this probability is 0, and the phase is known with certainty. We have the same situation as described in Chapter 5.

The overall likelihood of this pedigree is now more analogous to the phase-unknown situation in the lower generation of the pedigree. There are two possible phases for *father*, with Phase I $= D\ 1/+\ 2$, with P(Phase I) $= (1 + \mu)/(1 + 2\mu)$; Phase II $= D\ 2/+\ 1$, with P(Phase II) $= \mu/(1 + 2\mu)$. Now, consider the bottom generation. First, *dau1* has disease locus genotype $+/+$, having received the *2* allele from *father*. Under Phase I, this happens with likelihood $1 - \theta$, and likelihood θ under Phase II. Children *dau2* and *son1* are identical, having either disease locus genotype $D/+$ or D/D. Three possible scenarios can be considered here. The possibilities are that they received the D allele from *father*, and the $+$ allele from *mother* with a likelihood of

$$\left[\left(\frac{1}{2}\right)\theta + \left(\frac{1}{2}\right)\mu(1 - \theta)\right](1 - \mu)$$

under Phase I and

$$\left[\left(\frac{1}{2}\right)(1 - \theta) + \left(\frac{1}{2}\right)\mu\theta\right](1 - \mu)$$

under Phase II, that they received the $+$ allele from *father*, and a mutated D allele from *mother* with a likelihood of $(\frac{1}{2})(1 - \mu)(1 - \theta)\mu$ under Phase I and

$(\frac{1}{2})(1 - \mu)\theta\mu$ under Phase II; or that they received the D allele from both parents with a likelihood of

$$\left[\left(\frac{1}{2}\right)\theta + \left(\frac{1}{2}\right)\mu(1 - \theta)\right]\mu$$

under Phase I and

$$\left[\left(\frac{1}{2}\right)(1 - \theta) + \left(\frac{1}{2}\right)\mu\theta\right]\mu$$

under Phase II. Finally, for *dau3* and *son2* the received genotype is $+/+$. Clearly, they also received the *I* allele from *father*, making their likelihood just θ under Phase I, and $1 - \theta$ under Phase II. Putting all of this together, the overall likelihood of the pedigree is

$P(\text{Pedigree}|\text{Father is Phase I})P(\text{Phase I})$

$+ P(\text{Pedigree}|\text{Father is Phase II})P(\text{Phase II})$

In this case, it works out to be

$$L = \frac{1 + \mu}{1 + 2\mu}(1 - \theta)\,[\theta + \mu(2 - \mu)(1 - \theta)]^2\theta^2$$

$$+ \frac{\mu}{1 + 2\mu}\theta[(1 - \theta) + \mu(2 - \mu)\theta]^2(1 - \theta)^2$$

Again, if you set $\mu = 0$, this likelihood is identical to that for the same pedigree obtained in Section 3.4. The lod score is then $\log_{10}[L(\hat{\theta},\mu)/L(\hat{\theta} = \frac{1}{2},\mu)]$. To verify the calculations done by the LINKAGE programs above, please plug in the value of 0.01 for μ, and 0.797 for θ. The resulting lod score should be 0.4015, just as computed with LINKAGE. It is important to realize that 0.01 is an extremely high value to assume for μ, however, because the mutation rate must fit with certain conditions regarding mutation–selection equilibrium, which always requires that $\mu \leq p$, the frequency of the disease allele, as you will see in the following sections.

21.3 Mutation–Selection Equilibrium

In the previous example, we looked at the effect of various mutation rates on the lod score in our pedigree. However, we failed to consider whether or not they were meaningful estimates. In determining the mutation rate for a given disease, we need to select a value that is appropriate. If we assume that the disease allele frequency is stable and equal to p, then the mutation rate and selection coefficient must balance out, so that the frequency of the disease gene remains constant from generation to generation. Most genetic diseases have negative effects on the fitness of an individual, and thus a certain proportion s of affected individuals do not reproduce in a given generation (s can also be interpreted as the relative reproductive fitness of any one individual). To establish equilibrium of the allele frequency, these lost disease alleles must be replaced somehow. The only way to increase the frequency of the disease is through new mutations. At equilibrium, therefore, the number of new mutations must equal the number of lost alleles in a given generation (Wright, 1968). For example, if we are dealing with an autosomal recessive disease, and a proportion s of affected individuals are lost due to selection, then sp^2 genes are lost in each generation, and the new gene frequency is $p_2 = p_1(1 - sp_1)$. If there were no new mutations, then over time, the gene frequency would continually decrease. These alleles lost due to selection must be replaced continually for the gene frequency to be maintained. Clearly, then, the mutation rate must replace all of the alleles lost from selection, so $\mu = sp^2$, whenever p is presumed to be small. Therefore, the general equilibrium condition can be specified by $p = \sqrt{\mu/s}$ for a recessive disease. Similarly, it can be shown that for an autosomal dominant disease, $p = \mu/s$. For more details about mutation–selection equilibrium, consult Cavalli-Sforza and Bodmer (1971).

21.4 Sex-linked Lethal Recessive Disease

The simplest and most important situation is that of sex-linked recessive lethal diseases, that is, ones for which no affected people live to reproduce. This situation is complete selection against the disease phenotype. Unchecked, such diseases lead inexorably to the loss of the disease allele. However, many such diseases are known to exist with constant prevalence. The best explanation is that the alleles are maintained in mutation–selection equilibrium (Haldane, 1935). In linkage analysis, the important allele frequency is that of the mating population. Because the disease is lethal at a young age and sex-linked recessive, all males in the mating population carry the normal allele, and the disease allele frequency in females is p. Let us consider the distribution of genotypes in the next generation. Clearly, the possible matings (and offspring) are

$$(+/+ \, ♀ \times + \, ♂) \rightarrow \tfrac{1}{2} \, +/+ \, ♀, \tfrac{1}{2} \, + \, ♂$$

and

$$(D/+ \, ♀ \times + \, ♂) \rightarrow \tfrac{1}{4} \, D/+ \, ♀, \tfrac{1}{4} \, +/+ \, ♀, \tfrac{1}{4} \, D♂, \tfrac{1}{4} \, + \, ♂$$

In this generation, half of the disease alleles went to $D/+$ females, and the other half went to the D males. Because all of the D males are lost due to selection, half of the disease alleles are lost in this generation, and $p_2 = p_1/2$ in the mating population, where p_1 is the gene frequency in the parental generation, and p_2 in the offspring generation. To maintain a stable equilibrium, a mutation rate of $p_1/2$ is required, to replace the lost alleles (Haldane, 1935). In practice, therefore, whenever analyzing a sex-linked recessive lethal disease, it is imperative to allow for $\mu = p_1/2$ in the linkage analysis, because in a nuclear family with one affected child, there is therefore a $\tfrac{1}{3}$ chance of his being a new mutation (the gene frequency in the parental generation being p, and the mutation rate being $p/2$). Then, the probability of any single disease allele in the next generation being a new mutation is $(p/2)/(p + p/2) = \tfrac{1}{3}$. This property can play a significant role in the linkage analysis. Consider the simple pedigree from Chapter 6 Figure 6–1 with an X-linked recessive disease segregating. Alter the marker locus genotype of *son4* to be *1* instead of *2*, remem-

Table 21–2. Analysis of Sex-linked Disease with and without Mutation Rate (Two Affected Sons)

θ	$Z(\theta, \mu = 0)$	$Z(\theta, \mu = p/2)$
0	$-\infty$	-1.2365
0.1	-0.2289	-0.2094
0.2	-0.0602	-0.0549
0.3	-0.0113	-0.0097
0.4	-0.0007	-0.0004

Table 21–3. Analysis of Sex-linked Disease with and without Mutation Rate
(One Affected Son)

θ	$Z(\theta,\mu=0)$	$Z(\theta,\mu=p/2)$
0	$-\infty$	-0.0980
0.1	-0.8874	-0.0837
0.2	-0.3876	-0.0549
0.3	-0.1514	-0.0265
0.4	-0.0355	-0.0069

bering that in allele numbers format hemizygous male phenotypes must be entered as if homozygous with two copies of the allele (i.e., *1* is coded as *1 1*). Now analyze this pedigree as you did in that chapter with this one marker typing change (no mutation rate). Then analyze the pedigree allowing for a mutation rate equal to *p*/2. The results should resemble those shown in Table 21–2.

In this example, there was little effect of allowing for the theoretical value for the mutation rate. However, if we make *son4* unaffected and redo the analysis, a much more pronounced effect occurs. Because there are two affected sons in this example, it is clearly much more likely that one gene is segregating in the family (likelihood *p* = 0.01) than that two mutations (likelihood = μ^2 = 0.005² = 0.000025) or one gene and one mutation (likelihood = $p\mu$ = (0.005)(0.01) = 0.00005) occurred. However, in the pedigree with only one affected son, the likelihood is of the order *p* = 0.01 for having the disease caused by a gene and μ = 0.005 for having the disease caused by a new mutation. For this reason, μ has a much greater effect on the second single-affected child pedigree than in the double-affected child pedigree, as shown in Table 21–3.

This result demonstrates that the mutation rate is much more important in pedigrees with small numbers of affected individuals, as explained above. The message is that you must always allow for mutation when there is selection against the disease, and in the case of sex-linked recessive lethal diseases the mutation rate should be *p*/2. Remember, that for most diseases, μ should not be estimated directly, but rather an appropriate value should be selected, using mutation–selection equilibrium conditions.

☐ Exercise 21

Reanalyze the pedigree from Exercise 6, assuming the disease is fully lethal, and no affected individuals live to reproduce. Then determine the appropriate mutation rate for the pedigree in Exercise 7, assuming that 50% of all affected individuals do not live to reproduce. Compute the appropriate mutation rate to ensure a stable mutation–selection equilibrium and then perform an appropriate linkage analysis on this pedigree.

Design a computer experiment to show which alleles are allowed to mutate into which other alleles given the implementation of mutation in the LINKAGE programs.

22 □

Gene Frequencies and LINKAGE

In the previous chapter, we discussed issues of mutation rates and population genetics. Here we discuss the relevance of gene frequency information in linkage analysis, the methods for estimating them, and the consequences of using incorrect gene frequency models in a linkage analysis.

22.1 How Are Gene Frequencies Used in the LINKAGE Programs?

In the LINKAGE programs, the population frequency of each marker and disease allele is required for the computation of the likelihood. If every genotype at a locus in a pedigree is uniquely known, then the gene frequencies for that locus have no effect on the value of the lod score. However, as soon as there is one founder whose genotype cannot be uniquely determined, the gene frequencies begin to affect the lod scores. This holds for both marker and disease loci—at disease loci, the gene frequencies are always important, because the correspondence between genotype and phenotype is rarely 1:1. The frequency of each allele can play a significant role in the analysis. For this reason, it is imperative to have good estimates for the gene frequencies of each allele at each locus, because in practice there is almost always some ambiguity in the genotypes of some individuals in almost every pedigree. Furthermore, it is crucial that investigators uniquely identify each allele, so that, for example, the *1* allele is the same allele in each pedigree, whenever some individuals are untyped at a locus. Otherwise the gene frequency estimates will not really be appropriate.

Any deviations from the true gene frequencies can have major effects on the results and conclusions drawn from any given linkage analysis. To demonstrate this dependency, let us reconsider the example pedigree from Chapter 7 about homozygosity mapping (Figure 7–2). This pedigree showed a recessive disease with only one affected individual typed, with genotype *1 1* at the marker locus. Based on the information obtained from the consanguinity in this family, we were able to achieve a maximum lod score of 1.14 at $\theta = 0$. However, this result was certainly heavily dependent on the gene frequencies we selected. Reanalyze this pedigree with various gene frequencies for both

Table 22–1. Maximum Lod Scores Obtained for Homozygosity Mapping Problem with Different Disease and Marker Gene Frequencies

Frequency of *1* Allele	Frequency of Disease Allele				
	0.9	0.5	0.1	0.01	0.00001
0.9	0.00012	0.00338	0.01945	0.03859	0.04274
0.5	0.00102	0.02802	0.14323	0.25348	0.27468
0.1	0.00622	0.14860	0.53034	0.76720	0.80614
0.01	0.01473	0.29571	0.82723	1.10035	1.14338
0.00001	0.01706	0.32902	0.88315	1.16052	1.20401

disease and marker loci. Let the frequency of the disease allele and the *1* allele at the marker locus be 0.9, 0.5, 0.1, 0.01, and 0.00001, considering all possible combinations of disease and marker allele frequencies. The resulting maximum lod scores should be those shown in Table 22–1 (all with $\hat{\theta} = 0$).

It is obvious that when only a few individuals in a pedigree are typed, the gene frequency plays an important role. Table 22–1 shows that when the gene frequency of the disease allele is less than 90%, the gene frequency of the *1* allele has more effect on the analysis than the frequency of the disease allele. This is true because the penetrances at the disease locus tell us more about the untyped individuals' disease locus genotypes than we know about their marker locus genotypes. We know that the parents of the affected boy are each heterozygous for the disease allele and that one of each of their parents also must be heterozygous. However, at the marker locus, the parents could just as easily be homozygous for the *1* allele as heterozygous for it. The fact that we have less information about the genotypes of the untyped individuals makes the gene frequency particularly relevant. This example is quite extreme, and in practice if your families can show such drastically different lod scores when the gene frequencies alone are altered, the significance of your results must be highly questionable. In such a situation, the only reasonable solution may be to type additional pedigree members so as to reduce the dependency on gene frequency. In situations in which this is not possible, report the lod scores for all sets of p_i within their confidence intervals as done by Hsiao and co-workers (1989), for example. As an illustration of the lack of dependency on gene frequency in fully known pedigrees, reconsider the pedigree from Chapter 2: the phase-unknown nuclear pedigree (Figure 2–2). Analyze this pedigree with whatever gene frequencies you like, and the maximum lod score will always be 0.124929, at $\theta = 0.21$. The absolute values of the log likelihoods themselves change, but the value of the lod score does not.

22.2 The Consequences of Using Incorrect Gene Frequencies

From the results of the analysis above, it is clear that the gene frequencies can play an important role in linkage analysis. Nevertheless, if gene frequencies were selected randomly beforehand, it is not clear whether there would be a systematic effect on the lod score. Often investigators working with multiallelic CA repeat markers assume, for the purposes of the linkage analysis, that all alleles have equal gene frequencies. This is typically done because these markers have not been sufficiently well characterized, and accurate gene frequency estimates are unavailable. Also, it is often difficult to characterize the alleles in a population. For example allele *1* in family 1 may not correspond in general to allele *1* in family 2. This type of situation further complicates the problem of estimating gene frequency, because allele *1* may have a different meaning and a correspondingly different gene frequency in different families. In general, the only good solution to this problem is to characterize each allele uniquely. In this way, the *1* allele always refers to a specific allele, which should be invariant in different pedigrees. Only in this manner can we deal with the problem of estimating gene frequencies appropriately and avoid the bias associated with incorrect gene frequency modeling.

The effects of arbitrarily choosing to use equal gene frequencies in a linkage analysis was shown to lead to a systematic bias in favor of linkage when some individuals in a pedigree are untyped or when genotypes cannot be uniquely determined (Ott, 1992). In other words, setting the gene frequencies equal for all alleles tends to give false-positive evidence of linkage and even positive expected lod scores when there really is no linkage. To see this, look at the results of the homozygosity mapping exercise above. In this example, let us assume the actual gene frequency of the *1* allele was 0.9, and the gene frequency of the disease allele was 0.01. The maximum lod score with the assumed actual gene frequencies is only 0.03859. However, if there were 10 alleles at this locus, and we assumed erroneously that their frequencies were equal, the lod score would have jumped to 0.76720. In general, there is a systematic bias, which has been extensively studied by Ott (1992), through simulation and analytical means. The message here is that it is always important to have accurate gene frequency estimates when there are untyped individuals in your pedigrees, or when there is not a 1:1 correspondence between genotype and phenotype (i.e., dominance, recessivity, etc.).

22.3 Estimation of Gene Frequencies

Published estimates are available for the gene frequencies of many markers, based on a random sample of unrelated individuals. As a first approximation these readily available values may be used; however, the gene frequencies may differ strongly between populations at selectively neutral markers. Thus, it is advisable to estimate marker allele frequencies on your own from a cohort of unrelated individuals taken from the same genetic population as your disease pedigrees. If you consistently type 50 to 100 random individuals (depending on the number of alleles in your system) for each marker and estimate the allele frequencies from these observations, you would have an accurate source of information about your specific population. This is a very good approach to resolving this problem. There are, however, often situations in which this additional work is unfeasible or in which an investigator wishes to estimate the gene frequencies based on family data. Typically in a large pedigree there will be several founder individuals who are unrelated. These individuals are known to be from the appropriate genetic population and can be used as a cohort for investigating the frequency of marker alleles (though certainly not for the disease allele due to ascertainment problems). To do this, you could treat the unrelated individuals as an independent sample and apply counting methods, as has been described elsewhere (Hartl, 1988; Weir, 1990). Another approach, which is more powerful when some of the founders have not been typed, is to use the ILINK program of the LINKAGE package to estimate the allele frequencies from the pedigree data (Boehnke, 1991).

To estimate the gene frequencies with the ILINK program, it is essential to modify the parameter file manually, since PREPLINK is not equipped for this option. Let us start with a simple example. Consider the pedigree from

Exercise 2. In this pedigree there are eight founders, two of whom are untyped. Directly estimating the allele frequencies based on the six typed founders produces four copies of the *1* allele, two copies of the *2* allele, five copies of the *3* allele, and one copy of the *4* allele, giving gene frequency estimates of 0.3333, 0.1667, 0.4167, and 0.0833, respectively, for the four alleles. However, there is some information in the pedigree about the genotypes of the two untyped founder individuals. To take advantage of it, we use the ILINK program. Prepare the parameter file for this example, assuming the disease locus to be fully penetrant, autosomal dominant with gene frequency for the disease allele equal to 0.00001. At the marker locus there are four alleles, and you can assume the above estimated values as starting values for their gene frequencies. Now make this parameter file in ILINK format and write the file. It should resemble the following:

```
2 0 0 3   << NO. OF LOCI, RISK LOCUS, SEXLINKED (IF 1) PROGRAM
0 0.0 0.0 0   << MUT LOCUS, MUT MALE, MUT FEM, HAP FREQ (IF 1)
  1  2
1    2   << AFFECTION, NO. OF ALLELES
 9.99990E-01 1.00000E-05   << GENE FREQUENCIES
 1 << NO. OF LIABILITY CLASSES
 0 1.0000 1.0000 << PENETRANCES
3   4   << ALLELE NUMBERS, NO. OF ALLELES
0.3333  0.1667  0.4167  0.0833   << GENE FREQUENCIES
 0 0   << SEX DIFFERENCE, INTERFERENCE (IF 1 OR 2)
  0.1000 << RECOMBINATION VALUES
 1 << THIS LOCUS MAY HAVE ITERATED PARS
 0
```

Now, you must make a few changes to this file. First, the next to last line reads

```
1 << THIS LOCUS MAY HAVE ITERATED PARS
```

Because you wish to iterate the parameters (gene frequencies) for the second locus, change the 1 to a 2. Next consider the bottom line of this file, which now contains a 0. In general, the final line of this file tells the program which parameters to iterate and which ones to keep fixed. A zero means that parameter should remain fixed, and a 1 means the corresponding parameter should be estimated. If there are n loci in your parameter file, the first $n - 1$ parameters are the $n - 1$ recombination fractions. So, if you wish to estimate all recombination fractions, you need $(n - 1)$ 1's on the last line. If you only want to estimate the first recombination fraction and keep the others fixed, you need a 1 followed by $(n - 2)$ 0's on the last line, and so on. If you specify a constant ratio of male-to-female map distance, the next parameter corresponds to this ratio. If you want to estimate it, you must add an additional 1. Otherwise, add a 0 to keep it fixed. Similarly, if you specify variable ratios of male-to-female map distance in each interval, you must add an additional $n - 1$ 1's to estimate (or 0's to fix) the $n - 1$ female recombination fractions for each interval as well. If you specify m alleles at the locus on the next to last line of the file, the next $m - 1$ parameters are the gene frequencies of the first $m - 1$ alleles at that locus (the last gene frequency being set equal to $1 - \Sigma p_i; \ i < m$).

So, for our problem, we want to fix the recombination fraction between the two loci as 0.079, as found in Exercise 2 (modify the third line from the bottom to ensure that the recombination value is correct), and estimate the gene frequencies for the four alleles at the second locus. Thus, the last line of the parameter file should be 0 1 1 1, because we want to fix the recombination fraction, there is no sex-difference parameter, and we wish to estimate the three free gene frequencies, with $p_4 = 1 - p_1 - p_2 - p_3$. When you have made these changes, save this file as DATAFILE.DAT. It should look like this:

```
2 0 0 3  << NO. OF LOCI, RISK LOCUS, SEXLINKED (IF 1) PROGRAM
0 0.0 0.0 0 << MUT LOCUS, MUT MALE, MUT FEM, HAP FREQ (IF 1)
  1 2
1  2  << AFFECTION, NO. OF ALLELES
 9.99990E-01 1.00000E-05  << GENE FREQUENCIES
 1 << NO. OF LIABILITY CLASSES
 0 1.0000 1.0000 << PENETRANCES
3  4  << ALLELE NUMBERS, NO. OF ALLELES
0.3333  0.1667  0.4167  0.0833  << GENE FREQUENCIES
 0 0  << SEX DIFFERENCE, INTERFERENCE (IF 1 OR 2)
  0.079 << RECOMBINATION VALUES
  2 << THIS LOCUS MAY HAVE ITERATED PARS
  0 1 1 1
```

Then, call up the UNKNOWN program. The version of UNKNOWN you use *must* be dated after July, 1993, and distributed by us at Columbia University, because earlier program versions had a bug that affected allele frequency estimation and all analyses with linkage disequilibrium. These earlier versions of the UNKNOWN program had one peculiarity that drastically affected the estimation of allele frequencies from pedigree data. If everyone in a pedigree was untyped at a given locus, the UNKNOWN program assigned everyone the genotype *1 1* at that locus, which also represents absence of linkage information. However, it caused all founder individuals to have genotype *1 1*, leading inexorably to an overestimation of the frequency of the *1* allele whenever some pedigrees were completely uninformative. Therefore, we recently modified the UNKNOWN program by setting the variable makehomozygous = false (which will cause these pedigrees to be left with genotype *0 0* rather than making them homozygous *1 1*) whenever linkage disequilibrium is used *or* allele frequencies are estimated. To make valid estimations of allele frequencies in general pedigree data sets, it is imperative to run the UNKNOWN program immediately before doing such an analysis.

Then call up the ILINK program to analyze the pedigree and estimate the allele frequencies for locus 2. Note again that LCP cannot be used because it rewrites the bottom of the parameter file. The FINAL.DAT file should look like the following:

```
CHROMOSOME ORDER OF LOCI:
 1 2
**************** FINAL VALUES **************
PROVIDED FOR LOCUS  2 (CHROMOSOME ORDER)
*********************************************
GENE FREQUENCIES :
0.333383 0.199991 0.399935 0.066691
*********************************************
THETAS:
0.079
*********************************************
-2 LN(LIKE)  =  1.192555040143E+002
LOD SCORE  =  1.820979412697E+000
NUMBER OF ITERATIONS  =  6
NUMBER OF FUNCTION EVALUATIONS  =  37
PTG  =  -1.875727167222E-006
*********************************************
*********************************************
```

So you see that the gene frequency estimates were somewhat refined. Rerun the ILINK program, using the newly refined estimates of gene frequency as starting values, to see if they can be refined further. In this case, they cannot be refined further, and the program should return the same estimates. At this point, two questions immediately pop into mind. First of all, we did this estimation conditional on there being linkage between marker and disease. What happens to the estimates if we assume that the recombination fraction between disease and marker is 50%? This involves estimating marker allele frequencies ignoring all information about linkage. To do this, alter the DATAFILE.DAT such that the recombination value is set to 0.5 and rerun the ILINK program. This time, the estimates change slightly to 0.366901, 0.200645, 0.365811, and 0.066643, respectively, which can be further refined to 0.366830, 0.200045, 0.366430, and 0.066695. The final thing to consider is the possibility of jointly estimating recombination fraction with the gene frequencies. This can be done by setting the bottom line of the parameter file to be 1 1 1 1, such that all four parameters be estimated. Using the original starting values, as shown in the parameter file above, the first estimates should be $\theta = 0.078$, $p_i = 0.333419, 0.200082, 0.399984$, and 0.066515, which can be further refined to $\theta = 0.078$, $p_i = 0.333366, 0.200032, 0.399933$, and 0.066669. Table 22–2 summarizes the results of these analyses.

Here we see that estimating the gene frequencies based solely on the marker genotypes leads to slightly different estimates than when the gene frequencies are estimated jointly with linkage to a second locus (here the disease). Fortunately, the difference is not huge, though it may have a significant influence on the lod scores in some situations. One way to correct for this difference is to treat the marker allele frequencies as nuisance parameters in the analysis and compute your lod score as

$$Z(\hat{\theta}) = \log_{10}\left[\frac{L(\hat{\theta},\hat{p}_i)}{L(\theta = \frac{1}{2},\hat{p}_i)}\right]$$

where the p_i's are estimated separately under linkage (in the numerator) and under no linkage (in the denominator). The numerator and denominator can be separately determined from the ILINK output. In this case, the FINAL.DAT files created by ILINK for the two appropriate analyses show that $-2 \ln[L(\hat{\theta},\hat{p}_i)] = 119.255$, so $\log_{10}[L(\hat{\theta},\hat{p}_i)] = -25.925$. Similarly, $-2 \ln[L(\theta = \frac{1}{2},\hat{p}_i)] = 127.559$, so $\log_{10}[L(\theta = \frac{1}{2},\hat{p}_i)] = -27.730$. Therefore,

$$Z[\hat{\theta}] = -25.925 - (-27.730) = 1.8052$$

This is not much different from the original lod score (assuming equal gene frequencies) of 1.78 or from the lod score when gene frequencies were estimated assuming linkage (1.82), with said estimates used in both numerator and denominator of the lod score (Of course, this last statistic has 4 df, because four parameters are estimated in the numerator and none in the denominator). Because most pedigree members were typed in this example, the gene

Table 22–2. Gene Frequency Estimates Under Different Hypotheses

	$\theta = 0.079$	$\theta = 0.500$	$\theta = \hat{\theta}$	Counting
p_1	0.333383	0.366830	0.333666	0.333333
p_2	0.199991	0.200045	0.200032	0.166667
p_3	0.399935	0.366430	0.399933	0.416667
p_4	0.066691	0.066695	0.066669	0.083333

frequencies are not very crucial, whereas in other examples, the results may vary dramatically. If there is sufficient data, it is safest and most conservative to estimate the gene frequencies *separately* in numerator and denominator of the likelihood ratio as this statistic properly retains only 1 d.f.

In conclusion, we have learned how to estimate gene frequency parameters in the LINKAGE programs and why it is important to do so. We have also examined the ramifications of using improper gene frequencies to do a linkage analysis in practical situations.

☐ Exercise 22

Go back to Exercise 8 and estimate gene frequencies for the ABO blood group in this same pedigree. Does the lod score change when these frequencies are estimated instead of using population gene frequency estimates? Then, consider the incomplete penetrance model used in Exercise 9 on this same family. Does incorporating this reduced penetrance affect your estimates of marker allele frequencies? How does the gene frequency information affect the lod score between ABO and the disease?

23 □

Linkage Disequilibrium between Alleles at Marker Loci

Linkage disequilibrium is another population genetic phenomenon that can be useful in gene mapping. When the occurrence of pairs of specific alleles at different loci on the same haplotype is not independent, the deviation from independence is termed *linkage disequilibrium*. In this chapter, we introduce various methods for detecting and quantifying such linkage disequilibrium, and we demonstrate its use in linkage analysis with the LINKAGE programs.

23.1 What Is Linkage Disequilibrium?

For now, we restrict ourselves to the simplest case of linkage disequilibrium between alleles of two loci with two alleles each. In general, linkage disequilibrium is usually seen as an association between one specific allele at one locus and another specific allele at a second locus. Table 23–1 is a 2×2 table in which each cell represents one of the four possible haplotypes created by the two marker loci. The rows refer to the allele at the first marker, and the columns refer to the allele at the second marker. The number of observations in each cell, are represented by $X1$, $X2$, $X3$, and $X4$ where $X1 + X2 + X3 + X4 = n$. The probabilities given in each cell are the probabilities of any random individual in the same population having the haplotype indicated by that cell. The coefficient of gametic linkage disequilibrium between allele *1* at locus 1 and allele *1* at locus 2, is D_{11} (often denoted by δ), and is defined as $E[X1X4 - X2X3 \mid n = 1]$.

In general, we can extend this concept to multiple alleles and estimate haplotype frequencies for the $n_1 n_2$ possible haplotypes, but this usually requires a much larger sample size than the two-marker/two-allele case, with the corresponding analytical approaches being analogous.

23.2 Population-based Sampling and the EH Program

First we need to select a random cohort of individuals from one genetic population, meaning that the individuals should be from one (hopefully) randomly mating interbreeding unit. For example, assume that all of the individuals on

Table 23–1. Linkage Disequilibrium Coefficient Definitions

Marker 1	Marker 2	
	Allele *1*	Allele *2*
Allele *1*	$X1$ $\\ p_1p_2 + D_{11}$	$X2$ $\\ p_1(1 - p_2) - D_{11}$
Allele *2*	$X3$ $\\ (1 - p_1)p_2 - D_{11}$	$X4$ $\\ (1 - p_1)(1 - p_2) + D_{11}$

p_1 = gene frequency of allele *1* at marker 1; p_2 = gene frequency of allele *1* at marker 2; and D_{11} = coefficient of linkage disequilibrium between allele *1* at locus 1, and allele *1* at locus 2.

a given Pacific island with minimal immigration constitute one homogeneous interbreeding population. Likewise, one could consider French-Canadians, or Bavarian Germans, or Transylvanian Magyars to be approximately homogeneous. Often people extend this concept with reasonable accuracy to larger groups that appear to be randomly mating.

Let us assume we wish to test the absence of disequilibrium between allele *A* at locus 1, and allele *B* at locus 2, ($D_{AB} = 0$). Our sample of individuals consists of genotypic data, however, making it typically impossible to fully distinguish all of the haplotypes in each individual. Each individual can be classified uniquely in terms of his or her two-locus genotype and can be placed into one of the cells of Table 23–2. If the individual falls into cell 1, then you know it is made up of two identical A B haplotypes. Similarly, a person in cell 4 has one A B haplotype, and one A b haplotype. In almost every cell, this haplotype determination can be done uniquely, with the notable exception of cell 5, in which case there can be either of two phases, A B/a b, or A b/a B. These individuals present a difficulty, but omitting them from consideration in an analysis of this type can lead to a bias and a loss of information for the test, despite what you might think. Methods have been developed, however, to allow these individuals to be used in the analysis via likelihood methods. We maximize the log likelihood of the data observed, in which

$$\ln[L(\text{data})] = \sum_{i=1}^{a_1a_2} k_i \ln(p_i)$$

k_i = number of observations of two-locus genotype *i*; p_i = probability of observing two-locus genotype *i*. The only remaining question is how to compute the p_i. For most cases this is straightforward. In cell 1, we know that there are two A B haplotypes, so $p_1 = [P(\text{A B})]^2$. Similarly, in cell 4, there is one A B haplotype, and one A b haplotype, so the probability of being in this cell is $p_4 = 2P(\text{A B})P(\text{A b})$. For cell 5, however, there is some ambiguity about the phase, so

$$P(Aa,Bb) = P(\text{A B/a b}) + P(\text{A b/a B})$$

$$= 2P(\text{A B})P(\text{a b}) + 2P(\text{A b})P(\text{a B})$$

The computation of all cell probabilities is shown in Table 23–3.

Then, we maximize the likelihood above over the possible haplotype frequencies or, equivalently, over the three parameters $p(\underline{\text{A}})$, $p(\underline{\text{B}})$, and D_{AB} that make up the haplotype frequencies in the two-allele/two-locus case. This likelihood can then be compared with the maximum likelihood when D_{AB} is set equal to 0 (i.e., absence of linkage disequilibrium). This forms the basis of a test of linkage equilibrium and has been implemented in the linkage utility program EH (for estimate haplotype frequencies). Similar programs are given in Weir (1990).

Table 23–2. Table of All Possible Two-locus Genotypes

	Locus 1		
Locus 2	*AA*	*Aa*	*aa*
BB	k_1	k_2	k_3
Bb	k_4	k_5	k_6
bb	k_7	k_8	k_9

Let us assume the following data set, in the notation of Table 23–2: $k_1 = 10$, $k_2 = 10$, $k_3 = 3$, $k_4 = 15$, $k_5 = 50$, $k_6 = 13$, $k_7 = 5$, $k_8 = 13$, and $k_9 = 10$. In every case, except k_5, all the haplotypes can be uniquely determined, and counting we find 45 A̲ B̲ haplotypes, 29 a̲ B̲ haplotypes, 38 A̲ b̲ haplotypes, and 46 a̲ b̲ haplotypes. Assuming this is an exhaustive population sample of haplotypes, we can perform a chi-square test of independence of the 2 × 2 table shown below:

	A	*a*
B	45	29
b	38	46

In this case, $\chi^2_{(1)} = 3.83$, with a corresponding *p*-value of 0.05. The corresponding haplotype frequency estimates are as follows:

	A	*a*
B	0.284810	0.183544
b	0.240506	0.291140

Parametrizing these haplotype frequencies in terms of $p(A)$, $p(B)$, and D_{AB}, we determine that $p(A) = 0.284810 + 0.240506 = 0.525316$; $p(B) = 0.284810 + 0.183544 = 0.468354$; $D_{AB} = p(\text{A̲ B̲}) - p(A)p(B) = 0.284810 - (0.525316)(0.468354) = 0.038776$. However, this sample was biased due to the elimination of the 50 observations in k_5. The EH program can be used as described above to perform the appropriate analysis on all the data together. Let us set up our input file for EH as follows:

```
Line 1: Number of alleles at each of the two loci
Line 2: k₁ k₄ k₇
Line 3: k₂ k₅ k₈
Line 4: k₃ k₆ k₉
```

Table 23–3. Table of Probabilities of Each Cell in Table 23–2, Parametrized by Haplotype Frequency

	Locus 1		
Locus 2	*AA*	*Aa*	*aa*
BB	$p(\text{A̲ B̲})^2$	$2p(\text{A̲ B̲})p(\text{a̲ B̲})$	$p(\text{a̲ B̲})^2$
Bb	$2p(\text{A̲ B̲})p(\text{A̲ b̲})$	$2p(\text{A̲ B̲})p(\text{a̲ b̲}) + 2p(\text{A̲ b̲})p(\text{a̲ B̲})$	$2p(\text{a̲ B̲})p(\text{a̲ b̲})$
bb	$p(\text{A̲ b̲})^2$	$2p(\text{A̲ b̲})p(\text{a̲ b̲})$	$p(\text{a̲ b̲})^2$

Create such a file and name it EH.DAT. The file should look like this:

```
2 2
10 15 5
10 50 13
 3 13 10
```

Then, call the EH program by entering EH at the DOS prompt. Respond *no* when the program asks if you wish to use the case-control sampling option. Then, specify the input file as EH.DAT and the output file as EH.OUT, because the defaults are already set up. Then, after the program runs, you should get an output file similar to the following:

```
Estimates of Gene Frequencies (Assuming Independence)
----\------------------------------------------------------------
locus\allele      1         2
-------\----------------------------------------------------------
     1 |        0.5155    0.4845
     2 |        0.4806    0.5194
------------------------------------------------------------------

# of Typed Individuals: 129

There are 4 Possible Haplotypes of These 2 Loci.
They are Listed Below, with their Estimated Frequencies:


-----------------------------------------------------------------
|   Allele     Allele  |       Haplotype Frequency          |
|     at         at    |                                    |
|   Locus 1    Locus 2 |   Independent    w/Association     |
-----------------------------------------------------------------
     1           1         0.247762        0.327684
     1           2         0.267742        0.187820
     2           1         0.232859        0.152937
     2           2         0.251638        0.331560
-----------------------------------------------------------------

# of Iterations =  16

                                      df    ln(L)   Chi-square
-----------------------------------------------------------------
H0: No Association                     2   -252.68    0.00
H1: Allelic Associations Allowed       3   -248.23    8.89
```

Table 23–4. Table of Haplotype Frequency Estimates Based on Both Methods, First by Censoring the Individuals with Ambiguous Haplotypes, and Secondly by Using All the Data, with the EH Program

| | Haplotype Frequencies | | | |
| | Without k_s | | With k_s | |
Haplotype	Independent	Associate	Independent	Associate
A B	0.246034	0.284810	0.247762	0.327684
A b	0.279282	0.240506	0.267742	0.187820
a B	0.222320	0.183544	0.232859	0.152937
a b	0.252364	0.291140	0.251638	0.331560
$p(A)$	0.525316		0.515504	
$p(B)$	0.468354		0.480621	
δ	0.038776		0.079922	

Table 23–5. Format for Entering Multiallelic Genotype Information in the EH Program for Two Loci

Locus 1	Locus 2					
	1/1	*1/2*	*2/2*	*1/3*	*2/3*	*3/3* . . .
1/1	*a1*	*b1*	*c1*	*d1*	*e1*	*f1*
1/2	*a2*	*b2*	*c2*	*d2*	*e2*	*f2*
2/2	*a3*	*b3*	*c3*	*d3*	*e3*	*f3*
1/3	*a4*	*b4*	*c4*	*d4*	*e4*	*f4*
2/3	*a5*	*b5*	*c5*	*d5*	*e5*	*f5*
3/3	*a6*	*b6*	*c6*	*d6*	*e6*	*f6*
.						
.						
.						

Of interest here is the chi-square statistic, which is the difference in 2 ln(likelihood) (which is 8.89). In this case, the chi-square statistic has 1 df, because under the hypothesis of allelic association, there are three free parameters (the haplotype frequencies), whereas under the hypothesis of no allelic association, there are only two free parameters (the two gene frequencies). The difference in free parameters is 1, so the distribution has 1 df. The *p*-value associated with $\chi^2_{(1)} = 8.8928$ is 0.002873. Furthermore, comparing the haplotype frequency and δ estimates from the two approaches, with and without censoring the k_5 individuals, it is clear that they contribute significant information about disequilibrium, even though the phase cannot be uniquely determined a priori, as shown in Table 23–4.

The EH program also is capable of estimating haplotype frequencies for loci with more than two alleles; however, the format for data entry is more complicated. In general, for two loci in the EH program, you must enter the data as follows:

Line 1:   Number of alleles at each locus

Subsequent Lines: The number of observations of each genotype as per Table 23–5 (just the numbers of observations, not the rest of the table. The table, and column and row headers are given to indicate the format in which you should enter the numbers of observations, not as something to be entered as well). The EH program can also be used analogously for estimating haplotype frequencies at more than two loci.

Table 23–6. Format for Entering Multilocus Genotypic Data in the EH Program

Locus 1	Locus 2	Locus 3		
		1/1	*1/2*	*2/2*
1/1	1/1	*a1*	*b1*	*c1*
	1/2	*a2*	*b2*	*c2*
	2/2	*a3*	*b3*	*c3*
1/2	1/1	*a4*	*b4*	*c4*
	1/2	*a5*	*b5*	*c5*
	2/2	*a6*	*b6*	*c6*
2/2	1/1	*a7*	*b7*	*c7*
	1/2	*a8*	*b8*	*c8*
	2/2	*a9*	*b9*	*c9*

Here two alleles per locus are assumed. Additional alleles could be dealt with in the manner outlined in Table 23–5.

To do this, the appropriate genotype entry format for three loci is demonstrated in Table 23–6 (Of course, on line 1 you now have three numbers of alleles instead of two to tell the program there are three loci in the data file). Additional loci are added in an analogous manner.

23.3 Estimating Disequilibrium from Pedigree Data

The EH program incorporates a powerful and robust way of testing and estimating deviations from linkage equilibrium between alleles at marker loci, based on a random sample of unrelated individuals in a fixed homogeneous population. It allows the user to include those individuals with no phase information in a disequilibrium analysis. However, if you have family pedigree information, it is possible to incorporate the phase information obtained from such data in your analysis.

In the literature, some attempts have been made to look at family data by using the founders and married-ins as the set of unrelated individuals for conducting the disequilibrium analysis (Kerem et al., 1989). The advantage here is that the phase can be determined in the doubly heterozygous individuals, allowing haplotypes to be counted directly without relying on the EH algorithm. However, in determining the phase of the haplotypes in these cases, researchers generally ". . . have assumed that there were no recombinants in our family material" (Chakravarti et al., 1984). As pointed out by Chakravarti and associates (1984), this is going to lead to biased results, because there is no basis for making such an assumption in all circumstances. The probability of a recombination is equal to the recombination fraction between the two loci, which is usually not zero! However, the phase information from such family information could be taken advantage of by using the ILINK program to estimate haplotype frequencies from the pedigree data. This method still uses the founders but takes into account the recombination fraction between the loci, along with other factors. Let us consider the pedigree drawn in Figure 23–1.

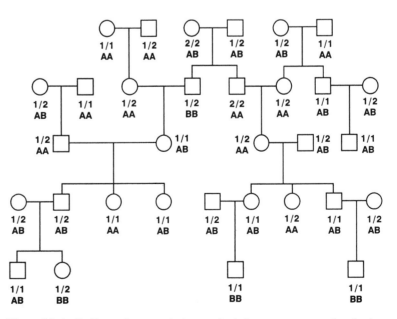

Figure 23–1. Pedigree for association analysis between two marker loci

First consider the founders and married-in individuals as a cohort of unrelated individuals from this population and analyze them with the EH program. The results should resemble the following:

```
Estimates of Gene Frequencies (Assuming Independence)
----\-----------------------------------------------------
locus\allele     1         2
--------\--------------------------------------------------
    1 |         0.5769    0.4231
    2 |         0.6538    0.3462
-----------------------------------------------------------

# of Typed Individuals: 13
```

There are 4 Possible Haplotypes of These 2 Loci.
They are Listed Below, with their Estimated Frequencies:

Allele at Locus 1	Allele at Locus 2	Haplotype Frequency	
		Independent	w/Association
1	1	0.377219	0.576921
1	2	0.199704	0.000002
2	1	0.276627	0.076925
2	2	0.146450	0.346152

```
# of Iterations = 8
```

	df	ln(L)	Chi-square
H0: No Association	2	−22.01	0.00
H1: Allelic Associations Allowed	3	−16.00	12.02

Clearly, there is overwhelming evidence for disequilibrium in this example ($\chi^2_{(1)} = 12.02$, $p = 0.0005$), with a strong association between the *1* and *A* alleles. Now, use the full amount of information at your disposal to estimate haplotype frequencies with the ILINK program. Enter the pedigree above in a LINKAGE format pedigree file (both markers in allele numbers format). Then, call up the PREPLINK program and specify the two allele–numbers loci (NO DISEASE LOCUS!) with the gene frequency estimates as obtained from the EH program above. Now, refine the gene frequency estimates using the ILINK program, as explained in Chapter 22. Do this first for locus 1 and then for locus 2, updating the frequencies for locus 1 as per your ILINK estimates. In this case, because there are no untyped people at either locus, it may be advisable to estimate the gene frequencies independently of the recombination fraction (Remember that θ should have no effect on the gene frequency estimates). Then compute the lod score for this pedigree. You should find that the gene frequency estimates do not change and are already maximized by the EH program. The maximum lod score for this pedigree, then, occurs at $\theta = 0$, with $Z(\theta = 0) = 1.2$, with a corresponding -2 ln(like) value of 99.48.

Now, use ILINK to maximize the likelihood over haplotype frequencies to see if there is significant evidence for disequilibrium when the entire pedigree is used to establish phase for the doubly heterozygous individuals. In addition we can see what the effect is on the haplotype frequency estimates. First, read the parameter file back into the PREPLINK program, this time selecting option (e) Haplotype Frequencies. You are prompted with the following screen:

```
*******************************************
(a) SEE HAPLOTYPE FREQUENCIES
(b) CHANGE HAPLOTYPE FREQUENCIES
(c) HAPLOTYPE FREQUENCIES DEFINED  :  N
(d) RETURN TO MAIN MENU
*******************************************
```

Select option *(c)* to define haplotype frequencies, and for starting values give the haplotype frequencies estimated by the EH program (under independence, because under the hypothesis of allelic association, the frequency of the 1 B haplotype is too close to zero) as follows:

```
ENTER NEW FREQUENCY AFTER EACH ''?''
NOTE THAT HAPLOTYPES ARE GIVEN USING CHROMOSOME ORDER OF LOCI
LOCUS   :     1  2
ALLELES :     1  1 0.000000E+00
  ?
0.377219
ALLELES :     1  2 0.000000E+00
  ?
0.199704
ALLELES :     2  1 0.000000E+00
  ?
0.276627
ALLELES :     1  1 0.000000E+00
  ?
0.146450
ENTER c TO CONTINUE
```

Now, return to the main menu and write the new parameter file. Then, bring the file into your word processor and examine it. It should now resemble the following:

```
2 0 0 3  << NO. OF LOCI, RISK LOCUS, SEXLINKED (IF 1) PROGRAM
0 0.0 0.0 1 << MUT LOCUS, MUT MALE, MUT FEM, HAP FREQ (IF 1)
  1  2
3  2    << ALLELE NUMBERS, NO. OF ALLELES
3  2    << ALLELE NUMBERS, NO. OF ALLELES
 0.377219 0.199704 0.276627 0.146450 << HAP FREQ
 0 0 << SEX DIFFERENCE, INTERFERENCE (IF 1 OR 2)
 0.5000 << RECOMBINATION VALUES
2 << THIS LOCUS MAY HAVE ITERATED PARS
0
```

Now alter the bottom of the parameter file by adding three 1's after the 0 on the last line to indicate that the three haplotype frequencies are to be estimated (the fourth being equal to $1 - p_1 - p_2 - p_3$) while fixing the recombination fraction at $\theta = \frac{1}{2}$. Run UNKNOWN (again, you must have the version dated after July, 1993 from Columbia University, which sets the variable makehomozygous = false). Then run the ILINK program, and your FINAL.DAT file should resemble the following:

```
CHROMOSOME ORDER OF LOCI:
  1   2
**************** FINAL VALUES *********
PROVIDED FOR LOCUS 2 (CHROMOSOME ORDER)
*******************************************
HAPLOTYPE FREQUENCIES:
 0.576458 0.000691 0.077266 0.345585
*******************************************
```

```
THETAS:
 0.500
*******************************************
-2 LN(LIKE)  =  9.302258802337E+001
LOD SCORE  =  0.00000000000E+000
NUMBER OF ITERATIONS  =    10
NUMBER OF FUNCTION EVALUATIONS  =    59
PTG  =  -7.504932736675E-005
*******************************************
*******************************************
```

Naturally, these haplotype frequency estimates are almost identical to those obtained from the EH program, because no information about phase is available from the rest of the family when the markers are assumed to be unlinked. However, if we jointly estimate the recombination fraction with the haplotype frequencies, additional phase information may be available. To do this, read the parameter file into your word processor and modify the bottom three lines to look like the following:

```
0.1000 << RECOMBINATION VALUES
2 << THIS LOCUS MAY HAVE ITERATED PARS
1 1 1 1
```

In this way, the recombination fraction is estimated along with the three haplotype frequencies. Now, rerun the ILINK program, and you should get the following quite different results:

```
haplotype frequencies  =  0.316321, 0.257770, 0.340819, 0.085091
θ = 0; -2 ln(Like) = 97.994
```

These results are very different. On looking at the family, it appears that in most of the heterozygous founders, the *1* allele is on the same haplotype as the *B* allele, but this is never seen in the individuals with unambiguous phase. Table 23–7 summarizes the results of the haplotype frequency estimates.

Interestingly, the gene frequency estimates are almost constant in each example, and the differences in haplotype frequency can be explained entirely in terms of D_{1A}, which is indicated in the last column above. It shows that although under the hypothesis of no linkage there is evidence for a strong association between the *1* and *A* alleles, when analyzed under the assumption of linkage, this association disappears, and in fact a slight association is noted between the *1* and *B* alleles. The question of how to use this output to develop a test for the presence of linkage disequilibrium remains. We have four likelihoods to consider, as indicated in Table 23–8.

Clearly, the bottom line should have a value of $-2 \ln(\text{likelihood})$ that is less than or equal to the value on the second to last line, because these are nested hypotheses. This means that our maximization must be stuck in some

Table 23–7. Haplotype Frequency Estimates Obtained from EH and from ILINK Based on Figure 23–1

Method of Estimation	Haplotype				D_{1A}
	1 A	1 B	2 A	2 B	
EH: Independence	0.377219	0.199704	0.276627	0.146450	0
EH: Association	0.576921	0.000002	0.076925	0.346152	0.200
ILINK: θ = 0.5	0.576458	0.000691	0.077266	0.345585	0.199
ILINK: θ = $\hat{\theta}$ = 0	0.316321	0.257770	0.340819	0.085091	−0.06

Table 23–8. Table of -2 ln(Likelihoods) under Different Hypotheses about θ and D_{1A}

D_{1A}	θ	-2 ln(Likelihood)
0	0.5	105.01
0	$\hat{\theta} = 0$	99.48
$\hat{D}_{1A} = \quad 0.199$	0.5	93.02
$\hat{D}_{1A} = -0.06$	$\hat{\theta} = 0$	97.99

local maximum. Let us maximize the likelihood at various fixed values of the recombination fraction θ. Set up a series of ILINK analyses to compute the values of -2 ln(likelihood) for values of θ between 0 and 0.5 in steps of 0.05. Also record what the FINAL.DAT file indicates as the "LOD SCORE" for each point. The results you obtain should be approximately the same as those in Table 23–9.

This is a very interesting result, because it shows a dichotomy of sorts between two very different local maxima for the likelihood over D_{1A}. For small θ, $D_{1A} = -0.07$ is about optimal, whereas for large θ, $D_{1A} = 0.200$ is optimal. It stands to reason that at some point the two must give an approximately equal likelihood, and that point should be somewhere between $\theta = 0.25$, and $\theta = 0.3$. It turns out that at $\theta = 0.275$, the value of -2 ln(likelihood) with $D_{1A} = -0.07$ is 103.05, and with $D_{1A} = 0.200$, it equals 103.05, so at this point the global maximum over D_{1A} switches over. This very interesting phenomenon occurs because in the founder individuals of this pedigree, there are seven observed 1 A haplotypes, two 2 A haplotypes, and one 2 B haplotype. This provides some evidence for a population association between the *1* and *A* alleles, as is the case when $D_{1A} = 0.2$. However, on closer examination of the pedigree, we find that in the eight doubly heterozygous individuals, under the hypothesis of tight linkage, the *1* allele occurs predominantly in association with the *B* allele. This apparent contradiction leads us to this dichotomy between two potential estimates of the disequilibrium coefficient. The "LOD SCORES" in Table 23–9 clearly follow a similar dichotomy, being very positive until $\theta = 0.275$ and suddenly becoming very negative. This is because these "LOD SCORES" are computed with the estimated haplotype frequencies used in both numerator and denominator. The more appropriate way to compute lod scores in such a situation is as $\log_{10} [L(\hat{\theta}, \hat{D}_{1A})/L(\theta = \frac{1}{2}, \hat{D}_{1A})]$, the values of which are indicated in the last column of Table 23–9 (with D_{1A} estimated separately in numerator and denominator). In this analysis, although

Table 23–9. Table of Likelihoods Maximized over D_{1A} for a Set of Fixed Values of θ in the Pedigree from Figure 23–1

Theta	D_{1A}	-2 ln(Likelihood)	"LOD SCORE"	Lod Score
0	-0.060	97.98	1.98	-1.08
0.05	-0.060	99.13	1.73	-1.33
0.1	-0.061	100.15	1.52	-1.55
0.15	-0.067	101.05	1.36	-1.74
0.2	-0.072	101.86	1.21	-1.92
0.25	-0.076	102.64	1.07	-2.05
0.3	$+0.200$	101.61	-1.87	-1.87
0.35	$+0.200$	99.09	-1.31	-1.32
0.4	$+0.200$	96.88	-0.84	-0.84
0.45	$+0.200$	94.88	-0.40	-0.40
0.5	$+0.200$	93.02	0.00	0.00

Table 23–10. Table of Observations for Analysis with the EH Program in Exercise 23

Locus 1	Locus 2									
	1/1	*1/2*	*1/3*	*1/4*	*2/2*	*2/3*	*2/4*	*3/3*	*3/4*	*4/4*
1/1	10	5	6	4	1	2	3	1	2	0
1/2	6	3	3	3	1	2	1	1	2	1
2/2	12	9	8	11	3	2	5	1	0	3
1/3	1	2	2	1	1	1	1	0	4	2
2/3	0	2	2	8	2	2	9	3	6	8
3/3	8	6	4	10	3	3	8	5	9	13

ILINK tells you the "LOD SCORE" is 1.98, correctly treating the haplotype frequencies as nuisance parameters results in a lod score at $\theta = 0$ of -1.08, when the analysis is done properly. This exercise points out just how important it is to do the linkage analysis carefully. When using haplotype frequency information, one *must* be careful about reestimating the frequencies under the hypotheses of linkage and no linkage, respectively. In this case, it is also interesting to consider the effect of using the haplotype frequency estimates obtained from the EH program and computing lod scores based solely on these estimates. In this case, using those estimates gives you a lod score at $\theta = 0$ of $-\infty$, with an exclusion region extending through $\theta = 0.275$, whereas in the appropriate ILINK analysis, the lod scores started increasing again from $\theta = 0.275$ to $\theta = 0$. This result indicates that in this analysis, you make false exclusions, whereas by following the "LOD SCORE" values given in the ILINK program, you make false assumptions of a positive linkage finding.

□ Exercise 23

Compute the genotype probabilities for all possible genotypes for use in the EH program, assuming one four-allele locus, and one three-allele locus. Then, analyze the observations in Table 23–10 with the EH program and separately by censoring individuals with ambiguous haplotype phase.

Next, consider the pedigree from Exercise 8, and look for linkage disequilibrium between alleles of the ABO blood group and the other marker locus. Analyze this pedigree with ILINK to estimate haplotype frequencies for each θ in steps of 0.1 from $\theta = 0.1$ to $\theta = 0.5$. (*Hint:* Be sure to eliminate the disease locus from the pedigree and parameter files before you commence this analysis.)

24.

Linkage Disequilibrium and Disease Loci

When looking for linkage disequilibrium between a disease allele and a marker allele, the methods explained in the previous chapter cannot be applied, due to ascertainment problems. The straight EH approach is not practical, because the population frequency of most genetic diseases is so small that in a random sample of individuals, you are not likely to encounter a single affected person. It is therefore imperative to devise directed ascertainment schemes, in which the sample is enriched for the disease. In this chapter, we introduce some basic approaches to this problem and the ways such disequilibrium can be used in a linkage analysis with the MLINK and ILINK programs.

24.1 Case-control Sampling

Perhaps the most obvious approach is to take a sample of unrelated individuals affected with a certain genetic disease, and compare the frequency of certain alleles with their frequency in a sample of unrelated normal individuals. If the mode of inheritance for the disease is known, it is possible to estimate haplotype frequencies. However, the primary object is to test whether there is an allelic association. If a sample of affected persons and a sample of normal individuals are collected from the same population, a chi-square test is performed to test the equality of the gene frequencies in the case and control samples. For example, consider the following set of observations:

	Marker allele	
	1	2
Case	60	40
Control	40	60

A simple chi-square test is performed on this 2 × 2 table and analyzed using the CONTING program, finding a value of 8.00 for the chi-square statistic with a corresponding two-sided *p*-value of 0.004. Another useful linkage utility program is 2BY2, which performs Fisher's exact test on a 2 × 2 table. In this case, you call up the 2BY2 program and enter the data as in the table above. The exact one-sided *p*-value in this case is 0.0035. Because this *p*-value is one-sided and the other is two-sided, this *p*-value should be doubled for an approximate comparison of the two approaches.

This is a simple approach. If we assume that the disease is fully penetrant recessive with very rare frequency of the disease allele, we can estimate haplotype frequencies for the disease marker haplotypes as follows. Clearly, we know that everyone in the disease sample carries two copies of the disease allele, so we can say that $P(\text{allele } 1|\text{disease allele}) = 0.4$, and $P(\text{allele } 2|\text{disease allele}) = 0.6$. Assuming we have a population-based estimate for the disease allele frequency (in this case, $p = 0.001$), we can compute the disease marker haplotype frequencies as $P(1\ \underline{D}) = P(\text{allele } 1|\text{disease allele})P(\text{disease allele}) = (0.4)(0.001) = 0.0004$. Similarly, $P(2\ \underline{D}) = 0.0006$. Because the disease allele is so rare, we can safely assume that the control population consists solely of homozygous normal individuals. In this case, then, by the logic outlined above, $P(1\ +) = 0.5994$ and $P(2\ +) = 0.3996$.

24.2 More Complicated Penetrance Models

If the disease is dominant, or phenocopies are allowed for, the situation is more complicated. We use the case-control option of the EH program to allow for these types of diseases, to compute haplotype frequencies more accurately, and to test linkage equilibrium given various specific disease models when the data are sampled according to a case-control strategy, as above. The basic idea behind this program is that samples of individuals with and without the disease are collected separately. Then, according to the penetrances and gene frequencies (which must be user-specified for the disease locus only), each individual is assigned a probability of having each possible disease locus genotype. For example, if we have $f_1 = P(\text{Aff}|DD)$; $f_2 = P(\text{Aff}|Dd)$; $f_3 = P(\text{Aff}|dd)$; and $p = P(D)$; then we have the prevalence

$$\phi = f_1 p^2 + 2f_2(1 - p)p + f_3(1 - p)^2 \text{ in the population.}$$

Then, for each affected individual, we compute $P(DD|\text{Aff}) = f_1 p^2/\phi$, and so on. Each observation of an affected individual is then partitioned among the three possible genotypes according to these conditional probabilities. For example, if we have one affected individual with marker genotype *1/1*, he is partitioned into three observations: $P(DD|\text{Aff})$ observations of disease locus genotype *DD*, marker locus genotype *1/1*; $P(Dd|\text{Aff})$ observations of disease locus genotype *Dd*, marker locus genotype *1/1*; and $P(dd|\text{Aff})$ observations of disease locus genotype *dd*, marker locus genotype *1/1*. Similar decomposition is done with the unaffected individuals (who have penetrances $P(\text{NA}|DD) = 1 - P(\text{Aff}|DD)$, etc.), and the resulting data are combined across disease locus phenotypes. Thus, if we have m_1 observations of affected persons with marker genotype *1/1*, and m_2 observations of unaffected individuals with marker genotype *1/1*, we have genotype-decomposed observations of $m_1 P(DD|\text{Aff}) + m_2 P(DD|\text{NA})$ observations of disease locus genotype *DD*, marker locus genotype *1/1*, and so on, for the other possible disease locus genotypes. This genotype-based data can then be analyzed with the EH program, with the restriction that the disease allele frequency must remain equal to p throughout. Because of the case-control ascertainment scheme involved

Table 24–1. Data Set for Case-control Study of Disequilibrium with EH

	Marker Locus Genotype									
Sample	*1/1*	*1/2*	*1/3*	*1/4*	*2/2*	*2/3*	*2/4*	*3/3*	*3/4*	*4/4*
Case	13	5	11	4	0	3	2	8	10	9
Control	2	4	5	7	2	6	5	5	18	14

here, the disease allele frequency would generally be vastly overestimated if it were estimated from the data.

To use this version of the EH program, prepare your data in exactly the same form as in Chapter 23, with the exception that you must have separate files for the case data (CASE.DAT) and the control data (CONTROL.DAT). In these files, indicate the numbers of observations of each genotype at the marker locus (or loci) in exactly the same format as shown in the previous chapter. The one difference is that you must now additionally specify the gene frequency of the disease allele and penetrance values for each disease locus genotype (always assuming the disease-predisposing allele to be the first allele at the disease locus). As an example, consider the data shown in Table 24–1. The CASE.DAT file, for example, should resemble the following:

```
4
13 5 0 11 3 8 4 2 10 9
[EOF]
```

To run the program, type EH at the DOS prompt, and when the program prompts you with

```
Do you wish to use the case–control sampling option? [Y/N]
```

Respond by entering Y. Then, you need to tell the program the names of the separate input files for the CONTROL sample genotypes and the CASE sample genotypes. Because we created these two files with the appropriate default names, you need only hit the ⟨Enter⟩ key when prompted with

```
Enter control data file [CONTROL.DAT], and
Enter case data file [CASE.DAT].
```

The output file can also be left at the default EH.OUT. The next phase requires that various parameters of the disease locus be specified. In this case, the gene frequency of the disease allele is 0.01; then the penetrances for each of the three possible disease-locus genotypes must be specified, in this case assuming a dominant disease with 80% penetrance and 0.1% penetrance for phenocopies as follows: $+/+$ ($= 0.001$), $+/D$ ($= 0.80$), D/D ($= 0.80$). The output file EH.OUT should resemble the following:

```
Estimates of Gene Frequencies (Assuming Independence)
(Disease gene frequencies are user specified)
----\-------------------------------------------------
locus\allele    1         2         3         4
--------\---------------------------------------------
Disease |     0.9900    0.0100
      1 |     0.2481    0.1090    0.2970    0.3459
------------------------------------------------------
# of Typed Individuals: 133

There are 8 Possible Haplotypes of These 2 Loci.
They are Listed Below, with their Estimated Frequencies:
```

Allele at Disease	Allele at Marker1	Haplotype Frequency	
		Independent	w/Association
+	1	0.245602	0.189420
+	2	0.107895	0.138740
+	3	0.294060	0.286691
+	4	0.342443	0.375149
D	1	0.002481	0.004356
D	2	0.001090	0.000060
D	3	0.002970	0.003216
D	4	0.003459	0.002367

# of Iterations = 23

	df	Ln(L)	Chi-square
H0 : No Association	3	−294.40	0.00
H1 : Markers and Disease Associated	6	−287.89	13.02

The likelihood ratio test of linkage equilibrium between the marker and disease then is $-2 \ln[L(H_0)/L(H_1)] \sim \chi^2$, with $6 - 3 = 3$ df. In this case, this statistic has a value of 13.02 with an associated *p*-value of 0.0046, which is significant evidence for linkage disequilibrium between the disease and marker alleles with the estimated haplotype frequencies shown above. Apparently the strongest association is between the disease allele and allele *1* at the marker locus.

One additional point of interest is that contrary to the situation in which sampling is random with respect to both markers, in this case, the estimated frequencies of the marker alleles are different under the assumption of linkage disequilibrium. For example, under the hypothesis of no disequilibrium, the frequency of the *1* allele is estimated to be 0.2481, whereas under the hypothesis of linkage disequilibrium, its frequency is estimated to be $P(1) = P(1 \ +) + P(1 \ D) = 0.189420 + 0.002367 = 0.191787$, which is much smaller. This decrease is a result of the fact that the *1* allele is associated with the *D* allele, which is overrepresented in the sample because the case-control sampling scheme overrepresents haplotypes that carry the *D* allele.

This approach can be used just as well to estimate haplotype frequencies with two or more marker loci, but it is important to be careful about what you consider a significant result. Although linkage disequilibrium at more than two loci is beyond the scope of this book, we caution the unwary user to not misuse this method in such situations. Consider the following simple example with two marker loci. Assume that we observe the genotypes shown in Table 24–2. Clearly, there is no association between any of the marker alleles and the disease, yet there is a strong association between the alleles of the two markers. If you run the EH program on these data, you should find that there are now three likelihood values given at the bottom, $\chi^2(H_0) = 0.00$; $\chi^2(H_1) = 29.67$; and $\chi^2(H_2) = 29.67$. These values are

$$-2 \ln[L(H_0)/L(H_i)] = 2 \ln[L(H_i)] - 2 \ln[L(H_0)]$$

and therefore provide the appropriate test statistic for comparing either hypothesis against the overall null hypothesis of no association between any alleles at any of the loci. Thus, there is highly significant ($p < 0.000001$) evidence for an association between alleles of the two markers, independent of the disease, and highly significant evidence for an overall association

Table 24-2. Data Set for Case-control Study of Disequilibrium with a Disease and Two Marker Loci

	Marker 1					
	Case			*Control*		
Marker 2	*1/1*	*1/2*	*2/2*	*1/1*	*1/2*	*2/2*
1/1	10	5	2	10	5	2
1/2	5	10	5	5	10	5
2/2	2	5	10	2	5	10

($p = 0.000006$). However, the most appropriate test for association between disease and alleles at one or more of the markers is to compare H_2 with H_1. You may question the use of H_1 as the appropriate null hypothesis in general, especially if there is no significant evidence for rejecting H_0 in favor of H_1. In fact, we are not interested in whether the markers are associated with each other (and typically in such a study, we assume this to be the case), but are solely interested in whether the disease is associated with one or more of the markers. In this case the desired test is $-2 \ln[L(H_1)/L(H_2)]$, which is equivalent to

$$\chi^2(H_2) - \chi^2(H_1) = [2 \ln L(H_2) - 2 \ln L(H_0)] - [2 \ln L(H_1) - 2 \ln L(H_0)]$$

$$= 2 \ln L(H_2) - 2 \ln L(H_1) = -2 \ln[L(H_1)/L(H_2)]$$

and can thus be easily determined. In this case, there is clearly no significance, because $\chi^2(H_2) - \chi^2(H_1) = 29.67 - 29.67 = 0$, so there is absolutely no evidence for any association between the disease allele and any allele at any of the marker loci.

24.3 The Theory behind the Haplotype Relative Risk

In many case-control studies of allelic association, people question the meaning of the results, because it can be difficult to find well-matched case and control samples from the same **genetic** population. As a possible remedy to this problem, Rubinstein and associates (1981) proposed their genotype-based haplotype relative risk (GHRR) design to obtain matched case and control samples in an association study. The basic idea of their method is to collect a random sample of affected individuals, and their parents, and base the analysis solely on these small nuclear families. The affected child's marker genotype is considered as the "case" sample, and the two parental alleles that were not transmitted to the affected child are considered as an artificial "control" sample, obviously well matched from the same genetic population. For example, consider a family with parental genotypes G/H, and H/J, with affected son H/H, as shown in Figure 24-1.

In this family, the "case" genotype is H/H, and the artificial "control" genotype is G/J—the two alleles (one from each parent) that were not transmitted to the affected child. The original formulation by Rubinstein and colleagues looked at whether a given allele was present or absent from each "genotype." For our case, we look at the H allele. Clearly, there are two H alleles in the transmitted (case) sample and no H alleles in the nontransmitted sample (control). Hence, this family contributes one observation of H transmitted and one observation of $\overline{H}$ nontransmitted. We then collect n such nuclear families

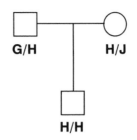

Figure 24–1. Sample HRR pedigree

and obtain two such observations from each family (one transmitted and one not-transmitted). Filling in Table 24–3 with these observations, we test linkage equilibrium by a simple chi-square test of independence on this table, as

$$\chi^2 = \frac{2N(WZ - XY)^2}{(W + X)(W + Y)(X + Z)(Y + Z)}$$

It is important to point out that the theory that has been developed for the HRR is based on the rather restrictive assumption that families are singly ascertained and that the affected child in the analysis must be the proband in each family. It is unclear what the effect of violating these rather strict rules may be, so it is suggested that if you are planning to start an association study using this approach, that you collect families based solely on this criteria. Granted that for many complex diseases with high rates of sporadic cases, you may have a large number of sporadic cases in your sample, but if some association exists, then if you collect a sufficiently large sample, you should be able to detect it anyway. Please refer to Terwilliger and Ott (1992b) for further details about sample size and power considerations.

24.4 The Application of the HRR and the CONTING Program

This test of linkage equilibrium is very simple to apply, because any fully typed family of this type can be uniquely classified according to whether a given allele (here denoted *H*) is transmitted and not-transmitted. This can be done easily by hand, and no complicated computer software is needed. Further, there is a linkage utility program called CONTING, which can be used to compute the chi-square statistic for any such 2 × 2 table. Let us assume that we have collected 50 such families, with $W = 40$, $X = 10$, $Y = 20$, and $Z = 30$. Now, call up the CONTING program. It prompts you with

```
Interactive use? [Y/n]
```

Table 24–3. Haplotype Relative Risk 2×2 Table

	H	$\overline{H}$	Total
Transmitted	W	X	(W + X)
Nontransmitted	Y	Z	(Y + Z)
	(W + Y)	(X + Z)	2N

to which you respond Y. Then it asks

```
NEW TABLE:
Number of rows (0 to stop)  =
```

to which you respond 2. Similarly, tell the program that there are 2 columns (because we have a 2 × 2 table). You are then asked (Your responses are indicated in italics)

```
Enter observed numbers rowwise
Row 1- 40   10
Row 2- 20   30
```

The program then recreates the 2 × 2 table to allow you to verify that you have entered the data correctly, as follows:

```
The observed figures are:
       1       2
1    40.     10.
2    20.     30.
Use Yates' correction for continuity (y/N)?
```

If the sample size is large, as in this case, you do not need to correct for continuity, so hit ⟨Enter⟩ (the uppercase N indicates that this is the default). You then see the following screen:

```
Frequencies expected under independence:
       1        2
1    30.00    20.00
2    30.00    20.00
To continue, press ⟨return⟩ key.
```

These values are the expected counts in each cell, assuming independence of the 2 × 2 table. When you hit the ⟨enter⟩ key, the results of the chi-square calculation appear as follows:

```
The contributions to chi-square are:
       1       2
1    3.33    5.00
2    3.33    5.00
Chi-square = 16.67 1 degree of freedom
2-sided p-value = 0.000045
```

```
Collapse some rows or columns to form a new table (screen input)?
```

to which you should respond N, followed by

```
NEW TABLE:
Number of rows (0 to stop)  =
```

You may now enter 0 to exit the program. As you can see, the null hypothesis of equilibrium is rejected by this test at the 0.000045 level, so we have very significant evidence for linkage disequilibrium. As an exercise, use your calculator and substitute the appropriate values of *W*, *X*, *Y*, and *Z* in the chi-square formula above to verify that this result is correct. You should get

$$\chi^2 = \frac{2(50)[(40)(30) - (20)(10)]^2}{(40 + 10)(40 + 20)(10 + 30)(20 + 30)} = 16.67$$

which matches the result obtained using the CONTING program.

24.5 Paired Sampling and the CHIPROB Program

It is also possible to consider each family as contributing one observation to Table 24–4, in which each family is classified in terms of both its transmitted and nontransmitted genotypes. For the sample pedigree described above, the one observation is in cell B (H transmitted, $\overline{H}$ not transmitted). Looking further at this table, we see that the marginals of Table 24–4 provide the data on which the haplotype relative risk statistic is based.

We base our tests of equilibrium on this table as well, by performing a McNemar test. Clearly, the null hypothesis of the HRR test (from the previous section) is that $W = Y$. But, if we consider the actual familial source of the data in the paired sampling case, we see that this hypothesis is equivalent to $(A + B) = (A + C)$, which implies $B = C$. A simple and straightforward test of this sort is a McNemar test on this paired sampling table. The Mc-Nemar test is

$$\chi^2 = \frac{(B - C)^2}{B + C}$$

as described in Terwilliger and Ott (1992b). This test is easy to apply and intuitively appealing, but it has uniformly lower power than tests of the HRR variety. However, as pointed out by Spielman and co-workers (1993), the McNemar test has the advantage that we needn't assume the presence of Hardy-Weinberg equilibrium, which is not present when there is population stratification. Furthermore, the power of this test is minimally lower than the HRR tests in general, making it a preferable option when population stratification is likely.

Let us apply this test to our sample data from Section 24.4. Fill in the missing data in Table 24–4 as $A = 15$, $B = 25$, $C = 5$, $D = 5$ (*Note: $W = A + B = 40$, etc.*). Applying the simpler McNemar test, we use our calculators to obtain the value

$$\chi^2 = \frac{(25 - 5)^2}{25 + 5} = 13.33$$

To determine the associated p-value, we must either consult a chi-square table or use the linkage utility program CHIPROB. When you call up this program, you are prompted with

`Enter χ² and df`

At this point, you enter 13.33 1, because the value of your statistic is 13.33, and there is 1 df. The program then provides the appropriate two-sided p-value of 0.000263. To exit the CHIPROB program, enter a 0 at the next prompt. This p-value is still highly significant but less significant than the HRR statistic applied to the same data.

Table 24–4. Paired Sampling HRR Table

Transmitted	Nontransmitted		Total
	H	$\overline{H}$	
$\underline{H}$	A	B	W
$\overline{H}$	C	D	X
	Y	Z	N

24.6 Haplotype-based Haplotype Relative Risk

Terwilliger and Ott (1992b) developed a way to use this HRR experimental design to glean much additional information from the same data set. In the case of the original GHRR statistic, Rubinstein and colleagues (1981) lumped together H/H homozygotes, and $H/\overline{H}$ heterozygotes as H genotypes. However, Terwilliger and Ott (1992b) noticed that because under the null hypothesis the two parental genotypes are independent, the transmitted and nontransmitted alleles from each parent can be treated as independent observations and thus supply us with four observations per family, in what they termed the haplotype-based haplotype relative risk (HHRR) statistic. Returning to the sample pedigree above, we see that it now contributes two observations of H transmitted (H/H), and two observations of $\overline{H}$ nontransmitted (G/J). In this case, the same statistic can be applied, only now N refers to the total number of parents, as opposed to the total number of families, and is thus twice as large as it was under the GHRR method. If we break down our sample data set of 50 families into haplotypes, we may find the following data (In form of Table 24–4 above) $A = 19$; $B = 42$; $C = 10$; and $D = 29$. This means that $W = 61$; $X = 39$; $Y = 29$; and $Z = 71$. If we then compute the chi-square statistic associated with this table (as described above for the GHRR), we would find that the HHRR is equal to

$$\chi^2 = \frac{2(100)[(61)(71) - (39)(29)]^2}{(61 + 39)(61 + 29)(39 + 71)(29 + 71)} = 20.69$$

The p-value obtained from CONTING (or equivalently from CHIPROB) is 0.000005, which is much stronger than the result obtained from the GHRR approach. Analogously, if we apply the McNemar test to this data as well to give the result

$$\chi^2 = \frac{(42 - 10)^2}{42 + 10} = 19.69$$

Again, this test gives somewhat lower significance than the HHRR statistic but higher than the genotype-based McNemar test. In general, Terwilliger and Ott (1992b) showed that the HHRR approach provides better power than the GHRR approach almost uniformly and is thus more useful generally for both HRR and McNemar type statistics.

It is also important to be careful about multiple comparisons (cf. Ott (1991), sec. 4.7) in evaluating the significance of any given test result, because researchers often consider each marker allele separately against the disease allele. In these cases, divide the critical p-value by the number of comparisons done to allow adequately for the multiple testing problem (Anderson and Sclove, 1986).

24.7 Using ILINK to Estimate Linkage Disequilibrium with Disease

Of course, the ILINK program can be used to estimate haplotype frequencies, as we saw in Chapter 23. However, there are problems with this estimation when one of the loci involved is the disease locus. The basic problem is that the disease allele is necessarily overrepresented in the pedigree data set. Haplotype frequencies $\hat{P}(\underline{D}\ i)$ can be estimated and then normalized a posteriori to disease allele frequency for the known population as

$$P(\underline{D}\ i) = p_D\left[\frac{\hat{P}\ (\underline{D}\ i)}{\Sigma_i\hat{P}\ (\underline{D}\ i)}\right]$$

for example. Still, the estimates may not be accurate, because the constraint on disease allele frequency was made after the maximization process, not before it. The limitation of the ILINK program makes this approach somewhat unreliable. Furthermore, it is generally better to estimate your haplotype frequencies from one data set, and then use this information in subsequent pedigree analysis. The method for using the ILINK program to estimate haplotype frequencies in general was illustrated in Chapter 23, and the normalization process is analogous to what was done in the EH program.

24.8 Using Linkage Disequilibrium in the LINKAGE Programs

It is possible to use information about linkage disequilibrium in the LINKAGE programs to do a standard linkage analysis. The use of such haplotype frequency information can have a strong effect on the linkage analysis results because it makes the prior probabilities of the possible parental phases unequal in an otherwise phase-unknown mating. Let us consider the two pedigrees shown in Figure 7–3 from the section on marriage loops. Remember that these pedigrees are completely uninformative for linkage, because they are both phase-unknown matings with only one offspring each. What happens to this analysis if we allow for the presence of linkage disequilibrium?

In these pedigrees, we know the disease is recessive and that each parent is heterozygous at the disease locus. So, let us consider the first pedigree: with parents *2/3* and *1/1*. In this pedigree, the only potentially informative meiosis is from *father:* the *2/3* individual. There are two possible phases for this parent: $\underline{2\ D/3\ +}$ and $\underline{2\ +/3\ D}$. The likelihoods of these two phases are $L_1 = P(\underline{2\ D})P(\underline{3\ +})$ and $L_2 = P(\underline{2\ +})P(\underline{3\ D})$, respectively. Under Phase I the affected daughter is a recombinant, and under Phase II she is a nonrecombinant, so the likelihood of this pedigree is $L_1\theta + L_2(1 - \theta)$. Under the assumption of no linkage disequilibrium, $L_1 = L_2$ by definition, so the overall likelihood of this pedigree is L_1, which is independent of θ and thus provides no information about linkage. However, whenever there is linkage disequilibrium and $L_1 \neq L_2$, this likelihood is a function of θ and therefore provides information about linkage. For the second pedigree, by analogy, we have phases for *father* of $\underline{1\ D/2\ +}$ or $\underline{1\ +/2\ D}$, with corresponding likelihoods $L_3 = P(\underline{1\ D})P(\underline{2\ +})$ and $L_4 = P(\underline{1\ +})P(\underline{2\ D})$ and overall pedigree likelihood of $L_3(1 - \theta) + L_4\theta$. Our lod score for the two pedigrees together is therefore equal to

$$Z(\theta) = \log_{10}[L_1\theta + L_2(1 - \theta)] - \log_{10}\left[\frac{1}{2}(L_1 + L_2)\right]$$

$$+ \log_{10}[L_3(1 - \theta) + L_4\theta] - \log_{10}\left[\frac{1}{2}(L_3 + L_4)\right]$$

Consider the haplotype frequency information given in Table 24–5. Under these four models (the first of which represents no linkage disequilibrium, and the others which represent extremely strong associations between the disease allele and one of the marker alleles), the lod scores are very different owing

Table 24–5. Haplotype Frequency Models for Analysis of Pedigrees from Figure 7–3, where $k = p(1-p)$

Haplotype	Model 1	Model 2	Model 3	Model 4
D 1	$0.25p$	$0.01p$	$0.98p$	$0.01p$
D 2	$0.40p$	$0.98p$	$0.01p$	$0.01p$
D 3	$0.35p$	$0.01p$	$0.01p$	$0.98p$
+ 1	$0.25(1-p)$	$0.25(1-p)$	$0.25(1-p)$	$0.25(1-p)$
+ 2	$0.40(1-p)$	$0.40(1-p)$	$0.40(1-p)$	$0.40(1-p)$
+ 3	$0.35(1-p)$	$0.35(1-p)$	$0.35(1-p)$	$0.35(1-p)$
L_1	$k(0.40)(0.35)$	$k(0.98)(0.35)$	$k(0.01)(0.35)$	$k(0.01)(0.35)$
L_2	$k(0.40)(0.35)$	$k(0.40)(0.01)$	$k(0.40)(0.01)$	$k(0.40)(0.98)$
L_3	$k(0.25)(0.40)$	$k(0.01)(0.40)$	$k(0.98)(0.40)$	$k(0.01)(0.40)$
L_4	$k(0.25)(0.40)$	$k(0.25)(0.98)$	$k(0.25)(0.01)$	$k(0.25)(0.01)$

to the incorporation of phase information. Let us compute the lod scores at various values of the recombination fraction. Note that the constant k can be dropped from each of the L_i because they are likelihoods, each divided by the same constant $k = p(1 - p)$. Under model 1, the lod score is

$$\log_{10}[(0.40)(0.35)\theta + (0.40)(0.35)(1 - \theta)] - \log_{10}\left\{\frac{1}{2}[(0.40)(0.35)\right.$$

$$\left. + (0.40)(0.35)]\right\} + \log_{10}[(0.25)(0.40)\theta + (0.25)(0.40)(1 - \theta)]$$

$$- \log_{10}\left\{\frac{1}{2}[(0.25)(0.40) + (0.25)(0.40)]\right\} = \log_{10}[(0.40)(0.35)]$$

$$- \log_{10}[(0.40)(0.35)] + \log_{10}[(0.25)(0.40)] - \log_{10}[(0.25)(0.40)] = 0$$

for all θ. For the other models, the analytically computed lod scores are given in Table 24–6. To analyze the same pedigrees with the LINKAGE programs, it is necessary to specify haplotype frequencies in the parameter file. To do this, use the pedigree and parameter files from Chapter 7, files EX6A.*. Read the EX6A.DAT file into PREPLINK and select the (e) Haplotype frequencies option followed by (c) HAPLOTYPE FREQUENCIES DEFINED. You are then prompted with the following screen:

```
ENTER NEW FREQUENCY AFTER EACH ''?''
NOTE THAT HAPLOTYPES ARE GIVEN USING CHROMOSOME ORDER OF LOCI
LOCUS  :  1 2
ALLELES :  1 1 0.0000000000000E+00
   ?
```

Table 24–6. Lod Scores Computed for Various Values of θ on Pedigrees from Figure 7–3 with Haplotype Frequency Models Given in Table 24–5

θ	Lod Scores			
	Model 1	*Model 2*	*Model 3*	*Model 4*
0	0.000	−3.130	0.326	0.387
0.1	0.000	−1.307	0.275	0.325
0.2	0.000	−0.761	0.219	0.258
0.3	0.000	−0.428	0.156	0.182
0.4	0.000	−0.188	0.084	0.097

You now have to input the appropriate frequency for the haplotype containing allele *1* at locus 1 and allele *1* at locus 2. In this case, locus 1 is the disease locus, and at the disease locus allele *2* is the disease allele, with frequency 0.00001. From Table 24–5, you can see that this haplotype frequency 1 1 (under model 1) is $(0.25)(0.99999) = 0.2499975$. Enter the appropriate frequencies for each of the other haplotypes. It is imperative to realize that the order of loci (for haplotype frequency computation purposes) is not the order of loci in the parameter file but is rather the user-specified locus order. For example, if we specify locus order 2 1, we then treat the marker as locus 1 and the disease as locus 2, even though the disease was still the first locus in the parameter file. When you have entered the appropriate haplotype frequencies, set up the file to analyze the pedigrees in MLINK format, starting a recombination fraction of 0, in steps of 0.1, stopping at $\theta = 0.4$. Then save this file as EX6A1.DAT. Note that LCP cannot be used when you are using linkage disequilibrium in the analysis. You must therefore copy EX6A.PED to PEDFILE.DAT, and EX6A1.DAT to DATAFILE.DAT, and run the UNKNOWN and MLINK programs. Again, UNKNOWN versions from Columbia University dated after July 1993 must be used, especially when dealing with multipoint data, because homozygous *1 1* individuals have different disease locus genotype probabilities from unknown individuals, based on the linkage disequilibrium information. If you are considering multipoint analysis, and the other loci are informative, making all individuals in a pedigree *1 1* affects the results of the multipoint linkage analysis. Furthermore, in risk calculations the homozygosity at the marker locus *can and does* affect the genetic risk to the proband in the presence of linkage disequilibrium. All the lod scores for each of the four models should be identical to those shown in Table 24–6.

In this small example, you can see the potential effect of allowing for disequilibrium in your linkage analyses. An example in which this was applied with greatly increased power was the recent investigation of myelin basic protein and multiple sclerosis (Tienari et al., 1992). In this case the lod score rose from 1.64 to 3.42 when linkage disequilibrium was allowed for. Of course, these investigators first had to prove that linkage disequilibrium existed and then had to estimate the haplotype frequencies.

☐ Exercise 24

Consider the data from the HHRR analysis above and suppose we want to estimate haplotype frequencies on this data set. Assume the disease is a fully penetrant recessive disorder with gene frequency 0.01 for the disease allele. Design an experiment using this parametric information to test linkage equilibrium and to estimate the haplotype frequencies in this data set.

25 □

Parametric Analysis of Complex Diseases

In this chapter, we introduce the most basic approaches to linkage analysis of complex diseases. We briefly consider how to select a model to use in the analysis. Furthermore, we discuss methods of affecteds-only analysis and the benefits of this type of analysis. We also introduce the problem of inflation of the maximum lod score due to maximizing the lod score over different models for the disease.

25.1 Complex Diseases

Complex disease is a broad designation that basically covers any disease we cannot accurately define or explain. This designation covers a large range of possible problems or complexities. Complex disease generally refers to diseases with unknown mode of inheritance, especially polygenic models, or other modes of inheritance that cannot be simply fit to a reasonable single-locus model. A disease can also be considered complex when we don't really know who is affected, or at least who is a potential carrier of a specific genetic defect. This is commonly the case with psychiatric disorders, in which a single genetically relevant phenotype cannot really be distinguished from another with any great accuracy. It is often hoped that discovery of the genetic cause or causes of these diseases will allow for better definition of the disease phenotypes and allow researchers to determine better what affection really means. This is in a sense "reverse genetics" carried to an extreme. Genetic heterogeneity (both allelic and nonallelic), which will be discussed later, and the possibility of large rates of sporadic nongenetic causes of the same (or similar) disease phenotypes (among other things) also make a disease complex. All such factors have the basic effect of making fully parametrized likelihood analysis very difficult and error-prone. Numerous possible methods for dealing with these problems have been proposed, but none is completely satisfactory, and much work will likely be required to develop more efficient approaches to these problems. At least these approaches give us a starting point for gross-scale localization of genes that play some role in the etiology of these diseases.

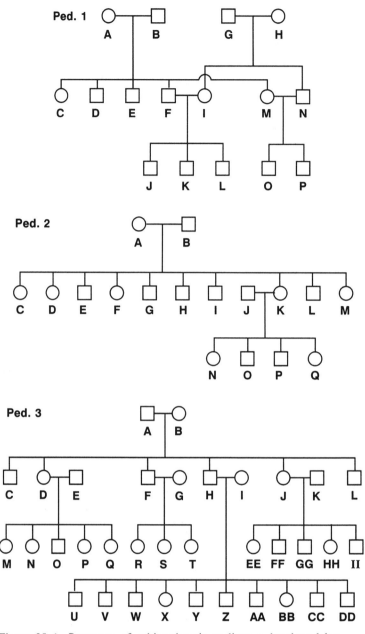

Figure 25–1. Structure of schizophrenia pedigrees developed by Sherrington and associates (1988)

In this chapter, we consider some simple approaches to the problem. The analyses are done on a well-known data set—the schizophrenia pedigrees of Sherrington and colleagues (1988)—with two markers on chromosome 5 as shown in Figure 25–1 and with disease and marker phenotypes indicated in Table 25–1. We use this example to explain various potential analysis techniques for linkage with complex diseases. We selected this data set to illustrate some techniques for the analysis of complex diseases and not to be critical of the analyses performed in the original study. We do not try to recreate the analyses performed by Sherrington and colleagues but rather start from scratch, and illustrate some potential methods for the analysis of such a data set. We feel it is useful to demonstrate these techniques with a real data set.

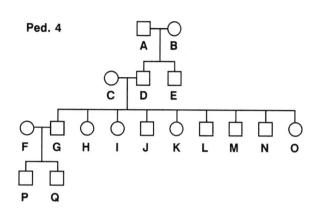

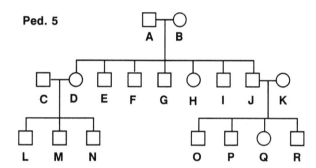

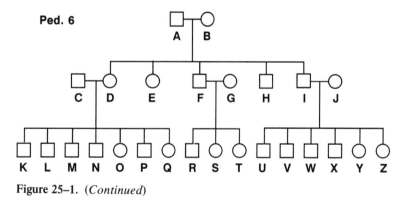

Figure 25–1. (*Continued*)

Moreover, in this example the disease is truly complex, because we have no real knowledge about the mode of inheritance or the correct diagnostic criteria. This data set, therefore, serves as a useful vehicle for illustrating the primitive approaches we consider in this chapter.

25.2 Entering Data for Multiple Diagnostic Schemes

Our first task is to devise a way to enter the data on these pedigrees in LINK-AGE format. The problem is that in this data set three possible diagnostic schemes are to be considered. To make the analysis as simple as possible, we

Table 25–1. Disease and Marker Phenotypes for People in Schizophrenia Pedigrees from Figure 25–1

		Diagnosis Under Scheme			Marker Phenotype	
Pedigree	Person	*1*	*2*	*3*	*M1*	*M2*
1	A	Aff	Aff	Aff	1 2	1 3
1	B	N/A	N/A	N/A	1 2	3 3
1	C	N/A	N/A	Aff	2 2	3 3
1	D	Aff	Aff	Aff	2 2	3 3
1	E	Aff	Aff	Aff	2 2	3 3
1	F	Aff	Aff	Aff	2 2	3 3
1	G	???	???	???	0 0	0 0
1	H	???	???	???	0 0	0 0
1	I	N/A	N/A	N/A	1 2	1 3
1	J	N/A	N/A	N/A	1 2	3 3
1	K	N/A	N/A	N/A	1 2	3 3
1	L	Aff	Aff	Aff	1 2	3 3
1	M	Aff	Aff	Aff	1 2	3 3
1	N	N/A	N/A	N/A	2 2	1 3
1	O	N/A	N/A	N/A	1 2	1 3
1	P	Aff	Aff	Aff	2 2	1 3
2	A	Aff	Aff	Aff	0 0	0 0
2	B	N/A	N/A	N/A	0 0	0 0
2	C	N/A	Aff	Aff	1 1	0 0
2	D	N/A	N/A	N/A	1 1	0 0
2	E	Aff	Aff	Aff	1 2	2 3
2	F	N/A	N/A	N/A	1 2	1 3
2	G	N/A	N/A	N/A	1 2	2 3
2	H	Aff	Aff	Aff	1 1	1 3
2	I	Aff	Aff	Aff	1 1	1 3
2	J	N/A	N/A	N/A	0 0	0 0
2	K	N/A	Aff	Aff	1 1	2 3
2	L	Aff	Aff	Aff	1 1	1 3
2	M	N/A	N/A	N/A	1 2	1 3
2	N	N/A	N/A	N/A	0 0	0 0
2	O	N/A	Aff	Aff	0 0	0 0
2	P	N/A	Aff	Aff	0 0	0 0
2	Q	N/A	N/A	N/A	0 0	0 0
3	A	N/A	N/A	N/A	1 1	1 3
3	B	N/A	N/A	N/A	0 0	0 0
3	C	Aff	Aff	Aff	1 1	1 3
3	D	N/A	Aff	Aff	1 1	1 3
3	E	N/A	N/A	N/A	1 2	1 3
3	F	Aff	Aff	Aff	1 1	1 1
3	G	N/A	N/A	N/A	1 2	1 1
3	H	N/A	N/A	Aff	1 1	1 3
3	I	N/A	N/A	N/A	1 1	3 3
3	J	N/A	Aff	Aff	1 1	1 3
3	K	N/A	N/A	N/A	1 1	1 2
3	L	N/A	Aff	Aff	1 1	1 3
3	M	N/A	N/A	N/A	1 1	1 3
3	N	N/A	N/A	N/A	1 1	1 3
3	O	N/A	N/A	Aff	1 1	3 3
3	P	N/A	N/A	Aff	1 1	1 3
3	Q	Aff	Aff	Aff	1 1	3 3
3	R	N/A	N/A	N/A	1 1	1 1
3	S	N/A	N/A	N/A	1 1	1 1
3	T	N/A	N/A	Aff	1 2	1 1
3	U	Aff	Aff	Aff	1 1	3 3
3	V	N/A	N/A	N/A	1 1	1 3
3	W	Aff	Aff	Aff	0 0	0 0
3	X	N/A	N/A	N/A	1 1	1 3
3	Y	Aff	Aff	Aff	0 0	0 0
3	Z	N/A	N/A	N/A	1 1	1 3
3	AA	Aff	Aff	Aff	1 1	3 3
3	BB	Aff	Aff	Aff	1 1	3 3
3	CC	N/A	Aff	Aff	1 1	3 3
3	DD	Aff	Aff	Aff	1 1	1 3
3	EE	N/A	N/A	N/A	1 1	2 3
3	FF	N/A	N/A	Aff	1 1	2 3
3	GG	N/A	N/A	N/A	1 1	1 3

Table 25–1. (*Continued*)

| Pedigree | Person | Diagnosis Under Scheme | | | Marker Phenotype | |
		1	*2*	*3*	*M1*	*M2*
3	HH	N/A	N/A	Aff	1 1	2 3
3	II	N/A	N/A	N/A	1 1	2 3
4	A	N/A	Aff	Aff	0 0	0 0
4	B	N/A	N/A	N/A	0 0	0 0
4	C	N/A	N/A	N/A	0 0	0 0
4	D	N/A	N/A	Aff	0 0	0 0
4	E	N/A	N/A	Aff	0 0	0 0
4	F	N/A	N/A	N/A	0 0	0 0
4	G	Aff	Aff	Aff	1 1	3 3
4	H	N/A	N/A	N/A	1 2	3 3
4	I	Aff	Aff	Aff	1 2	3 3
4	J	Aff	Aff	Aff	1 1	3 3
4	K	Aff	Aff	Aff	0 0	0 0
4	L	N/A	N/A	N/A	1 2	3 3
4	M	N/A	N/A	N/A	1 2	3 3
4	N	N/A	N/A	N/A	1 2	3 3
4	O	N/A	N/A	N/A	2 2	3 3
4	P	Aff	Aff	Aff	1 2	1 3
4	Q	Aff	Aff	Aff	1 2	1 3
5	A	N/A	N/A	N/A	0 0	0 0
5	B	N/A	N/A	N/A	0 0	0 0
5	C	N/A	N/A	N/A	1 2	2 3
5	D	Aff	Aff	Aff	0 0	0 0
5	E	N/A	N/A	N/A	1 2	2 2
5	F	N/A	N/A	N/A	1 2	2 2
5	G	N/A	N/A	N/A	0 0	0 0
5	H	Aff	Aff	Aff	1 1	2 3
5	I	N/A	N/A	N/A	0 0	0 0
5	J	N/A	N/A	N/A	0 0	0 0
5	K	N/A	N/A	N/A	1 1	2 3
5	L	N/A	N/A	N/A	1 1	2 3
5	M	N/A	N/A	N/A	1 1	3 3
5	N	Aff	Aff	Aff	1 2	2 3
5	O	Aff	Aff	Aff	1 1	2 2
5	P	N/A	N/A	N/A	1 2	2 3
5	Q	N/A	N/A	N/A	1 2	2 3
5	R	Aff	Aff	Aff	1 1	2 3
6	A	N/A	N/A	N/A	0 0	0 0
6	B	N/A	N/A	N/A	0 0	0 0
6	C	N/A	N/A	N/A	0 0	0 0
6	D	Aff	Aff	Aff	1 1	1 3
6	E	Aff	Aff	Aff	1 1	1 3
6	F	N/A	N/A	N/A	1 1	1 3
6	G	N/A	N/A	N/A	0 0	0 0
6	H	N/A	N/A	N/A	1 1	1 1
6	I	N/A	N/A	N/A	1 1	1 3
6	J	N/A	N/A	N/A	1 2	3 3
6	K	N/A	N/A	N/A	1 2	1 2
6	L	Aff	Aff	Aff	1 2	2 3
6	M	Aff	Aff	Aff	1 2	2 3
6	N	Aff	Aff	Aff	1 2	3 3
6	O	N/A	N/A	N/A	1 2	1 3
6	P	Aff	Aff	Aff	1 2	1 3
6	Q	N/A	N/A	N/A	1 2	1 2
6	R	N/A	N/A	Aff	1 2	1 3
6	S	N/A	N/A	N/A	0 0	0 0
6	T	N/A	Aff	Aff	1 1	3 3
6	U	Aff	Aff	Aff	1 2	3 3
6	V	N/A	N/A	N/A	0 0	0 0
6	W	N/A	N/A	N/A	1 2	1 3
6	X	N/A	N/A	N/A	1 1	1 3
6	Y	N/A	N/A	N/A	1 2	1 3
6	Z	N/A	N/A	N/A	1 1	1 3

At the disease locus, ??? = Unknown; N/A = Not affected; Aff = Affected. Marker locus phenotypes are given in allele numbers format.

recommend entering the data so the different diagnostic schemes can be taken into account solely by making modifications to the parameter file without modifying the pedigree file. (It may be useful to review the affection status locus type before continuing to ensure you fully understand the definition of the 2 phenotype [see Chapter 10]).

You must define the trait as an affection status locus so that the same trait definition for each individual can be used under each model. This can be difficult, for example, when you wish to consider an individual to be affected under one diagnostic criteria and unaffected under another. To this end, we propose the following approach. In the present case, we have three diagnostic schemes (and any number of penetrance models), so we can set up an affection status locus with multiple liability classes. For example, consider the eight possible cross-scheme phenotype vectors for each individual shown in Table 25–2.

Under this classification scheme, if an individual is considered affected under diagnostic scheme 1, yet unaffected under schemes 2 and 3, he would be coded *2 1,* or presence of the phenotype defined in liability class 1. Then, you define the penetrances accordingly for each model, as you will see below. In general, it is not necessary to have liability classes corresponding to phenotypes that do not exist in your data set. Because "affected" and "not affected" are complementary phenotypes (i.e., $P(\text{Aff}|\text{genotype}) = 1 - P(\text{N/A}|\text{genotype})$), you can immediately cut in half the number of liability classes required. Consider the rearrangement of Table 25–2 shown in Table 25–3.

As you can see in Table 25–3, we matched up pairs of complementary phenotype definitions in order to define both of them with one liability class. Consider liability class 1, the phenotype for which is defined by (Aff, N/A, N/A) [The ordered triplet refers to the diagnosis of an individual in this liability class under (diagnostic scheme 1, diagnostic scheme 2, diagnostic scheme 3)]. Therefore under each diagnostic class, phenotype 2 means the presence of the indicated phenotype (Aff or N/A) for each scheme. Similarly, phenotype 1 means the absence of the indicated phenotype (Aff or N/A) for *each* scheme. Thus, because Aff is the indicated phenotype for diagnostic scheme 1, N/A is the absence of the indicated phenotype in diagnostic scheme 1. This same rule must hold for *all* diagnostic schemes. In this case, the complementary phenotype to (Aff, N/A, N/A) is (N/A, Aff, Aff) as indicated in Table 25–3. Remember that the phenotype 2 **does *not* generally mean affected** but merely indicates that the phenotype is defined by the given penetrances, whereas 1 means the phenotype is defined by the complement of the given penetrances.

Table 25–2. List of All Possible Diagnostic Categories for a Disease with Three Diagnostic Schemes, and Its Liability Class Representation

Scheme 1	Scheme 2	Scheme 3	Affection	Liability Class
Aff	N/A	N/A	2	1
Aff	Aff	N/A	2	2
Aff	N/A	Aff	2	3
Aff	Aff	Aff	2	4
N/A	Aff	N/A	2	5
N/A	Aff	Aff	2	6
N/A	N/A	Aff	2	7
N/A	N/A	N/A	2	8

Aff = Affected; N/A = Not affected.

Table 25–3. All Possible Diagnostic Categories for Three Diagnostic Schemes Expressed in Terms of Four Liability Classes

			Original		New	
Scheme 1	Scheme 2	Scheme 3	*Affection*	*Liability Class*	*Affection*	*Liability Class*
Aff	N/A	N/A	2	1	2	1
N/A	Aff	Aff	2	6	1	1
Aff	Aff	N/A	2	2	2	2
N/A	N/A	Aff	2	7	1	2
Aff	N/A	Aff	2	3	2	3
N/A	Aff	N/A	2	5	1	3
Aff	Aff	Aff	2	4	2	4
N/A	N/A	N/A	2	8	1	4

Aff = Affected; N/A = Not affected.

Let us go back to Figure 25–1. Note that three diagnostic schemes are to be considered, with the phenotypes given in Table 25–1 in separate columns for each individual for each diagnostic scheme. In this case, the *only* four categories to be considered (because only four occur) are (Aff, Aff, Aff), (N/A, Aff, Aff), (N/A, N/A, Aff), and (N/A, N/A, N/A). We must now determine the number of liability classes needed to define these models. Because there are four categories present in the data, let us start out by allowing for the four classes shown in Table 25–4 (You may, of course, allow for eight liability classes, but it is more efficient to streamline the analysis and allow for the minimum required number).

At first glance, it is clear that diagnostic classes 1 and 4 are complementary, so we can eliminate class 4 and code those individuals as 1 1. You should only have three diagnostic classes remaining, 1 = (Aff, Aff, Aff), 2 = (Aff, Aff, N/A), and 3 = (Aff, N/A, N/A). Then (Aff, Aff, Aff) is the complement of (N/A, N/A, N/A), which would be coded as phenotype 1 1, as shown in Table 25–4.

Now, create the required pedigree file for these pedigrees, SCHIZO.PED. Remember that for each individual in Figure 25–1, the following information is given in Table 25–1: their diagnostic status under each diagnostic criterion, in order (first column = scheme 1 diagnosis; second column = scheme 2 diagnosis; third column = scheme 3 diagnosis; fourth column = marker 1 phenotype; fifth column = marker 2 phenotype). Again, we are not trying to emulate the original analysis, and the diagnostic assignments in Table 25–1 may not correspond exactly to what was used in the original study.

The next task—of defining the penetrances—is difficult because we have different meanings for our phenotypes under each diagnostic scheme. For the sake of illustration, let us consider a dominant disease with penetrance 0.6 and no phenocopies. The penetrances for such a trait are shown in Table 25–5.

As you can see, affected and unaffected are complementary phenotypes, and "unknown" is model-independent. Now, how do we combine penetrance models and diagnostic schemes to create an appropriate data file? In diagnostic scheme 1 in liability classes 1, 2, and 3, the 2 phenotype defines the *affected* phenotype. Thus, our penetrances for the three liability classes are shown in Table 25–6. Similarly, for diagnostic scheme 2 for a recessive disease

Table 25–4. All Observed Diagnostic Categories for the Schizophrenia Pedigrees of Sherrington et al., and Their Liability Class Representation

Scheme 1	Scheme 2	Scheme 3	Phenotype	Liability Class
Aff	Aff	Aff	2	1
N/A	Aff	Aff	2	2
N/A	N/A	Aff	2	3
N/A	N/A	N/A	2	4 (or 1 1)

Aff = Affected; N/A = Not affected.

Table 25–5. Penetrances for Different Phenotypes for a Dominant Disease with 60% Penetrance

Phenotype	Penetrances for Genotypes		
	D/D	$D/+$	$+/+$
Affected	0.6	0.6	0.0
Unaffected	0.4	0.4	1.0

Table 25–6. Liability Class Definitions for the Dominant Disease with 60% Penetrance in Diagnostic Scheme 1

Liability Class	D/D	$D/+$	$+/+$
1	0.6	0.6	0.0
2	0.4	0.4	1.0
3	0.4	0.4	1.0

Table 25–7. Liability Class Definitions for a Recessive Disease with 40% Penetrance for Genetic Cases and 1% Penetrance for Phenocopies in Diagnostic Scheme 2

Liability Class	D/D	$D/+$	$+/+$
1	0.4	0.01	0.01
2	0.4	0.01	0.01
3	0.6	0.99	0.99

Table 25–8. Liability Class Definitions for a Dominant Disease with 20% Penetrance for Genetic Cases and 5% Penetrance for Phenocopies in Diagnostic Scheme 3

Liability Class	D/D	$D/+$	$+/+$
1	0.2	0.2	0.05
2	0.2	0.2	0.05
3	0.2	0.2	0.05

with 40% penetrance for homozygous gene carriers and 1% penetrance for everyone else, the liability class penetrance definitions are shown in Table 25–7. Finally, for diagnostic scheme 3 for a dominant disease with 20% penetrance for gene carriers and a 5% penetrance for nongene carriers, the penetrances are shown in Table 25–8.

25.3 Choosing an Appropriate Single-locus Parametric Model

In general, the selection of model parameters is best left to the segregation analyst. We do not discuss this complicated topic in this book but refer you to other more appropriate sources on segregation analysis modeling (Elston et al., 1986; Elandt-Johnson, 1971). In selecting analysis models, we assume you know some simple population parameters from other sources, including segregation analyses and the like. As we've pointed out already, if there is linkage, and your model is reasonably correct, you should be able to detect it (notwithstanding somewhat reduced power). Also, there is no increase in Type I error rates when an analysis is done under an incorrect model (Clerget-Darpoux et al., 1986), with few exceptions (e.g. Terwilliger et al., 1991). With a complex disease, we generally try a dominant model and a recessive model, because usually we are unclear about the overall mode of inheritance and because multiple loci (some dominant, some recessive) are possibily working epistatically to cause some disease phenotype, and you are interested in detecting any of the loci involved. Therefore, we typically try at least one model of each variety. The selection of the penetrance values is the only remaining variable. The most important thing in choosing an appropriate penetrance model is knowing the ratio of penetrances for phenocopies to genetic cases ($k = f_p/f$ from Chapter 9). If the penetrance is assumed to be age-dependent, then the penetrance ratio is most likely variable with respect to age as well. (Typically, we assume that those affected individuals with a later age of onset have a greater ratio than those with low age of onset, who are more likely to be genetic cases.) For the moment, assume that the ratio k is constant (if it is not, use some lifetime penetrance ratio for the remainder of the computations in this chapter). If k is constant, then our population prevalence ϕ of the disease should satisfy the equation

$$\phi = f\,[P(\text{Susceptible genotype}) + kP(\text{Nonsusceptible genotype})]$$

(see Chapter 10). If we are considering a dominant disease, $\phi_d = f[p\,(2 - p) + k(1 - p)^2]$, and if the disease is recessive, $\phi_r = f[p^2 + k(1 - p^2)]$. The gene frequency p and the overall penetrance for susceptible genotypes f are the only parameters to be specified. For any given value of p, f can be uniquely determined, and vice versa. Quantities like f can often be obtained approximately from segregation analysis, whereas p is typically more easily estimable from population data. The value of k can be estimated either through segregation analysis or through some population-based analysis. If we estimate, for example, that ($R =$) 50% of all cases of a disease are nongenetic, then we can use this information as well, because it means that

$$\frac{kf[P(\text{Nonsusceptible genotype})]}{\phi} = R = 0.50$$

so

$$kfP(\text{Nonsusceptible genotype}) = \phi R \qquad \text{and}$$

$$\phi = fP(\text{Susceptible genotype}) + \phi R$$

Table 25–9. Penetrance Models Based on Prevalence, and Ratio of Prevalences for Genetic Cases and Nongenetic Cases

Diagnostic Scheme	R	ϕ	p	k	f_{DD}	f_{D+}	f_{++}
Dominant							
1	0.35	0.01	0.01	0.010909	0.33	0.33	0.0036
2	0.50	0.015	0.01	0.020263	0.38	0.38	0.0077
3	0.65	0.025	0.01	0.037727	0.44	0.44	0.0166
Recessive							
1	0.35	0.01	0.1	0.005385	0.65	0.0035	0.0035
2	0.50	0.015	0.1	0.010133	0.75	0.0076	0.0076
3	0.65	0.025	0.1	0.018636	0.88	0.0164	0.0164

or

$$\phi = \frac{fP(\text{Susceptible genotype})}{(1 - R)}$$

which can be another useful parametrization of the prevalence, in which $f_p = \phi R/P(\text{Nonsusceptible genotype})$. In most cases, it is easier to obtain an estimate of R, the proportion of all cases in the population due to nongenetic causes (e.g., Merette et al., 1992). Given this value and the overall prevalence of the disease, we can determine either the gene frequency p from a given value of f or the penetrance f from a given value of p using the equations above.

We assume certain values of p and then determine f from them. Clearly, when the diagnostic criteria are changed, the prevalence values ϕ and prevalence ratios R change as well. In our example, let us assume values of ϕ for each diagnostic level as follows: $\phi_1 = 0.01$, $\phi_2 = 0.015$, and $\phi_3 = 0.025$; with prevalence ratios of $R_1 = 0.35$, $R_2 = 0.5$, and $R_3 = 0.65$; and $p_{\text{dom}} = 0.01$; and $p_{\text{rec}} = 0.1$. For each diagnostic model, determine the appropriate penetrance values for the analysis from the above equations, assuming the disease to be alternatively dominant ($p = 0.01$) and recessive ($p = 0.1$). The analysis parameters should match those in Table 25–9. Then make parameter files SCHIZO#.DAT, in which # ranges from 1 to 6 for the six models to be considered from Table 25–9. For the first marker use gene frequencies of 0.33 for the *1* allele and 0.67 for the *2* allele; at the second locus use gene frequencies of 0.32 for the *1* allele, 0.16 for the *2* allele, and 0.52 for the *3* allele. Then perform the appropriate two-point linkage analyses with the disease versus each of the two markers separately. The analysis results should match those in Table 25–10. Remember, that one should *not* do multipoint analysis with a complex trait (see Chapter 18) because of the increased propensity for false-negative results when there are model misspecifications (as there always are with analyses of a complex trait).

25.4 Interpreting Lod Scores Maximized over Models

In this exercise, the maximum lod score maximized over the models was 2.65 between marker 1 and disease (under dominant model with diagnostic scheme 3) and 2.22 between marker 2 and disease (with the same model). It has been repeatedly demonstrated that although analysis of a pedigree set under one

Table 25–10. Results of Analysis of Schizophrenia Pedigrees under Six Selected Penetrance Models

Model	Diagnostic Scheme 1		Diagnostic Scheme 2		Diagnostic Scheme 3	
	θ	*Lod Score*	θ	*Lod Score*	θ	*Lod Score*
Dominant						
Marker 1	0.0	1.640431	0.0	2.266583	0.0	2.652390
	0.1	1.255017	0.1	1.831763	0.1	2.122298
	0.2	0.815333	0.2	1.216497	0.2	1.433496
	0.3	0.395659	0.3	0.609274	0.3	0.742590
	0.4	0.098284	0.4	0.159752	0.4	0.203170
ILINK:	0.001	1.638094	0.001	2.265304	0.001	2.650069
Marker 2	0.0	−0.590675	0.0	0.942746	0.0	1.815745
	0.1	0.633358	0.1	1.666246	0.1	2.197464
	0.2	0.760761	0.2	1.422284	0.2	1.752781
	0.3	0.506081	0.3	0.854349	0.3	1.008521
	0.4	0.161641	0.4	0.255371	0.4	0.294816
ILINK:	0.171	0.778730	0.104	1.666898	0.078	2.217621
Recessive						
Marker 1	0.0	0.155426	0.0	0.812548	0.0	1.658007
	0.1	0.940155	0.1	1.765145	0.1	2.124254
	0.2	0.751805	0.2	1.371401	0.2	1.652050
	0.3	0.393696	0.3	0.740799	0.3	0.923150
	0.4	0.101407	0.4	0.205094	0.4	0.267005
ILINK:	0.105	0.940433	0.090	1.770275	0.077	2.148463
Marker 2	0.0	−3.638244	0.0	−2.800846	0.0	−3.993544
	0.1	−1.409702	0.1	−0.843994	0.1	−1.311147
	0.2	−0.540226	0.2	−0.255292	0.2	−0.494319
	0.3	−0.171925	0.3	−0.067066	0.3	−0.164924
	0.4	−0.033334	0.4	−0.013796	0.4	−0.035273
ILINK:	0.5	0.000000	0.5	0.000000	0.5	0.000000

fixed wrong model does not lead to an increased false-positive rate (Clerget-Darpoux et al., 1986), maximizing the lod score over different models does lead to "inflation" of the maximum lod score (Weeks et al., 1990a). It has been suggested that to appropriately correct for this maximization we should no longer accept a lod score of 3 as a critical value for declaring a linkage result significant but rather use 3 + log(n), where n is the number of models tested (Kidd and Ott, 1984). Weeks and associates (1990a) did a complex simulation study on this same set of pedigrees and found that the inflation of the maximum lod score corresponded almost exactly to this theoretical approximation. In light of this, it seems prudent to adopt this criterion for the declaration of linkage in a complex disease. Thus, for our example, we need a lod score greater than 3 + log(6) = 3.78.

An additional problem remains, however. In a normal, well-characterized mendelian disease, the critical value of $Z_{max} > 3$ as a test for linkage is robust to multiple testing, because as we find negative test results with more markers, the prior probability of linkage to the remaining markers increases sufficiently to offset the increased probability of finding a significant result by chance. In other words, if we eliminate 50% of the genome, the prior probability of linkage is twice as high for the remaining markers than it would have been before any of the genome had been excluded. This is true because it is known with certainty that the gene is somewhere and that the model is correct, so the disease gene would be detected if you examined a truly linked marker. This increased prior probability of linkage offsets the effect of testing multiple markers. Of course if you test 20 markers and each has a probability of 0.001 of having a significant linkage result by chance, then the probability that at least 1 of the 20 markers has a significant result by chance is approximately 0.02. However, although the prior probability of linkage of one marker is low, the probability that 1 of 20 markers is truly linked is somewhat larger, to such a degree that the phenomena of increased prior probability of linkage and multiple testing tend to offset each other. In a complex disease, in contrast to the situation above, there is no guarantee either that a disease gene truly exists, nor that it would be detected in our analysis, because we are knowingly using incorrect models in the analysis. As a matter of fact, linkage analyses of complex traits are often carried out with the stated purpose of showing the existence of major genes by virtue of significant evidence for linkage (i.e., How could there be linkage if there isn't really a gene?). In light of this, it may be prudent to allow for some correction for multiple testing. Given the past history of linkages with psychiatric diseases with very "significant" lod scores that "disappeared" under further scrutiny, it may be prudent to insist on such a correction for multiple markers. On average, 100 independent markers should be enough to cover most of the genome. If we assume the genome is approximately 4–5000 cM long (Weissenbach et al., 1992) and presume that markers that are 40–50 cM apart are approximately independent, then 100 independent markers would cover most of the genome. Of course more markers may be used in an analysis, but additional markers are no longer independent of one another. If we apply the correction for 100 markers by the $3 + \log(m)$ criterion, where m now refers to the number of markers, we start out in a genome-wide search with a critical value of $3 + \log(100) = 5$. If we allow adequately for the multiple models as well, we have a conservative critical value of $5 + \log(n)$, where n is the number of models tested. This may seem like a very strict criterion to declare a linkage test significant, in these diseases where the power of the test is going to be reduced significantly to begin with, due to the complexity of the diseases involved, but given the history of psychiatric genetics and the multiple sources of random error involved, it is arguable that this is a reasonable correction factor to apply in general for complex diseases, since when one starts a linkage study, they are typically planning to go until they find the gene, meaning that basically they would test all 100 markers, barring a significant finding. For example, for the study by Sherrington and associates (1988), if we allow for the 18 models used in the analysis and use a baseline threshold of 5, the critical value for declaring a linkage significant is $5 + \log(18) = 6.25$. The actual maximum lod score in that study was 6.49, which is still marginally significant but much less so than when it was compared with a critical value of 3.

25.5 Combining Diagnostic Criteria in a Single Model

It may be possible to combine the three diagnostic criteria in a single analysis model to reduce the number of models used in the analysis (*Note:* Any analysis attempted *must be included in the total* number of models considered, even if its results are not reported in the publication!). Looking back to Section 10.4, we understand how the penetrances were modeled for a disease with uncertainty of diagnosis. We can combine these three diagnostic schemes by

Table 25–11. Penetrance Model for Multiple Diagnostic Schemes in One Analysis Based on Probability (from Prior Belief) That People in a Certain Diagnostic Class Are Truly Affected by the Same Genetic Disease

Liability Class	Dominant Model			Recessive Model		
	DD	*D*+	++	*DD*	*D*+	++
1	0.38	0.38	0.0077	0.75	0.0076	0.0076
2	0.416	0.416	0.1554	0.675	0.1553	0.1553
3	0.476	0.476	0.4015	0.55	0.4015	0.4015

saying that people in diagnostic class 1 are definitely affected, those in diagnostic class 2 have a particular certainty p_2 of being affected (this should be based on some prior belief about the true nature of these spectrum phenotypes), and those in diagnostic class 3 have another probability p_3 of having their disease caused by the same genetic defect (cf. Ott, 1993b). In this way, we construct a penetrance model for the disease, giving greater weight to those in the first diagnostic level and lower weight to the diagnoses for the remaining individuals. Let us assume that $p_2 = 0.85$, and $p_3 = 0.70$ and consider the dominant and recessive penetrance models obtained in Table 25–9 under diagnostic scheme 2. In this case, for each genotype in each of our three liability classes, we have penetrances

$$f = p_i P(\text{Aff}|\text{genotype}) + (1 - p_i)P(\text{N/A}|\text{genotype})$$

for each genotype. Our final liability class models are indicated in Table 25–11. Note that the basic effect is to increase the penetrance ratios f_p/f toward 1 as more diagnostic uncertainty is introduced.

Clearly if there were a 50% chance that an individual were affected, the penetrance ratio would be 1. Can you show this mathematically? The results of this analysis are presented in Table 25–12. In this analysis, our maximum lod score with marker 1 was only 2.16, and with marker 2 it was 1.83. This may seem to be a loss of information, but consider this value relative to the critical limit for declaring a linkage significant under each situation. In the first

Table 25–12. Analysis Results of Penetrance Models in Table 25–11

Marker	Dominant Model		Recessive Model	
	θ	Lod Score	θ	Lod Score
1	0.0	2.162044	0.0	1.095595
	0.1	1.747951	0.1	1.807159
	0.2	1.164273	0.2	1.365761
	0.3	0.583685	0.3	0.730016
	0.4	0.152360	0.4	0.200834
ILINK:	0.001	2.160694	0.080	1.828390
2	0.0	0.743953	0.0	−3.568465
	0.1	1.428744	0.1	−1.103271
	0.2	1.221847	0.2	−0.428977
	0.3	0.726209	0.3	−0.153162
	0.4	0.218206	0.4	−0.033850
ILINK:	0.108	1.430856	0.5	0.000000

case, we had maximum lod scores of 2.65 and 2.22, respectively. If we assume the critical value to be 5 + log(n), the critical limit would have been 5 + log(6) = 5.78, whereas in the example with multiple diagnostic criteria combined in one analysis model, the critical limit would have been only 5 + log(2) = 5.30. Thus, with marker 1, we gained 0.49 units of lod score by trying three diagnostic models. However, the critical value when all three models were used was 0.48 units higher. Therefore, you can see that when the diagnoses are combined into one model, in this specific weighting of the different diagnostic models, there is no overall loss in significance, and yet the actual analysis is simplified substantially.

25.6 Affecteds-only Analysis

It has been thought that many of these so-called complex diseases are actually produced by a combination of different genes working together to produce a phenotype. If this is the case, then many unaffected individuals may possess the disease-predisposing genotype at one of the loci but lack the required second disease locus genotype necessary for development of the disease. For this reason, it is often advisable to consider all unaffected individuals to actually have "unknown" phenotype when doing linkage analyses. In this way, one bases the linkage analysis solely on the marker status of the affected individuals in the pedigree and doesn't apply any disease locus genotypic information to the unaffected individuals.

There are two ways to perform such a linkage analysis. The first way is to alter your pedigree file so all unaffected individuals are given the unknown phenotype. In the parameter files, then, for phenotypes that would have corresponded to unaffected (i.e., in diagnostic scheme 2, people with phenotype 2 3 would be unaffected), we replace the penetrances with those for unknown individuals (0.5 for all three genotypes, for example). To do this, an astronomical amount of file manipulation is necessary. All 1 1 individuals in the pedigree file must be changed to 0 1, and the penetrances for liability classes 2 and 3 must be changed, such that when these individuals are unaffected, the penetrances in the parameter files are equal for all three genotypes. There is a simpler way to do it, however. Simply reduce the maximum penetrance values for affection to 0.001 and keep the penetrance ratios the same as they were in the original files, as shown in Table 25–13 for the penetrance values shown in Table 25–9. In this way, for affected individuals the likelihoods remain the same, down to a constant multiplier, which disappears in the likelihood ratio (see Section 9.2) for each individual affected. However, for unaffected individuals, the penetrances are essentially equal for all three genotypes, with a

Table 25–13. Penetrances for Affected Individuals Only (for Affected f and Unaffected $1-f$) for the Models Outlined in Table 25–9, with Penetrance Ratios for Affected and Unaffected Individuals Indicated

Diagnostic Class	k	f_{DD}	f_{D+}	f_{++}	$(1-f_{DD})$	$(1-f_{D+})$	$(1-f_{++})$	$\frac{(1-f_p)}{(1-f)}$
Dominant	1 0.010909	0.001	0.001	(.001)k	0.999	0.999	0.99999	1.001
	2 0.020263	0.001	0.001	(.001)k	0.999	0.999	0.99998	1.001
	3 0.037727	0.001	0.001	(.001)k	0.999	0.999	0.99996	1.001
Recessive	1 0.005385	0.001	(.001)k	(.001)k	0.999	0.999995	0.999995	1.001
	2 0.010133	0.001	(.001)k	(.001)k	0.999	0.99999	0.99999	1.001
	3 0.018636	0.001	(.001)k	(.001)k	0.999	0.99998	0.99998	1.001

Table 25–14. Comparison of Results of the Two Methods of Analyzing Only Affected Individuals Using Diagnostic Scheme 3

Model	True Affected Individuals Only		Table 25–15 Penetrances	
	θ	*Lod Score*	θ	*Lod Score*
Dominant				
Marker 1	0.0	2.222397	0.0	2.223299
	0.1	1.683718	0.1	1.684594
	0.2	1.092772	0.2	1.093428
	0.3	0.544293	0.3	0.545285
	0.4	0.144506	0.4	0.144608
ILINK:	0.001	2.219163	0.001	2.220066
Marker 2	0.0	1.389189	0.0	1.389983
	0.1	1.355322	0.1	1.356693
	0.2	1.008209	0.2	1.009340
	0.3	0.549278	0.3	0.549901
	0.4	0.156570	0.4	0.156734
ILINK:	0.039	1.431084	0.039	1.432282
Recessive				
Marker 1	0.0	1.066889	0.0	1.068376
	0.1	1.019994	0.1	1.021295
	0.2	0.697922	0.2	0.698752
	0.3	0.351886	0.3	0.352275
	0.4	0.094701	0.4	0.094798
ILINK:	0.036	1.115353	0.036	1.116852
Marker 2	0.0	0.234950	0.0	0.233835
	0.1	0.280799	0.1	0.280290
	0.2	0.203024	0.2	0.202794
	0.3	0.104595	0.3	0.104506
	0.4	0.028112	0.4	0.028090
ILINK:	0.064	0.290322	0.064	0.289653

penetrance ratio in each case of 1.001. Remember that the penetrance ratio for unknown individuals is 1.000. This parametrization therefore is essentially equivalent to making all unaffected individuals unknown in the pedigree file, as described above. To see this, please apply both of these methods to the analysis of the schizophrenia pedigrees under diagnostic scheme 3, with both the dominant and recessive models. The results of these analyses are shown in Table 25–14. There are some differences in the lod scores between these two methods, but the change is only in the second or third decimal place, and as such has no important effect on the interpretation of the results. There are, of course, two possible sources of error here. The first is that our penetrance ratio in unaffected individuals is 1.001, not 1.000. Similarly, we have rounded off our penetrances to five significant digits for the nonsusceptible genotypes, altering this penetrance ratio to some degree as well. One potential method for making the two penetrance ratios even more accurate is to divide the penetrances by 1000, so that for the dominant model in diagnostic scheme 3, our penetrances are 0.00044, 0.00044, and 0.0000166. In this case we preserve the penetrance ratio among affected individuals exactly and reduce the penetrance ratio for unaffected persons to only 0.9999834/0.99956 = 1.0004. Dividing the penetrances by 1000 provides more than sufficient accuracy in any realistic situation.

□ **Exercise 25**

Consider these pedigrees again, using different starting information. Repeat the linkage analyses in this chapter, assuming prevalences $\phi_1 = 0.005$, $\phi_2 = 0.01$, $\phi_3 = 0.03$; prevalence ratios of $R_1 = 0.10$, $R_2 = 0.35$;, $R_3 = 0.50$; and gene frequencies of $p_{dom} = 0.01$ and $p_{rec} = 0.125$. Please determine the appropriate penetrance models for an affecteds-only analysis with each model (divide the true penetrances by 1000), and perform the linkage analysis with it.

Consider weighting the diagnostic criteria accordingly so that those in class 1 are considered to be affected with 99% certainty, those in diagnostic class 2 are affected with 80% certainty, and those in diagnostic class 3 are affected with 65% certainty. Then perform a regular linkage analysis, using as baseline penetrances those derived from the population characteristics of intermediate diagnostic model 2 above, under both recessive and dominant models. Do whatever analyses are needed to compare these results with the results obtained when the lod score is maximized over models.

26 □

Nonparametric Methods of Linkage Analysis

In this chapter we introduce nonparametric approaches to linkage analysis, so-called affected sib-pair, and affected pedigree member (APM) methods. These methods are based on the concepts of identity by descent and identity by state. The basic methods of sib-pair and affected pedigree member analysis are introduced, followed by the extended sib-pair analysis (ESPA) computer program. Power considerations are also discussed in terms of study design.

26.1 Identity by Descent versus Identity by State

Any two copies of allele *1* at a given locus are considered to be *identical by state* (IBS), but only copies of allele *1* that are inherited from a common ancestral source are said to be *identical by descent* (IBD). Of course, if two alleles are IBD, they are definitely also IBS, but the converse is not necessarily true. Consider pedigree I in Figure 26–1, with father *1/2,* and mother *1/3.* If they had children with marker genotypes *1/2* and *1/1,* then clearly there is one allele identical by descent, because the latter child had to receive a *1* allele from each parent, one of which is IBD with the *1* allele the first child received. However, if the children were *1/2* and *1/3,* then no alleles are IBD, because the first child received the *1* allele from his mother, and the second child received the *3* allele from his mother. Similarly, the first child must have received the *2* allele from his father, and the second child received the *1* allele from his father. Thus, although the two children share a *1* allele IBS, the *1* alleles in question came from different ancestral sources and thus are not IBD. In pedigree II in Figure 26–1, mother is *1/2,* and father is *1/1* with sons *1/1,* and *1/1.* The sons share two alleles IBS. Also, they must both have received the same *1* allele from their mother and therefore share one allele IBD. However, there is no information about the IBD status of the paternally derived alleles, because there is no way to differentiate one of the *1* alleles from the other. There is, therefore, a 50% chance that the *1* alleles are IBD and a 50% chance that they are not. We can either delete the paternal information (scoring the sib-pair as one IBD out of one opportunity) or give it a 50–50 weighting, labeling the sib-pair as having 1.5 IBD alleles out of 2 opportunities.

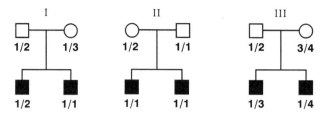

Figure 26–1. Example pedigrees for sib-pair analysis

Clearly there are advantages to each approach. The first allows us to give the most accurate interpretation of what we know, but the second allows us to use our full sample size. Even further complications can arise in situations where you have two parents, each with genotype *1/2*. If the children are homozygous, then IBD counts can easily be determined accurately. However, if the children are *both* heterozygous, then we cannot tell whether there are two alleles IBD or none. As long as at least one sib in each pair is homozygous there is no ambiguity, but when they are heterozygous there is ambiguity, and effectively no information is available about the sib-pair's IBD status.

26.2 Affected Sib-pair Analysis

Affected sib-pair analysis supposes that if a given marker is cosegregating with a disease-predisposing allele, then affected siblings of affected persons are more likely to receive the same allele identical by descent at a closely linked marker locus than if the marker locus was segregating independently (i.e., is unlinked) of the disease-predisposing allele. This method may seem very similar to the parametric idea of counting recombinants and nonrecombinants; the main difference is that this type of analysis requires no assumptions about the mode of inheritance. In this sense, sib-pair type methods are more robust than parametric methods because we do not have to rely on as many potentially erroneous model assumptions in the analysis. Moreover, the problem of trying multiple models and correcting for inflation of the lod score (as is often required in such cases), is avoided in sib-pair approaches, although we must still correct for multiple diagnostic schemes. The fundamental idea is that any two siblings are expected to have one allele identical by descent (IBD). However, when the sibs are both affected with a given disease and the analysis is done with a marker tightly linked to the disease-predisposing gene, then we expect the siblings to share more than one allele IBD. Let us consider the third example shown in Figure 26–1.

In this family, the two parents have marker genotypes *1/2* and *3/4*. They have two sons affected with a given disease, the first son having marker genotype *1/3* and the second having genotype *1/4*. It is clear that both sons got the *1* allele from their father, but one son got the *3* and the other got the *4* from their mother. Hence, these two children share one allele IBD. All possible combinations of sibling marker genotypes are shown in Table 26–1.

If there is no association between the disease and the marker locus, then each of these genotype combinations is equally likely. There are four combinations with two alleles shared IBD, eight combinations with one allele shared IBD, and four combinations with no alleles shared IBD. If we compute the expected (average) number of alleles shared IBD, the result is $(4 \cdot 2 + 8 \cdot 1)/16 = 1$. However, if there is complete linkage at $\theta = 0$ and the disease is dominant, then assuming, without loss of generality, that the disease came from the father, and is on the same haplotype with the *1* allele, the only pos-

Table 26–1. Possible Arrangements of Marker Genotypes of Two Affected Sons with Parents 1/2 and 3/4

SON1	SON2	IBD	SON1	SON2	IBD	SON1	SON2	IBD	SON1	SON2	IBD
1/3	*1/3*	2	*1/4*	*1/4*	2	*2/3*	*2/3*	2	*2/4*	*2/4*	2
1/3	*1/4*	1	*1/4*	*1/3*	1	*2/3*	*2/4*	1	*2/4*	*2/3*	1
1/3	*2/3*	1	*1/4*	*2/4*	1	*2/3*	*1/3*	1	*2/4*	*1/4*	1
1/3	*2/4*	0	*1/4*	*2/3*	0	*2/3*	*1/4*	0	*2/4*	*1/3*	0

sibilities are cases in which both sons carry a *1* allele. So, we have (*1/3, 1/3*), (*1/3, 1/4*), (*1/4, 1/3*), and (*1/4, 1/4*) as possible genotypes for the two sons. Each of these is equally likely, and our expected number of alleles IBD is $(2 \cdot 2 + 1 \cdot 2)/4 = 1.5$. Clearly, this is greater than 1 and can be detected in a sib-pair analysis with a large enough sample size. Similarly, if the disease is recessive, with the maternal disease allele on the same haplotype with the *3* allele and the paternal disease allele in coupling with the *1* allele, and $\theta = 0$, we have only the combination (*1/3, 1/3*) possible. Thus, we expect to find two alleles IBD. This is a complete association, which could be picked up in the analysis. Clearly most real situations are somewhere between these two extremes, and often we do not even know what the true disease model is. It can be demonstrated that when the model is known correctly, parametric analysis is more powerful than sib-pair methods, but when the disease model is not known and we are studying some complex disease, sib-pair methods can perform as well as or better than linkage analysis with an incorrect model. However, the power of a sib-pair test is always greatest when the disease is recessive. Simple sib-pair analysis can be done by hand, but more complicated variations of the technique need to be analyzed with such programs as ESPA (Sandkuyl, 1989) and SAGE (Elston et al., 1986), for example. Practical examples of how to perform affected sib-pair analysis with the ESPA program are presented in Section 26.5

26.3 Affected Pedigree Member Method

In the affected sib-pair method, we base our statistical analysis on how many alleles a given sib-pair shares IBD. Because each sib-pair shares either 0, 1, or 2 (a fact that can often be determined with little difficulty), the statistical analysis is quite simple. This is true because regardless of the gene frequencies or the mode of inheritance of the disease, when linkage is absent, you expect every sib-pair to share, on average, one allele IBD. In extended pedigrees, however, the situation is much more complicated, and it has been proposed that IBS rather than IBD relationships be examined for more distantly related individuals (Weeks and Lange, 1988). Again, these sibs tend to share alleles IBS at loci linked to disease-predisposing loci, because of an increased probability that they inherit the marker locus IBD with the disease locus or because the marker locus itself is contributing to the disease phenotype in some manner. Because some individuals are more distantly related, it is not typically possible to determine whether alleles are inherited IBD or not, so we must resort to comparing IBS status. This can be much more complicated, however, in a statistical sense.

Weeks and Lange (1988) proposed the similarity statistic (Z_{ij}) for two affected relatives. This statistic allows you to order the alleles for any individual without loss of generality in either direction. We do this for both affected relatives, such that the genotype of the first affected relative is (A_1, A_2), and the genotype of the second affected relative is (B_1, B_2). The pairs of alleles from the two relatives produce four options: (A_1,B_1), (A_1,B_2), (A_2,B_1), and (A_2,B_2). We then define a function $\delta(x,y)$ such that if x and y represent the same allele IBS, then $\delta(x,y) = 1$, otherwise $\delta(x,y) = 0$. For example, if the first affected relative has ordered genotype *(2,3)* and the second relative had ordered genotype *(1,3)*, then $\delta(A_1,B_1) = \delta(2,1) = 0$; $\delta(A_1,B_2) = \delta(2,3) = 0$; $\delta(A_2,B_1) = \delta(3,1) = 0$; and $\delta(A_2,B_2) = \delta(3,3) = 1$. The similarity statistic Z_{ij} is then defined as the average of these four possible δ functions for the two affected relatives in question

$$Z_{ij} = \frac{1}{4} \sum_{a=1}^{2} \sum_{b=1}^{2} \delta(A_a,B_b)$$

For our sample affected relative pair, the similarity statistic is $\frac{1}{4}(0 + 0 + 0 + 1) = \frac{1}{4}$. We then sum the similarity statistics for all possible affected relative pairs in an extended pedigree to compute an overall similarity statistic

$$Z = \sum_{i=1}^{s-1} \sum_{j=(i+1)}^{s} Z_{ij}$$

This statistic is simple and easy to compute for any given pedigree; however, it lacks one desirable property. Clearly, it is much more striking for two relatives (especially distant relatives) to share a very rare allele IBS than it is for them to share a very common allele IBS. Some allowance should be made for this, and it was proposed that a weighted average be used to make this contrast possible within the APM method. Weeks and Lange (1988) proposed altering the statistic by adding in a weight term as follows:

$$Z_{ij} = \frac{1}{4} \sum_{a=1}^{2} \sum_{b=1}^{2} \delta(A_a,B_b)\,f(A_a)$$

where $f(A_a)$ is the weight and is based on the gene frequency of allele a in person A. Three main weights have been proposed by Weeks and Lange:

$$f_1(A_a) = 1 \text{ (equal weights)}; \qquad f_2(A_a) = \frac{1}{p_{A_a}}; \qquad f_3(A_a) = \frac{1}{\sqrt{p_{A_a}}}$$

The latter two weights give more strength to any observed sharing of rare alleles than sharing of common alleles and alleviate the intuitive problem of the sharing of common alleles being equally significant with the sharing of rare ones. In our sample statistic, assuming gene frequency of 0.3 for allele *3* (the only one shared IBS by our two affected relatives), our weighted similarity statistics are

$$Z_1 = \frac{1}{4}(0 + 0 + 0 + 1) = 0.25$$

$$Z_2 = \frac{1}{4}(0 + 0 + 0 + 1(1/0.3)) = 0.833$$

$$Z_3 = \frac{1}{4}(0 + 0 + 0 + 1/\sqrt{0.3}) = 0.456$$

As shown above, the similarity statistics are simple and easy to compute. However, it is more difficult to determine the expected value under the null hypothesis for each of these similarity statistics. It is necessary to go through a complicated series of calculations, based on the theory of extended pedigree IBD relationships, to determine the null hypothesis mean and variance for each weighted similarity statistic. Then, these similarity statistics must be converted into standard normal random variables, so they can be easily combined across pedigrees and the results can be interpreted in a straightforward manner. The details of these transformations and calculations are beyond the scope of this book, and you are referred to Weeks and Lange (1988) for a more complete description of the mathematics of this nonparametric method of linkage analysis. The reliability and robustness of this method is unclear, because it is much more dependent on good gene frequency estimates than standard linkage analysis is. This was shown to be of major concern in Chapter 22. Given the strong dependency of this method on gene frequency and the complexities involved in using the program, we do not detail its usage. We felt the method should be introduced, however, because it is a popular approach to nonparametric analysis in pedigrees with structures that are not conducive to affected sib-pair analysis (i.e., not many affected sib pairs).

26.4 When to Use Nonparametric Methods

Nonparametric methods can be very powerful tools in linkage analysis, especially when you are trying to localize a disease gene to a given region and have little reliable information about the mode of inheritance. Moreover, they are very rapid, and affected sib-pair methods are both simple to apply and interpret. Although they have lower power than parametric analyses when the model is well characterized, nonparametric methods are not as susceptible to possible modeling errors. In general, if a complex disorder is being analyzed, it is advisable to use sib-pair or other nonparametric methods, either in lieu of or in addition to parametric analyses, to be more confident that an observed result is not spurious.

26.5 How to Do Sib-pair Analysis

In many cases, it is possible to do sib-pair analysis without complicated computer programs. You merely count the number of IBD alleles in all affected sibling pairs in your sample. Interestingly, Suarez and Van Eerdewegh (1984) showed that all possible pairs of affected sibs in a large sibship can be treated separately, with no effect on the mean or variance of the statistic under the null hypothesis. Moreover, according to Blackwelder and Elston (1985), forming all possible pairs from any given sibship is in most cases the most powerful approach, although they recommend that an appropriate weighting of the contribution of such large sibships might be obtained by dividing it by $s(s - 1)/2$. The relative power of such weighted versus unweighted measures, however, depends on the particular model for the disease in question. A good overview of the various test statistics for affected sib-pair analyses is given in Blackwelder and Elston (1985). The ESPA program employs the mean test, which is a chi-square test comparing the number of observed alleles IBD with the number expected under the null hypothesis of no linkage. In this test, the number of shared alleles is compared with the number expected to be shared under the null hypothesis (50% shared, 50% unshared). The statistic, therefore is a standard chi-square test

$$\chi^2 = 2 \frac{[S - E(S)]^2}{E(S)} = 4 \frac{[S - (S + NS)/2]^2}{S + NS}$$

where S = number of observed alleles shared IBD, and NS = number of observed alleles not shared IBD.

26.6 Extended Sib-pair Analysis and the ESPA Program

It is often the case that one or more affected sibs are untyped at a given locus or their parents are untyped. The extended sib-pair analysis (ESPA) program of Sandkuyl (1989) uses the MLINK program of the LINKAGE package to compute the probability of each possible marker genotype for untyped individuals, thus computing the IBD count for each sib-pair based on these probabilities. In this way, the user is able to use pedigrees that would've been uninformative in a straight sib-pair analysis, in which IBD cannot be uniquely established based on the available marker typings in the family.

Basically, the program uses MLINK in a single-locus analysis to compute genetic risks for each possible genotype of each untyped parent or sib in a family. The analysis is based on the gene frequencies of each allele and the information available from other typed members of the pedigree, without considering the disease locus at all (a requirement for the analysis of disease to be nonparametric). Purists might contend that this analysis is no longer truly nonparametric because the mode of transmission and gene frequencies at the marker locus must be defined uniquely, but the important thing is that the disease locus is never even considered in the parametric phase of this analysis to allow the test of linkage to retain its essential nonparametric quality vis-a-vis the disease locus. Furthermore, the parametrization is only used in ambiguous cases to assign values to the expected number of alleles IBD in any given sib-pair, and it involves no parametrization of the degree of association (i.e., θ), therefore, still providing a nonparametric test of linkage.

The ESPA program computes an expected IBD count for each such ambiguous situation by computing the probability of each possible family configuration and the corresponding IBD counts and forming a weighted average of the IBD counts as follows:

$$\sum_{i=0}^{2} i P(i \text{ alleles IBD}) = P(1 \text{ allele IBD}) + 2P(2 \text{ alleles IBD})$$

with the $P(i$ alleles IBD) being the sum of the probabilities of all family configurations in which i alleles are IBD for the sib-pair in question. The ESPA program incorporates an efficient algorithm for doing these computations in the dBASE programming language. At the present time, ESPA works only for families with no consanguinity loops and autosomal linkage and is currently restricted to loci with five or fewer alleles. For loci with more than five alleles, ESPA can still be used to do a traditional sib-pair analysis, making any sib-pairs uninformative when IBD status cannot be uniquely determined.

26.7 Using the ESPA Program

The ESPA program (version 2.2) uses a straight LINKAGE format pedigree file, in which the first locus must correspond to the disease status, and the second locus must be the marker to be analyzed in allele numbers format. No parameter file is required, because the number of alleles and their gene frequencies must be entered interactively. For the schizophrenia pedigrees from the previous chapter, you created one pedigree file in which the different diagnostic categories were allowed for by altering the liability class of an individual: *2 1* individuals were affected under all three models, *2 2* individuals were affected under models 2 and 3, and *2 3* individuals were only affected under model 3. The unaffected individuals were coded as *1 1*, meaning they were unaffected under all three models of diagnosis. The parameter files were then written such that for diagnostic class 2, for example, *2 1* and *2 2* individuals were given the penetrance values for affected individuals, and *2 3* individuals were defined to be unaffected via the penetrance model indicated in the previous chapter. Unfortunately, the ESPA program ignores all liability class information and considers code *2* to mean affected, and *1* to mean unaffected. This occurs because ESPA is nonparametric with respect to the disease (therefore penetrance values are meaningless anyway). So, if you use the pedigree file as it currently exists in the ESPA program, you are doing the analysis with *2 1, 2 2,* and *2 3* individuals all considered to be affected, which corresponds to diagnostic model 3. Copy the SCHIZO.PED file to DIAG3.PED. Then, modify the file so all the *2 3* individuals are changed to *1 3*. Save this file as DIAG2.PED (since now only individuals in liability classes 1 and 2 are considered to be affected). Finally, change all the *2 2* individuals to *1 2*, so the only affected people remaining in the pedigree are coded *2 1*. Save this final file as DIAG1.PED, corresponding to the first diagnostic criterion. Now, you can run the ESPA program to do the sib-pair analysis under each of the three diagnostic models. There are two markers for which marker locus phenotypes are provided in this pedigree. Unfortunately, the ESPA program only considers the disease (locus 1 in every case) and the first allele numbers marker in the file. To analyze each of the two loci, use the LSP program to extract the disease and locus 2 in one pedigree file, then do the same for the disease and locus 3, as in Chapter 4. Create these six files with LSP (DIAG#M1.PED, and DIAG#M2.PED, etc., for example, where # is replaced by the diagnostic scheme number), by copying the PEDFILE.DAT file to the appropriate file name. This means that the PEDFILE.DAT file in which you extracted loci 1 (the disease) and 2 (marker 1) from DIAG1.PED should be renamed DIAG1M1.PED.

We take you through the analysis for the first example (with file DIAG1M1.PED) step by step. First call up the ESPA program by typing RUN at the DOS prompt (assuming, of course, that you are working in the directory containing the ESPA program or that ESPA is in the path on your machine). Then, the program asks you

```
Name of pedigree file:
```

to which you respond DIAG1M1.PED. Then, it prompts you with

```
More than one liability class (Y/N):  N
```

Here, you must change the N to a Y, because in your pedigree file there is a separate column for the liability classes. Even though this program doesn't use the liability class information, it has to know if there is going to be an extra column in the pedigree file containing this information, so it doesn't treat the liability class as if it were the first allele at the marker locus. Next, the program asks:

```
Completely known sibships only (Y/N):  Y
```

This option refers to whether the program should try and infer identity by descent in situations in which it is unclear due to untyped parents or even one of the affected sibs being untyped. As was mentioned earlier, if you say No to this option, you are restricted to a maximum of five alleles at the marker locus. If you answer Yes and do not ask the program to use partially informative sib-pairs, the number of alleles is no longer limited to five. Respond N to this question to take full advantage of this program's capabilities. Note that the output is broken down so the information from completely known sibships is available separately as well as combined with the total information from the entire pedigree set. If you answer Y, the program begins calculations at this

Table 26–2. Results of ESPA Analysis of DIAG1M1.PED

	Not Shared	Shared	χ	p	Total χ	Total p
Completely known:	3.00	9.00	3.00	0.0416		
Missing parent(s):	5.00	8.71	1.01	0.1580		
Missing sib(s):	0.00	0.88	0.88	0.1850	4.22	0.0200

point. Because we answered No, we are required to respond to the following questions defining the marker locus:

```
How many marker alleles? (maximum 5):  2
```

which we leave as it is because there are two alleles at the first marker locus in our pedigree file. Then we enter the gene frequencies

```
Frequency of allele 1        .0000
Frequency of allele 2        .0000
```

Using the cursor keys to move back and forth between lines, change these numbers to 0.33 and 0.67, respectively, for the two alleles. Then, hit the ⟨Enter⟩ key, and the program begins the analysis. The screen contains the following information when the analysis is complete:

```
Information content in 44 nuclear families
Completely known:              12 sib-pairs.   (27.3%)
One or both parents missing:   19 sib-pairs.   (43.2%)
One or both sibs missing:       1 sib-pairs.   (2.3%)
Not informative:               12 sib-pairs.   (27.3%)
```

This is the breakdown of the 44 affected sib-pairs detected in this family set, separated according to the information available in the pedigree about the sib-pairs. At the bottom of the screen are the results of the analysis, as shown in Table 26–2. In this analysis, if we had only considered sib-pairs with completely known IBD information, the value of χ^2 is 3.00, with a p-value of 0.0416. This is the most robust measure, because it is completely independent of our gene frequency estimates. However, if we take full advantage of our pedigree data combined with our gene frequency estimates for the marker locus, we are able to look at the total χ^2 of 4.22, with a corresponding p-value of 0.0200. Because we are trying to declare a linkage significant, we need a criterion as stringent as the lod score of 3 in linkage analysis. Because the largest p-value that can be associated with such a lod score is 0.001, we recommend that a p-value of no more than 0.001 be used as the cutoff point for declaring a sib-pair test significant. Similarly, if the disease is complex, from the arguments presented in Chapter 25 we should use the equivalent of a lod score of 5, which has a p-value of no more than 0.00001. Multiple comparisons should be allowed for in an analogous way. Although the result is interesting, it is not significant evidence of linkage.

☐ Exercise 26

Perform the ESPA analysis under all three diagnostic models with each of the two marker loci in the set of schizophrenia pedigrees from the previous chapter. Are the results consistent with our linkage analysis? Is there more or less significance in this nonparametric analysis? Why? Which result would you have more faith in, and how would you interpret this finding in practice?

27.

Genetic Heterogeneity

In this chapter, the most fundamental approaches to linkage analysis under genetic heterogeneity are introduced. The two most important questions are: (1) Given a positive linkage test result, is there significant evidence for a proportion of the families segregating the linked gene and another proportion segregating a putative unlinked gene for the same disease?; and (2) Although I do not have significant evidence for linkage assuming homogeneity of the disease gene, if I allow for a certain percentage of my families to be segregating an unlinked gene, is there significant evidence for linkage to a disease gene in a proportion of my families? It is typically assumed that only one of the two disease genes segregates per family, which is reasonable for rare diseases. An overview of some of the methods available to address these two questions is presented, followed by an introduction on how to use the HOMOG program to do the simple analyses discussed above.

27.1 Genetic Heterogeneity

When people talk of genetic heterogeneity, they refer to a situation in which any of a number of genetic causes can act independently to produce an identical disease phenotype. There are many different types of heterogeneity. The simplest type is *allelic heterogeneity,* in which multiple separate disease alleles at the same locus can each cause the same disease phenotype. An example of this is cystic fibrosis (CF), for which a number of different mutated alleles have been isolated, each of which can contribute to the CF phenotype. In general, these do not provide any significant hardship for the linkage analyst, with the exception of analyses involving linkage disequilibrium or genetic risk calculations.

Another form of heterogeneity, which is of greater significance to the linkage analyst, is *nonallelic* (or *locus*) *heterogeneity,* in which disease alleles at two or more independently acting loci could each cause the same disease phenotype. For example, a biochemical pathway might be disrupted by a defect in any of the enzymes required for the pathway to be completed. Typically, either mutation would cause the phenotype that prevents the end product of that biochemical pathway from being synthesized, causing the disease. An example of such a disease is Charcot Marie-Tooth disease (Chance et al., 1990). This nonallelic heterogeneity can be further subdivided into diseases with multiple genetic causes, with either the same or different modes of inheritance. For example, retinitis pigmentosa shows both forms of heterogeneity, with at least two separate loci for an X-linked recessive form, an autosomal recessive form, and an autosomal dominant form (McKusick, 1990). Heterogeneity is much easier to detect when there is a different mode of inheritance in some families from others, since this can typically be seen without the need for linkage analysis. However, when two forms of the disease share a common mode of inheritance (e.g., autosomal dominant), the only way to determine that more than one genetic locus is involved is by using a special form of linkage analysis that treats the heterogeneity as an additional parameter in the analysis. The remainder of this chapter discusses the application of some current methodologies for linkage analysis under nonallelic heterogeneity. For a comprehensive discussion of various theoretical approaches to this problem, please consult Ott (1991).

27.2 Test for Homogeneity Given Linkage

The simplest thing to test for, given a significant linkage test result (i.e., a lod score greater than 3), is whether there is significant evidence to support the hypothesis that some of the families in our pedigree set might be segregating a different unlinked gene for the same disease, and not the gene that is linked to the marker in question in this analysis. The method we apply in this chapter is the so-called *A-test* (Smith, 1963), or *admixture test*. The underlying assumption in this test is that there are two categories of families in the data: some with $\theta = \frac{1}{2}$, and some with $\theta = \theta_1 < \frac{1}{2}$, with a proportion α of families segregating the linked gene (i.e., $\theta = \theta_1$ in proportion α of the families, and $\theta = \frac{1}{2}$ in proportion $(1 - \alpha)$ of the families). The additional assumption is that unequivocal assignment of any family to one class or the other is impossible *a priori*. This is almost always the case, because we have no way other than through linkage analysis of assigning any given family to one category or the other. So, the likelihood for any given family can be written as $L(\alpha,\theta) = \alpha L(\theta) + (1 - \alpha)L(\theta = \frac{1}{2})$, which can be rewritten as $\alpha L(\theta)/L(\theta = \frac{1}{2}) + (1 - \alpha)$, because $L(\theta = \frac{1}{2})$ is a constant. Thus, for *n* families, the total likelihood is

$$\Pi_i \left[\alpha \frac{L_i(\theta)}{L_i(\theta = \frac{1}{2})} + (1 - \alpha) \right]$$

If we want to test the null hypothesis of linkage homogeneity (i.e., that all families are of the linked type), we form a likelihood ratio as

$$\frac{L(\alpha,\theta)}{L(\alpha = 1,\theta)} = \Pi_i \left[\alpha + (1 - \alpha) \frac{L_i(\theta = \frac{1}{2})}{L_i(\theta)} \right]$$

Then

$$2 \ln \Pi_i \left[\alpha + (1 - \alpha) \frac{L_i(\theta = \frac{1}{2})}{L_i(\theta)} \sim \chi^2_{(1)} \right]$$

However, because the test is of the form

$$\frac{L(\alpha < 1, \theta)}{L(\alpha = 1, \theta)}$$

that is, H_0: $\{\alpha = 1\}$ versus H_1: $\{\alpha < 1\}$, it is carried out in a one-sided manner, and therefore the p-values must be adjusted accordingly. In other words, we find the p-value associated with the $\chi^2_{(1)}$ value computed from the likelihood ratio test and divide the corresponding p-value in half to compute the appropriate p-value for this chi-square test of homogeneity. This is true for reasons outlined in Ott (1985).

27.3 Test for Linkage Given Heterogeneity

Another null hypothesis is possible for the likelihood ratio test of homogeneity described above. Consider a null hypothesis of no linkage against an alternative hypothesis of linkage and heterogeneity. Such a test is parametrized as

$$\frac{L(\alpha,\theta)}{L(\alpha = 1, \theta = \tfrac{1}{2})}$$

However, when considering this test, there are two fundamental problems in interpretation. First, we are trying to declare a linkage significant while allowing for heterogeneity as a sort of nuisance parameter. We therefore need a significance level at least equivalent to that of the lod score of 3 criterion in a straight linkage analysis. If we consider the maximum "lod score with heterogeneity" to be

$$\log_{10}\left[\frac{L(\hat{\alpha},\hat{\theta})}{L(\alpha = 1, \theta = \tfrac{1}{2})}\right]$$

and require that this value exceed 3 as a test of linkage, we are being slightly nonconservative, because there is an additional free parameter α in the numerator of this lod score. To allow for this additional degree of freedom, add approximately $\log_{10}(2) = 0.30$ to the critical value. This then makes a critical value of 3.30 for declaring the linkage test significant (corresponding to a likelihood ratio of 2000:1).

However, there is another problem with this likelihood ratio test. Under the null hypothesis $\theta = \tfrac{1}{2}$ in all families, the parameter α disappears. Notice that the likelihood of any given family is $L(\alpha,\theta) = \alpha L(\theta) + (1 - \alpha)L(\theta = \tfrac{1}{2})$. This makes

$$L\left(\alpha,\theta = \frac{1}{2}\right) = \alpha L\left(\theta = \frac{1}{2}\right) + (1 - \alpha)L\left(\theta = \frac{1}{2}\right) = L\left(\theta = \frac{1}{2}\right)$$

One could also parametrize this likelihood, making $\alpha = 0$, in which case θ disappears as a parameter, because

$$L(\alpha = 0,\theta) = 0L(\theta) + (1 - 0)L\left(\theta = \frac{1}{2}\right) = L\left(\theta = \frac{1}{2}\right)$$

Therefore, we have a completely degenerate situation under the null hypothesis, where $L(\alpha = 0,\theta) = L(\alpha,\theta = \tfrac{1}{2}) = L(\theta = \tfrac{1}{2})$. Thus there is one parameter under H_0, whereas under H_1 there are two (α and θ). This leads to a problem with the asymptotic distribution of the likelihood ratio, and

$$-2 \ln\left[\frac{L(\theta = \frac{1}{2})}{L(\alpha,\theta)}\right] \not\sim \chi^2$$

Hence, we have even further troubles. Several researchers have considered the asymptotic distribution of this statistic (M. Shoukri, Personal communication; Davies, 1977; Faraway, 1993), which can be extremely complicated. In light of all this, it seems that we should not in general apply any asymptotic theory to this test statistic but rather use a criterion of a likelihood ratio above 2000:1 to declare that significant evidence exists for linkage in some of the families in our data set. This criterion of 2000:1 odds is based on the normal 1000:1 odds required in a normal linkage test, and the allowance for the second free parameter (α) in the numerator of the odds ratio.

27.4 Using the HOMOG Program

Both of these tests are incorporated in the HOMOG program (Ott, 1991). To use this program, compute lod scores at a large number of recombination fractions in each pedigree separately. Let us consider the schizophrenia pedigrees from Chapter 25, under the recessive model with diagnostic scheme 3. Compute two-point lod scores between marker 2 and the disease, at θ values ranging from 0 to 0.45 in steps of 0.05. Use LCP as you did earlier to perform this analysis on all the pedigrees together. Then examine the FINAL.OUT file obtained from this analysis. The $\log_{10}$(likelihood) for each pedigree at each recombination is shown in Table 27–1. You should then compute the lod scores at each value of θ for each pedigree separately, using the formula $Z(\theta) = \log_{10}L(\theta) - \log_{10}L(\theta = \frac{1}{2})$ or by using the LINKLODS computer program. These lod scores are required for the input file for the HOMOG program. The format for the input file is as follows:

Line 1 :   Title of the problem

Line 2 :   N STEPSIZE LDIFF where N = the number of values of θ at which the lod scores are given in the input file (Note: values should not be given for $\theta = 0.5$, where $Z(\theta = 0.5) = 0$); STEPSIZE = the step size in which α should be incremented. By default this value should be set to 0.05, meaning that the likelihood is evaluated for values of $\theta = 0, 0.05, 0.1, 0.15, \ldots$; LDIFF is optional and can be omitted without a problem. It stands for the difference in natural log likelihood to be used as the basis for the support interval for α around its MLE. In other words if this value is equal to 2, the program gives you a 2-unit support interval for all parameters (Remember that these intervals are given in terms of *natural* log, not *common* log!).

Line 3: OUT ALOW LL,   where OUT refers to the output option. The program can give you, in the output file, a table of values of ln $L(\alpha,\theta)$ over all α and θ combinations. It can also give you a list of lod scores for each family separately. The value of the variable OUT identifies what combination of these options you wish to have in your output file, as indicated in Table 27–2; ALOW is the smallest value of α to be considered. For example, if you wished to consider only values of $\alpha \geq 0.1$, set ALOW = 0.1. In most situations,

Table 27–1. The $\log_{10}$(Likelihood) for Each Pedigree at Each Value of θ for the Schizophrenia Pedigrees with Recessive Model, Diagnostic Scheme 3

	Pedigree					
θ	*1*	*2*	*3*	*4*	*5*	*6*
0.00	− 27.088124	− 11.855281	− 28.836341	− 9.981559	− 14.330920	− 22.606300
0.05	− 26.760831	− 11.849109	− 28.469527	− 10.008431	− 14.209290	− 21.585746
0.10	− 26.564485	− 11.830223	− 28.337708	− 10.033840	− 14.145533	− 21.104337
0.15	− 26.431280	− 11.795900	− 28.292208	− 10.057423	− 14.112566	− 20.823790
0.20	− 26.335704	− 11.749105	− 28.289131	− 10.078831	− 14.097507	− 20.649023
0.25	− 26.265375	− 11.696470	− 28.307058	− 10.097721	− 14.093468	− 20.538287
0.30	− 26.213481	− 11.645108	− 28.333387	− 10.113758	− 14.096308	− 20.467862
0.35	− 26.176015	− 11.600649	− 28.360206	− 10.126625	− 14.103046	− 20.422618
0.40	− 26.150575	− 11.566824	− 28.382478	− 10.136040	− 14.111042	− 20.393293
0.45	− 26.135765	− 11.545810	− 28.397042	− 10.141784	− 14.117674	− 20.375567
0.50	− 26.130888	− 11.538696	− 28.402098	− 10.143715	− 14.120392	− 20.369191

however, it is safest to set ALOW = 0 and maximize the likelihood over all possible values of α; LL denotes the line length of the output file and is an optional variable. If it is omitted, the line length is assumed to be set to 80 characters. In some situations, you may wish to allow for longer lines, especially if OUT = 2 or 3, because the table of values of ln $L(\alpha,\theta)$ can become very long as the number of values of α and θ considered increases.

Line 4: θ_1, θ_2, . . . , θ_N where the θ_i are the values of θ for which the lod scores are going to be provided below. Generally, these should be in ascending order. Naturally, the finer the grid of points at which lod scores are computed, the more powerful the homogeneity test, because the maximization of the likelihood is thereby more accurate. (There is no need to provide the actual values of θ, because *no* interpolation scheme is used. You could just as easily provide integer values or map distance measures, as long as N real numbers are provided.)

Line 5 : NFAM   where NFAM is the number of families for which lod scores are provided.
Line 6 : $Z(\theta_1)$, $Z(\theta_2)$, ... , $Z(\theta_N)$ IN FAMILY 1
Line 7 : $Z(\theta_1)$, $Z(\theta_2)$, ... , $Z(\theta_N)$ IN FAMILY 2
. . .
Line (5 + NFAM) : $Z(\theta_1)$, $Z(\theta_2)$, ... , $Z(\theta_N)$ IN FAMILY NFAM

Note that any lod score less than − 80 is assumed to represent a lod score of − ∞, and in the output (and in the input files) log likelihoods of − ∞ should be indicated as − 99. The input file for this data set should be as follows:

```
Schizophrenia pedigrees – Recessive model – Diagnostic scheme 3
10 0.05
0 0
0 0.05 0.1 0.15 0.2 0.25 0.3 0.35 0.4 0.45
6
-0.957236 -0.629943 -0.433597 -0.300392 -0.204816 -0.134487 -0.082593 -0.045127 -0.019687 -0.004877
-0.316585 -0.310413 -0.291527 -0.257204 -0.210409 -0.157774 -0.106412 -0.061953 -0.028128 -0.007114
-0.434243 -0.067429 0.064390 0.109890 0.112967 0.095040 0.068711 0.041892 0.019620 0.005056
0.162156 0.135284 0.109875 0.086292 0.064884 0.045994 0.029957 0.017090 0.007675 0.001931
-0.210528 -0.088898 -0.025141 0.007826 0.022885 0.026924 0.024084 0.017346 0.009350 0.002718
-2.237109 -1.216555 -0.735146 -0.454599 -0.279832 -0.169096 -0.098671 -0.053427 -0.024102 -0.006376
```

Table 27–2. Table of Definitions of Output Options for HOMOG Programs in Variable OUT

OUT	Table of ln $L(\alpha,\theta)$	Lod Scores for Families
0	no	no
1	no	yes
2	yes	no
3	yes	yes

Save this file as HOMOG.DAT, the required input file name for the HOMOG programs, and type HOMOG at the DOS prompt to run the program and do the analysis. The output file should resemble the following:

```
Program  HOMOG  version 3.33  J. Ott
Heterogeneity: two family types, one with linkage, one without
  alpha = proportion of families with linkage (θ<1/2)
  1-alpha = proportion of families without linkage (θ=1/2)

>> Schizophrenia pedigrees - Recessive model - Diagnostic scheme 3 <<

    Table of conditional max. Ln(L) over α's, given θ or x
       θ or x    α max     Max.Ln(L)    Lik. ratio

    1   0.0000   1.0000    0.0000       1.0000
    2   0.0500   1.0000    0.0000       1.0000
    3   0.1000   1.0000    0.0000       1.0000
    4   0.1500   1.0000    0.0000       1.0000
    5   0.2000   1.0000    0.0000       1.0000
    6   0.2500   1.0000    0.0000       1.0000
    7   0.3000   1.0000    0.0000       1.0000
    8   0.3500   1.0000    0.0000       1.0000
    9   0.4000   1.0000    0.0000       1.0000
   10   0.4500   1.0000    0.0000       1.0000
```

The output above shows the maximum natural log likelihood for each value of θ maximized over α and normalized such that $\ln L(\theta = \frac{1}{2}) = 0$. In this case you note that for all α, when $\theta < \frac{1}{2}$, $\ln L(\theta,\alpha) < 0$, implying that the MLE of θ is 0.5 (or equivalently that the MLE of α is 1), meaning that all families are considered to be unlinked.

```
                                                 Estimates of
Hypotheses                      Max.ln L    Alpha      Theta
H2: Linkage, heterogeneity      0.0000      1.0000     99.0000
H1: Linkage, homogeneity        0.0000      (1)        99.0000
H0: No linkage                  (0)         (0)        (0.5)


Components of chi-square
Source                          df          Chi-square  L ratio
H2 vs. H1 Heterogeneity         1           0.000       1.0000
H1 vs. H0 Linkage               1           0.000       1.0000
H2 vs. H0 Total                 2           0.000       1.0000
```

The values in these tables are the crux of the analysis. The top table indicates the maximum natural log likelihood of the entire family set under each of the three hypotheses. The first line corresponds to $\ln L(\hat{\alpha},\hat{\theta})$; the second to $\ln L(\alpha = 1,\hat{\theta})$; and the third to $\ln L(\theta = \frac{1}{2})$. These three hypotheses are represented by H_2, H_1, and H_0, respectively and denote that in H_2 there is linkage and heterogeneity, in H_1 there is linkage and homogeneity, and under the true null hypothesis H_0 there is neither linkage nor heterogeneity. An estimate of 99.0000 for θ means the disease is unlinked ($\theta = \frac{1}{2}$). This value is used because when multipoint lod scores are utilized in a HOMOG analysis, the value of 0.5 may have some other meaning and because map distances are used instead of recombination fractions. The bottom table summarizes the three likelihood ratio tests possible with these three hypotheses. The first is the test of heterogeneity given linkage (H_2 vs. H_1), and the second is the standard test of linkage assuming homogeneity (H_1 vs. H_0), or just $L(\hat{\theta})/L(\theta=\frac{1}{2})$. The third is the joint test of linkage and heterogeneity, $L(\hat{\alpha},\hat{\theta})/L(\theta=\frac{1}{2})$, the properties of which are described above. Each of these values can be computed by finding the difference between the ln(likelihood) values for each hypothesis and multiplying it by 2. This then provides the quantity found under the chi-square column. The number of degrees of freedom is given in the first column, although the number of degrees of freedom in the test of H_2 versus H_0 is not really 2, and this statistic is not really distributed as a χ^2 random variable. The likelihood ratio in the last column provides the exact odds for the alternative hypothesis against the null hypothesis. By the criterion described above for considering the test of H_2 versus H_0 to be significant, this quantity must exceed 2000. In this example, there is absolutely no evidence for heterogeneity in the data, and as such the value of each likelihood ratio is 1, with $\chi^2 = 0$.

Family no.	Conditional prob. of linked type
1	1.0000
2	1.0000
3	1.0000
4	1.0000
5	1.0000
6	1.0000

Finally, the values in the table above are the conditional probabilities that each family is segregating the linked gene, assuming the values of α and θ estimated under H_2 from our observed family data. This conditional probability is described in Ott (1991). In general, the values found here should be taken with a grain of salt, and they cannot ever be validly used to separate families for the remainder of a linkage study. It should be required that any further marker typings be done on all the families combined and analyzed with these HOMOG programs, to compute the appropriate log likelihood ratio statistics on the entire data set. This thorough approach preserves the validity of the results and does not induce any potential bias that could lead to an increased false-positive rate. If additional linked markers are selectively typed solely in those families with high posterior probabilities of segregating a linked gene, families would be selected for further linkage analysis conditional on there being few observed recombinants, which could easily lead to false-positive evidence of linkage.

In general, all of the information required for a complete analysis of your data set, allowing for the presence of heterogeneity, is available from this output file. As a matter of practice you should always perform such an analysis with any complex disease, because nonallelic heterogeneity is usually assumed to be involved in the etiology of these diseases, and performing homogeneity tests can allow you to extract information from your data set more completely. Other programs (HOMOG2, HOMOG3, HOMOG3R), based on the same algorithm, are available to handle more complicated heterogeneity situations, but discussion of them is beyond the scope of this book.

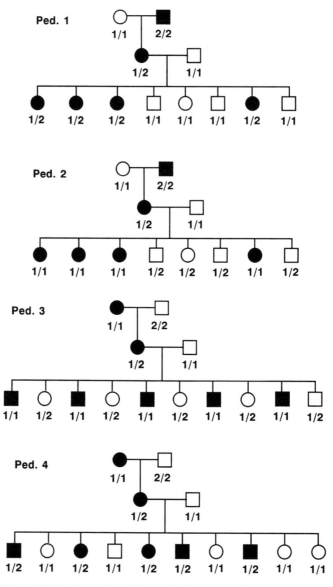

Figure 27–1. Example pedigrees for homogeneity test

☐ Exercise 27

For the four pedigrees shown in Figure 27–1, perform a complete linkage analysis, including homogeneity testing. Assume the disease to be inherited as an autosomal dominant disease with gene frequency of 0.00001 for the disease allele and assume a marker with two alleles with gene frequencies of 0.65 and 0.35, respectively.

28 □

Computer Simulation Methods

This chapter contains a brief overview of computer simulation and some of its many applications in human genetic linkage analysis. The various approaches to pedigree data simulation are introduced, as well as the various types of statistical information one can obtain from a simulation.

28.1 Random Numbers and Simulation

It is possible to write a computer program that generates so-called *pseudorandom* numbers based on an initial seed provided by the user. These routines approximate randomness using any of a large number of complicated mathematical functions designed to generate a series of numbers on the interval $(0,1)$ that are approximately uniformly distributed. This means that it is equally likely for any number on the interval $(0,1)$ to be chosen independent of the previously selected number.

Let us assume we wish to simulate one replicate of a coin toss. Because heads and tails have equal probability of 50%, we divide the interval in half and say that if a given random number is less than 0.5, it is heads, and if the number is greater than 0.5, it is tails. In this way, we can simulate the flipping of a fair coin by computer. If we think about it intuitively, flipping a coin can also be thought of as a primitive random number generator, and a sample simulation can be done solely by tossing a coin. To illustrate this technique, we consider the simple case of simulating a marker unlinked to the disease ($\theta = \frac{1}{2}$).

28.2 Pedigree Simulation by Tossing a Coin

Assume that for the pedigree shown in Figure 28–1 the disease is dominant with full penetrance, such that the disease phenotypes uniquely determine the corresponding disease locus genotypes. Then, let us simulate a two-allele marker, which is unlinked to the disease locus ($\theta = 0.5$), with equal gene frequency for each allele ($p_1 = p_2 = 0.5$). In this simple situation, we can sim-

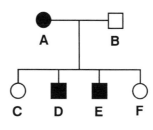

Figure 28–1. Pedigree for manual simulation example

ulate this pedigree solely by flipping a coin. As an example of how this works, let us first simulate marker locus genotypes for the parents in this pedigree (with phase). Because the marker locus has two alleles with equal gene frequency of 50%, we can simulate the alleles by coin toss. Assume for the founder individuals, that if the coin comes up heads we select allele *1,* and if the coin comes up tails we select allele *2.* WLOG, we first simulate the marker allele in phase with the disease allele in person *A.* The first flip of the coin comes up tails, so allele *2* is selected. Next, we simulate a marker allele in phase with the + allele in person *A.* The coin came up heads, so this haplotype is now assigned to carry allele *2.* Thus, this individual has genotype *1 2* at the marker locus. Similarly we must simulate the two marker alleles in individual *B.* Assume the coin comes up heads the first time and tails the second, giving this individual genotype *1 2.*

Next, we simulate the children of these parents. Let us first simulate the transmission of marker alleles from person *A* to her children. In this case, we know which disease locus allele was transmitted to each child. Thus, we need only simulate the recombination process from mother to child. If the marker is unlinked to the disease, the recombination probability is $\frac{1}{2}$ by definition. Assume that if the coin comes up heads a recombination occurred, and if it comes up tails no recombination event occurred. In the case of individual *C,* the coin comes up heads, so a recombination occurred in the meiosis from mother to child. Because this individual received the + allele from her mother, at the marker locus she must have received the *2* allele, which was in phase with the *D* allele in the mother, and a recombination event occurred. For individuals *D, E,* and *F,* assume the coin comes up tails. These individuals received marker alleles from their mother without recombination, meaning that they received alleles *2, 2,* and *1,* respectively. Finally, we need to simulate the alleles passed from individual *B* to his children. Because he is homozygous +/+ at the disease locus, we do not simulate recombination events; however, we still must simulate the segregation of the alleles from father to children. According to mendelian laws, there is a 50% chance that either allele was inherited at the marker locus from the father. Therefore, let us assign heads to the inheritance of allele *1,* and tails to the inheritance of allele *2* from the father. Flipping the coin, we come up with heads, heads, tails, and heads, meaning the alleles transmitted to individuals *C, D, E,* and *F* are *1, 1, 2,* and *1,* respectively. Thus, the final simulated replicate of our family is shown in Figure 28–2. The linkage analysis of this family yields a maximum lod score of 0.301029 at $\theta = 0$. We simulated one recombinant in this family, but because the analysis cannot make the phase assumption we made in our simulation, the recombination event goes unnoticed due to the marker alleles inherited from the unaffected parent. In fact, individuals *C* and *D* provide essentially no linkage information because they are heterozygous, and their

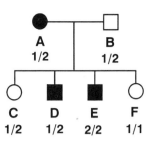

Figure 28–2. Manually simulated replicate of pedigree from Figure 28–1

parents are identical and heterozygous. It is equally likely that they received the *1* allele from *A* and the *2* allele from *B* as it is that they received the *1* allele from *B* and the *2* allele from *A*. Hence, there is essentially no information from such a situation. Thus, the only individuals who provide unequivocal information about recombination are *E* and *F*, who are homozygous at the marker, making it obvious which alleles were inherited from *A* with the disease. Because they were both nonrecombinants, we are left with a phase-unknown pedigree with two nonrecombinants, which yields a maximum lod score of $0.301029 = \log_{10}(2)$. What would have happened had both individuals in question been recombinants? Because the family is phase-unknown, the result of the analysis is the same as in this situation, due to the inheritance pattern being completely consistent with no recombination. In any event, this is a primitive example of how a pedigree simulation is conducted with the computer software we introduce in this chapter. The only difference is that our computer software allows us to simulate random numbers over the range of (0,1), such that probabilities other than 0.5 can be accurately simulated, which is not so simple using a coin toss as the random number generator.

28.3 The SIMULATE Program

It is a simple matter to simulate pedigree data based only on pedigree structure and not on any already known phenotypes, for in this case, one need not condition as one needs only to simulate based on straightforward population genetics and mendelian laws. Simulating a group of linked markers that are unlinked to the disease locus is equivalent to completely disregarding whatever information is known about the trait locus and is therefore model-free simulation.

The simulation is straightforward, using the concept of pseudorandom number generation introduced in the opening section of this chapter. We first simulate genotypes with phase at each marker independently in all founders (i.e., people without parents in the pedigree) according to the laws of population genetics, assuming Hardy-Weinberg equilibrium (HWE). The next step is to simulate marker segregation from the already simulated parents to their children. According to the law of independent segregation each child has a 50–50 chance of receiving either allele from each parent independently. However, if you are simulating multiple linked loci, the next locus no longer segregates independently, so you must simulate it according to the recombination fraction between itself and the first locus. Assume the recombination fraction (θ)

is 0.1; then if the random number generator selects a number below 0.1, a recombination is simulated, and the allele to be inherited from the parent in question must be selected from the other parental haplotype (this is why we must insist on simulating all genotypes with phase in the first step). We continue like this, switching parental haplotypes whenever a recombination is simulated across the chromosome, until we reach the final marker to be simulated. This process is repeated for each individual, from each of his parents. Once all individuals have been simulated, one simulated replicate is created of the linear set of multiple linked markers segregating through the pedigree (or set of pedigrees) independent of the predetermined trait locus (if one exists). These pedigree replicates are then saved in a form ready for analysis with the MSIM, LSIM, or ISIM programs of the SLINK package, as described below later in this chapter. The technical details of using SIMULATE are outlined in Section 28.5.

28.4 Possible Applications of Simulation under H_0

This simulation method can be useful in determining the *p*-value associated with a given observed maximum lod score in a pedigree (set). In other words, let us say that you found a lod score of 2.5 in your pedigree set with a given marker versus disease. In and of itself, this result is insignificant according to the traditional lod-score-of-3 criterion. However, it may be very unusual to observe such an extreme lod score in this particular family set. You could, for example, simulate the marker or markers in question in a large number of replicates of the family set and determine how often the observed lod score is reached or exceeded by chance. If this is extremely rare, you might want to report the simulated *p*-value associated with this result. However, it may also be easy to get such a high lod score in the pedigree set, in which case the significance should also be reported and used to guide your future plans. Knowing the *p*-value associated with given lod scores has many uses and applications. For the molecular biologist it is useful to know the null hypothesis distributions of maximum lod scores, because they can serve as a useful guide in the search for a new gene. In a pedigree that almost never (1/1000 replicates, for example) gives a lod score as high as 1, such a high lod score is much more significant than finding the same result in a pedigree that exceeds this threshold 10% of the time by chance. This kind of information can help the investigator decide whether or not to invest further energy in typing additional markers in a given region, to try and find the gene causing the disease in question. So, knowing these null hypothesis lod score distributions can be a useful tool for the linkage analyst throughout a given investigation. Furthermore, when maximizing the lod score over many different sets of genetic model parameters, the probability of exceeding a given lod score given no linkage and the exact set of models investigated needs to be computed. To compute these *p*-values, marker data needs to be simulated independent of the disease and then analyzed under various models. This unconditional method is ideally suited to such investigations.

Moreover, you can use this rapid approach to simulate the genotypes of any given set of markers segregating in the families to determine the power of your collection of pedigrees to order new markers against a known map of linked markers. This is useful if you are deciding how many families to type for a given new marker in order to accurately order it with the required 1000:1 odds. If for a given marker set you find that you have 80% power to order the markers accurately with 1000:1 odds using half of your total available pedigrees, and you have 90% power if you type them all, it may be advisable to type only half of the families to begin with and then to type the remaining families later only if no significant result is obtained from the first half. You might also find that you have no chance to order the markers with 1000:1 odds in your pedigree set, in which case it might not be advisable to bother trying until you have collected more or better families.

For the statistical geneticist, testing the properties of new statistical methods is perhaps the most common application of simulation. Whenever a new method is derived and you desire to compute its power and other properties, you often need to rely on simulation, because theoretical computations involving pedigrees can often be prohibitive in realistic situations. Therefore, a rapid way of generating data is needed to do a particular study. The SIMULATE program can create any type of locus describable in LINKAGE format; so a trait locus linked to a number of markers can be simulated, and by modifying the source code slightly you can incorporate whatever ascertainment restrictions you desire. In this way, the properties of new methods and novel statistics can be tested in situations in which theoretical analysis cannot be easily done.

28.5 How to Use the SIMULATE Program

Let us consider the set of schizophrenia pedigrees from Chapter 25 and simulate an unlinked marker with the properties of markers 1 and 2 from that data set, with the dominant model for the disease in diagnostic scheme 3. Our goal in this case is to determine the probability (when there really is no linkage) of getting a lod score at least as large as the 2.65 we observed, assuming we analyzed the pedigree under only this one model. Similarly, we want to test the linkage of disease to marker 2 and determine the probability of getting a lod score at least as large as the 2.22 we observed in our example for that comparison. To do this we simulate the two markers linked to each other at recombination fraction 0.12 (Sherrington et al., 1988) and unlinked to the putative disease locus.

Three input files are required for the SIMULATE program: SIMPED.DAT (a pedigree file), SIMDATA.DAT (a locus parameter file), and PROBLEM.DAT (a file containing simulation parameters). We introduce the basic format for each file in the context of the schizophrenia pedigrees.

The SIMPED.DAT file is a linkage format pedigree file (processed by MAKEPED) with some slight alterations. The first locus should be the disease (if there is one). If no affection status locus is present, the program simulates a set of linked markers, but if a disease is present, it simulates the remaining loci and keeps the disease locus phenotypes as given in this file. The only restriction is that the disease must be the first locus in the file, and it must be an affection status locus. Instead of providing marker locus phenotypes for the remaining loci, we need to enter a 1 if the first marker locus is to be simulated, and a 0 if it is to be left unknown. The next column then contains a 1 or a 0 to tell the program whether the second marker is to be simulated or left untyped. Thus, each line of the SIMPED.DAT file contains an affection status locus for the disease, followed by a series of 0's and 1's to tell whether each marker locus is to be simulated or left untyped. If an individual is untyped for a given marker in the original data set, assume that he is unavailable for the simulation as well (for the same marker) to ensure that simulation results are

consistent with our real data set. For the schizophrenia pedigree set, the
SIMPED.PRE file should resemble the following (information shown for pedigree 1 only, to save space, but you should complete the file for all pedigrees):

```
1   A   0   0 2   2 1     1       1
1   B   0   0 1   1 1     1       1
1   C   B   A 2   2 3     1       1
1   D   B   A 1   2 1     1       1
1   E   B   A 1   2 1     1       1
1   F   B   A 1   2 1     1       1
1   G   0   0 1   0 1     0       0
1   H   0   0 2   0 1     0       0
1   I   G   H 2   1 1     1       1
1   J   B   A 2   2 1     1       1
1   K   G   H 1   1 1     1       1
1   L   F   I 1   1 1     1       1
1   M   F   I 1   1 1     1       1
1   N   F   I 1   2 1     1       1
1   O   K   J 1   1 1     1       1
1   P   K   J 1   2 1     1       1
```

Process this file with MAKEPED to make the SIMPED.DAT file needed
for the analysis. You then need to add a header as the first two lines of this
file. The first line must indicate the number of pedigrees in the SIMPED.DAT
file (in this case, there are 6), and the second line must contain the number of
individuals in each pedigree (including doubled individuals). In this case, the
first two lines should be as follows:

```
6
17 17 35 17 18 26
```

There is one more important alteration that must be made to this input
file. It is imperative that the individuals be numbered consecutively from 1
through *n*, where *n* is the number of individuals in the pedigree. They must
also be presented in numerical order in the file. In pedigree 1, however, there
is a marriage loop, and when individual 6 is doubled a new individual with ID
number 17 is added directly after individual 6. You must move this individual
to the end of the first pedigree, directly following individual 16, so the
SIMPED.DAT looks like the following (only pedigree 1 shown).

```
6
17 17 35 17 18 26
1    1    0    0    3    0    0 2 0   2 1   1   1
1    2    0    0    3    0    0 1 0   1 1   1   1
1    3    2    1    0    4    4 2 0   2 3   1   1
1    4    2    1    0    5    5 1 0   2 1   1   1
1    5    2    1    0    6    6 1 0   2 1   1   1
1    6    2    1    0   10   10 1 2   2 1   1   1
1    7    0    0    9    0    0 1 1   0 1   0   0
1    8    0    0    9    0    0 2 0   0 1   0   0
1    9    7    8   12   11   11 2 0   1 1   1   1
1   10    2    1   15    0    0 2 0   2 1   1   1
1   11    7    8   15    0    0 1 0   1 1   1   1
1   12   17    9    0   13   13 1 0   1 1   1   1
1   13   17    9    0   14   14 1 0   1 1   1   1
1   14   17    9    0    0    0 1 0   2 1   1   1
1   15   11   10    0   16   16 1 0   1 1   1   1
1   16   11   10    0    0    0 1 0   2 1   1   1
1   17    0    0   12    0    0 1 2   2 1   1   1
```

The second required file is called SIMDATA.DAT and provides the locus parameters for the simulation, including penetrance, gene frequencies, locus types and definitions, and intermarker recombination fractions. This file should be in standard MLINK format. For the schizophrenia pedigrees in diagnostic scheme 3 with the dominant model, the file should be as follows:

```
3 0 0 5  << NO. OF LOCI, RISK LOCUS, SEXLINKED (IF 1) PROGRAM
0 0.0 0.0 0  << MUT LOCUS, MUT RATE, HAPLOTYPE FREQUENCIES (IF 1)
 1  2  3
1  2  << AFFECTION, NO. OF ALLELES
 0.010000 0.990000  << GENE FREQUENCIES
 3 << NO. OF LIABILITY CLASSES
 0.4400 0.4400 0.0166
 0.4400 0.4400 0.0166
 0.4400 0.4400 0.0166 << PENETRANCES
3  2  << ALLELE NUMBERS, NO. OF ALLELES
 0.330000 0.670000  << GENE FREQUENCIES
3  3  << ALLELE NUMBERS, NO. OF ALLELES
 0.320000 0.160000 0.520000  << GENE FREQUENCIES
 0 0  << SEX DIFFERENCE, INTERFERENCE (IF 1 OR 2)
 0.50000 0.12000 << RECOMBINATION VALUES
 1 0.10000 0.45000 << REC VARIED, INCREMENT, FINISHING VALUE
```

This is basically the same as the LINKAGE parameter file we used in Chapter 25, with the recombination fractions correctly specified on the next-to-last line of the file indicating the recombination fractions required for the simulation to work. Because this program assumes the disease is unlinked to the markers, if a number other than 0.5 is given for the first recombination fraction, the program ignores it and still sets this θ to 0.5.

The final required input file is PROBLEM.DAT and should contain two lines. The first line should contain three seeds for the random number generator (these should be numbers between 1 and 30,000, with higher numbers providing better (i.e., more random) results). The second line should contain the number of replicates of the set of pedigrees desired. In general, this number should be very large when you are attempting to compute *p*-values. The normal *p*-value associated with a lod score of 3, for example, is always less than 0.001, so you need a large number of replicates to get an accurate estimate of such small *p*-values. For our purposes, however, let us simulate only 50 replicates in the interest of saving time. It is important to remember that the larger the number of replicates, the greater the accuracy. In general, 50 replicates is not nearly enough to obtain reliable estimates of small *p*-values, but in the interests of time we limit our study to this level for this instructional example. For our purposes, use seeds of 24553, 29773, and 20142. In practice, whenever you use the same seeds, the results will be identical because the sequence of pseudorandom numbers is fully determined by the seeds. Whenever these values change, however, the entire sequence will be altered as well. The PROBLEM.DAT file should look like the following:

```
24553  29773  20142
50
```

Next, run the SIMULATE program by typing SIMULATE at the DOS prompt (assuming the SIMULATE program is accessible to DOS either by being in the directory where you are working, or in the path). The program then simulates 50 replicates of the pedigree with both linked markers segregating in it.

28.6 Analyzing the Simulated Replicates with MLINK and ILINK

The file containing the simulated replicates is called PEDFILE.DAT. However, we are only interested in the two-point lod scores, so we need to use LSP to extract two loci at a time from this file. Hence, we must change the name of the output file. Let us call the new file SCHIZSIM.PED by typing RENAME PEDFILE.DAT SCHIZSIM.PED. Then, you may also rename the SIMDATA.DAT file to SCHIZSIM.DAT.

First, confirm that the two simulated markers are actually separated by approximately $\theta = 0.12$ by evaluating the lod score over the entire set of $50 \times 6 = 300$ simulated pedigrees. To do this, use LCP as you have done throughout the book, selecting loci 2 and 3 with the MLINK program, starting from $\theta = 0.1$, proceeding in steps of 0.01, and stopping at $\theta = 0.15$. The resulting maximum lod score should be found at $\theta = 0.13$, with $Z(0.13) = 121.01$. The lod score at $\theta = 0.12$ is only 0.04 lower, which is highly insignificant on such a large data set. We hereby verified that the two markers were simulated at the appropriate recombination fraction.

It remains to verify that the disease locus is, in fact, simulated unlinked to both marker loci. To do this, use MLINK to compute lod scores for the disease versus each marker at recombination fractions 0.45 through 0.5 in steps of 0.01 to verify that the maximum lod score occurs at the true value of $\theta = 0.5$. For disease versus each of the markers, the maximum lod score is 0 at $\theta = 0.5$, as expected. When the ILINK program is used, the estimated recombination fractions are $\hat{\theta}_{D,M1} = 0.526$, $\hat{\theta}_{D,M2} = 0.516$, and $\hat{\theta}_{M1,M2} = 0.125$. So, we produced a set of pedigrees consistent with our simulation parameters. In addition, we can compute the *expected lod score* for the original set of six pedigrees quite simply from this data. The formula for approximating the expected lod score at a given value of the recombination fraction is

$$E[Z(\theta)] \approx \frac{1}{n} \sum_{i=1}^{n} Z_i(\theta)$$

where n is the total number of replicates simulated, and the sum goes from $i = 1$ to n, where $Z_i(\theta)$ is the lod score at recombination fraction θ in replicate i. Clearly, then, we have computed the lod score for the entire family set, and because the lod score is additive over families, the results obtained from MLINK are

$$\sum_{i=1}^{n} Z_i(\theta)$$

If we then divide by the number of replicates (50), for markers 2 versus 3 we get

$$E[Z(\theta = 0.12)] = \frac{119.97}{50} = 2.40$$

Because 0.12 was the simulated recombination fraction, the expected lod score at $\theta = 0.12$ is of particular interest, and is denoted the ELOD. Another statistic of particular interest that can be computed from this data is the maximum expected lod score, or MELOD. This is the lod score at the value of θ for which the expected lod score is maximized, or $\max_{\theta}\{E[Z(\theta)]\}$. Asymptotically, the maximum always occurs at the true value of θ (at which the simulation was carried out), but in small samples (such as 50 replicates), there is likely to be some deviation. In our case, the maximum occurs at $\theta = 0.125$, as determined by ILINK. The corresponding MELOD is 121.07/50 = 2.42, which is slightly larger than the ELOD. In general, MELOD ≥ ELOD, and asymptotically they are equal. The ELOD is important because it tells you what lod score on average you can expect to get from your data set at the true recombination fraction (if it were 0.12, in this case). The MELOD has less utility, because it is larger than the ELOD solely due to random fluctuations. Because it is not a very meaningful measure, we discourage the use of ME-LOD when simulating all the marker information in a pedigree set.

28.7 Analyzing the Simulated Replicates with MSIM

To analyze the entire set of pedigrees at once takes an enormous amount of computer power, and the programs must be compiled to handle enormous numbers of pedigrees which can rapidly use up your available computer memory. Neither is it a trivial thing to manipulate the output from MLINK so the properties of each pedigree (from the original pedigree set) can be determined individually to establish the relative contributions of each to the ELOD. Furthermore, you might like to compute some other statistical measures on your data set before starting a linkage study. For purposes of analyzing simulated data, Weeks and colleagues (1990b) developed modified versions of ILINK, MLINK, and LINKMAP, which they called ISIM, MSIM, and LSIM, respectively. These programs compute the lod scores one replicate at a time and keep track of various pieces of information about each replicate of each family in the original pedigree set. To use these programs, you need to have the simulated replicates in a file called PEDFILE.DAT (the same name as the output file from SIMULATE or LSP) that contains the simulated replicates and a parameter file called DATAFILE.DAT that specifies the analysis parameters. Keeping in mind that we still need to extract only two loci at a time from our original pedigree and parameter files (SCHIZSIM.*), use the LSP program to extract the disease and marker 1, with the parameter file set up for MLINK (for use in our MSIM analysis), with starting recombination fraction of 0, in steps of 0.10, stopping at $\theta = 0.5$, with no sex difference in recombination rates. The MSIM program also reads the file SIMOUT.DAT, which was created by the SIMULATE program, to identify the number of replicates simulated, and so on. One additional file, LIMIT.DAT, is required. The MSIM program computes the probability $P(Z(\theta) > x)$ of exceeding a given lod score in any replicate of the pedigree set for which the user can select three values of x. These three lod score thresholds must be entered in a file called LIMIT.DAT. By default, 1, 2, and 3 are often chosen. But, if you wish to evaluate the significance level of a given observed maximum lod score, input that value as one of the three thresholds. For the analysis of disease versus marker 1 in our original analysis, we found a lod score of 2.65, so we might want to use thresholds of 1, 2.65, and 3 for this analysis. In this way, we can find the *p*-value associated with our lod score of 2.65 in this pedigree set. The LIMIT.DAT file should then resemble the following:

```
1 2.65 3
[EOF]
```

To do the analysis, first run the UNKNOWN program and then the MSIM program by simply typing MSIM at the DOS prompt after UNKNOWN is completed. Then examine the MSIM.DAT file, which contains the results of the analysis. The segment of the output corresponding to $\theta = 0.10$ follows:

Pedigree	Average	StdDev	Min	Max
THETAS 0.100				
1	−0.165047	0.283531	−0.781806	0.428780
2	−0.027733	0.223751	−0.361404	0.977586
3	−0.099215	0.264000	−0.609994	0.753716
4	−0.094414	0.197641	−0.458361	0.438553
5	−0.048003	0.241983	−0.643913	0.561918
6	−0.130423	0.281867	−0.770454	0.536066
Study	−0.564834	0.695094	−2.409748	1.274584

The column headed Average contains the average lod score over all replicates for each family. In practice, this average lod score is usually referred to as the expected lod score, which it approximates as shown above. The rows correspond to each of the pedigrees in the initial pedigree set, and the row headed Study provides the information on the entire set of pedigrees taken together. So, in this case the overall expected lod score at $\theta = 0.10$ is −0.564834. The next column provides the standard deviation of the expected lod score, which gives you some idea of the variability of the lod scores across replicates. The last two columns indicate the smallest and largest lod scores found over all replicates in the study. These values are indicated to provide an additional measure of the variability of the lod score across replicates. Bear in mind that the value under Max has no easily interpretable statistical importance. If you find a lod score of 1.2 in the original pedigrees, it has no increased significance, because the largest observed lod score in the set of simulated replicates is 1.27. You must still obtain a lod score of 3 to declare a linkage significant.

The next segment of the MSIM.DAT file contains the following information:

Pedigree	Average	StdDev	Min	Max
Average Maximum Lod Scores based on quadratic interpolation				
1	0.046081	0.127706	0.000000	0.523855
2	0.072394	0.221885	0.000000	1.254722
3	0.082413	0.198594	0.000000	0.995219
4	0.058039	0.143175	0.000000	0.586752
5	0.098635	0.172257	0.000000	0.758645
6	0.064638	0.137281	0.000000	0.557189
Study	0.125075	0.297165	0.000000	1.339499

This table contains a somewhat different piece of information—the average maximum lod score based on quadratic interpolation. The average maximum lod score is an approximation to the expected maximum lod score

$$E[\max_{\theta} Z(\theta)] \approx \frac{1}{n} \sum_{i=1}^{n} \max_{\theta} Z_i(\theta)$$

where the lod score is maximized over θ separately in each replicate. To remain consistent with the notation ELOD and MELOD, this might appropriately be called the EMLOD for *expected maximum lod* score. The minimum for this value is always 0, because $\max_{\theta} Z_i(\theta) \geq 0$, (because $Z(\theta = 0.5) = 0$ by definition). Furthermore, in any given replicate, $\max_\theta Z_i(\theta) \geq Z(\theta_0)$ by definition, so EMLOD $\geq$ MELOD $\geq$ ELOD. Because it is always larger than the ELOD many researchers prefer this number. This measure is an indicator of the maximum lod score you can expect in your data set on average, wherever it may occur. In some sense, this quantity is some measure of power, in that it provides the average value of the test statistic across the set of replicates. However, one nice property of the ELOD is that it is additive across pedigrees, while the EMLOD is not. If your pedigree gives you an ELOD of 1, you know that if you had two additional pedigrees of equivalent size and structure, you would have an overall ELOD of 3. However, if you have an EMLOD of 1, there is no direct way of knowing how many additional pedigrees are required for an EMLOD of 3.

In this case, our unlinked marker still gives an EMLOD of 0.125 (It is not typically zero, as there is usually some variability in the value of the maximum lod score even under no linkage—hence the possibility of false-positives), whereas the ELOD is 0.000 (at $\theta = 0.5$). It is intuitively clear that for 60 pedigrees in a set, the EMLOD is not $10 \cdot 0.125 = 12.5$, and yet the ELOD is $10 \times 0.000 = 0.000$.

In this case, the EMLOD's had to be determined by quadratic interpolation. With the MSIM program, the lod scores are computed only at a predefined set of recombination fractions; however, by a technique called *quadratic interpolation*, the maximum of any lod score curve can be approximated (Ott, 1991, p. 183). To avoid the approximation element, the ISIM program can be applied, as we show below.

Finally, the remainder of the file contains information about the probability of finding a lod score greater than the constants you specified in the LIMIT.DAT file. In this example, there are only two replicates with $\max_\theta Z(\theta) > 1$ and none with $\max_\theta Z(\theta) > 2.65$. Because 2.65 was the observed lod score, the associated estimated *p*-value is $0/50 = 0$. To determine a confidence interval for the *p*-value, use the linkage utility program BINOM by selecting the CONFIDENCE INTERVALS (2) option. Then the program asks you to

```
Enter observed k and n [ + no. of decimal places] ( − 1 exits, ENTER
repeats k,n)
```

In this case, enter 0 50, because there are 0 observations of $Z(\theta) > 2.65$ out of 50 opportunities. Next, the program asks for the upper error probability. Because the estimate is $\hat{p} = 0$, you need only enter the significance level here. If you want a 95% confidence interval, enter $(1 - 0.95) = 0.05$. The confidence interval is [0,0.0582]. The 99% confidence interval is [0,0.0880]. The basic message is that from a simulation of only 50 replicates, we can only conclude that $P(\max Z(\theta) > 2.65) \leq 0.0582$, with 95% certainty.

28.8 ISIM

An additional analysis program is of use here: the ISIM program, which accurately computes the EMLOD. To use this program, modify the DATAFILE.DAT file so it is in ILINK format by reading the DATAFILE.DAT into PREPLINK and putting the file in ILINK format, specifying that the recombination fraction be iterated. First run the UNKNOWN program and then the ISIM program by typing ISIM at the DOS prompt. The ISIM program is much slower than the MSIM program, so in many cases, it may be advisable to use the latter, having MSIM compute the lod scores at a minimum of three recombination fractions and then approximate the EMLOD by quadratic interpolation. It can be a good bit less accurate, as you can see from the following excerpt from the ISIM.DAT output file.

```
Average Maximum    StdDev      Min         Max
0.148284           0.307969    -0.000478   1.339499
```

Comparing these results with those obtained from MSIM, you can see that the EMLOD rose from 0.125075 to 0.148284 when the appropriate analysis was done with ISIM. The other quantities are comparable. Note that the Min column gives a value that is less than zero. This is what we observed with the ILINK program, in which the lod score is not 100% maximized, but only to a specified tolerance. Clearly -0.0005 is almost the same as zero, so there is nothing to worry about from such results.

28.9 SLINK

The SIMULATE program provides a fast way of simulating pedigree data in a completely random fashion, but it does not allow the user to simulate marker loci conditional on previously known information, such as disease locus phenotypes or partially known marker information. To do a simulation under these more general conditions requires the use of far more sophisticated computer algorithms. The most versatile such program available to date is the SLINK program of Weeks and co-workers (1990b). This program employs an algorithm of Ott (1989) to simulate marker data by using complicated likelihood methods. Basically, SLINK uses the MLINK program to compute the conditional probabilities of each multilocus genotype (genotype risk) for any individual in a pedigree, given the known genotypes and phenotypes of the other pedigree members

$$P(g_i \mid x_1, \ldots, x_n) = P\frac{(x_1, \ldots, x_i, g_i; x_{i+1}, \ldots, x_n)}{P(x_1, \ldots, x_n)}$$

where the denominator is the likelihood of the entire set of pedigree data, and the numerator is the likelihood of the pedigree data given that individual i has genotype g_i. Both of these values can be computed with the MLINK program. The SLINK program uses the algorithm from the MLINK program to compute these probabilities for each multilocus genotype to be simulated in each individual, based on the model specified for each locus (including the disease and markers) and the recombination fractions between adjacent pairs of loci. Then, based on these conditional probabilities, the SLINK program selects pseudorandom numbers to simulate multilocus genotypes for each pedigree member, one at a time, each time conditioning the results on everything that has already been simulated. For example, for the second individual, the appropriate conditional probability is

$$P(g_j \mid x_1, \ldots, x_i, g_i, x_{i+1}, \ldots, x_n)$$

This conditioning procedure then continues iteratively for each successive individual, until the last individual is simulated according to the distribution of

$$P(g_n \mid x_1, g_1, x_2, g_2, \ldots, X_{n-1}, g_{n-1}, x_n)$$

In this way, the SLINK program can simulate multilocus genotypes conditional on all previously simulated or previously known genotypic information in a pedigree. Unfortunately, as a consequence of this repeated conditioning algorithm, the program can be very slow. Other approaches to simulating marker genotypes conditional on disease phenotypes have been implemented in the SIMLINK program (Boehnke, 1986) and the CHRSIM program (Terwilliger et al., 1993b; Speer et al., 1992). These programs are much faster than SLINK but are not as general; SLINK allows for the presence of partial marker typing, and the other methods do not. However, the CHRSIM program allows the user to perform simulations assuming map functions other than the Haldane function (i.e., allowing for interference), which is not possible with SIMLINK or SLINK. Furthermore, CHRSIM, SIMULATE, and SLINK allow the user to simulate the data under one model and analyze it under a different one; SIMLINK does not.

The SLINK program is easy to use and follows the same basic file format as SIMULATE with a couple of small differences. Because SLINK performs a simulation conditional on known phenotypes at any of the loci (including disease and/or marker loci, the pedigree file requires that you specify a genotype for each locus in each individual (specifying the UNKNOWN phenotype for all individuals to be simulated and the KNOWN marker or disease phenotype for individuals whom you wish to predetermine the phenotypes). Then, at the end of each line in the pedigree file, you must input a so-called *availability code,* which is an integer between 0 and 4, the meanings of which are indicated in Table 28–1. When the trait is selected to be AS INDICATED, the trait phenotypes will be fixed as they are indicated in the SIMPED.DAT file. Otherwise, they will be simulated according to the parameters in the SIMDATA.DAT file. Typically, the trait is assumed to be AS INDICATED, because you want to examine properties of the pedigrees as they have been collected, assuming linkage to a trait locus with known phenotypes. At the marker locus, there are two options as well. Either an individual will be considered unknown at ALL marker loci, including those for which phenotypes are given in SIMPED.DAT, or the individual will be assigned a phenotype at all marker loci. If a phenotype other than UNKNOWN is indicated in the SIMPED.DAT file for a given locus, that phenotype is used. Otherwise, the phenotype is simulated for that locus. These codes should be indicated after the last locus in the SIMPED.DAT file. For the schizophrenia data, if we wished to simulate the disease being between the two marker loci, we could make the disease locus the second locus in our SIMPED.DAT and SIMDATA.DAT files. Let us assume that the locus order is Marker 1-(0.08)-Disease-(0.057)-Marker 2. We wish to simulate conditional on known disease locus phenotypes, and to simulate marker genotypes for individuals who had *both* markers typed in the original data set, leaving all the markers unknown for individuals with zero or one marker typed in the original pedigrees. It is a limitation of SLINK that either all markers must be known or all markers unknown for a given individual, unlike in SIMULATE in which each marker can be specified independently. The individuals should have genotype *0 0* at

Table 28–1. Table of Definitions of Availability Codes for SLINK

Code	Trait	Markers
0	As indicated	Unknown (even if phenotypes are given)
1	Simulate	Simulate or use given phenotypes
2	As indicated	Simulate or use given phenotypes
3	Simulate	Unknown (even if phenotypes are given)

each of the marker loci (such that all genotypes would be simulated by SLINK). The SIMPED.DAT file also should not have the header lines required by the SIMULATE program, because they are not needed by SLINK. The SIMPED.DAT file should resemble the following (for pedigree 1):

```
1   1   0   0   3   0     0 2 0   0 0   2 1   0 0   2
1   2   0   0   3   0     0 1 0   0 0   1 1   0 0   2
1   3   2   1   0   4     4 2 0   0 0   2 3   0 0   2
1   4   2   1   0   5     5 1 0   0 0   2 1   0 0   2
1   5   2   1   0   6     6 1 0   0 0   2 1   0 0   2
1   6   2   1   0  10    10 1 2   0 0   2 1   0 0   2
1   7   0   0   9   0     0 1 1   0 0   0 1   0 0   0
1   8   0   0   9   0     0 2 0   0 0   0 1   0 0   0
1   9   7   8  12  11    11 2 0   0 0   1 1   0 0   2
1  10   2   1  15   0     0 2 0   0 0   2 1   0 0   2
1  11   7   8  15   0     0 1 0   0 0   1 1   0 0   2
1  12  17   9   0  13    13 1 0   0 0   1 1   0 0   2
1  13  17   9   0  14    14 1 0   0 0   1 1   0 0   2
1  14  17   9   0   0     0 1 0   0 0   2 1   0 0   2
1  15  11  10   0  16    16 1 0   0 0   1 1   0 0   2
1  16  11  10   0   0     0 1 0   0 0   2 1   0 0   2
1  17   0   0  12   0     0 1 2   0 0   2 1   0 0   2
```

Similarly, the SIMDATA.DAT file should be in standard MLINK format as shown below:

```
3 0 0 5   << NO. OF LOCI, RISK LOCUS, SEXLINKED (IF 1) PROGRAM
0 0.0 0.0 0 << MUT LOCUS, MUT MALE, MUT FEM, HAP FREQ (IF 1)
  1  2  3
3  2   << ALLELE NUMBERS, NO. OF ALLELES
 0.33 0.67
1  2   << AFFECTION, NO. OF ALLELES
 0.010000 0.990000   << GENE FREQUENCIES
 3 << NO. OF LIABILITY CLASSES
0.44 0.44 0.0166
0.44 0.44 0.0166
0.44 0.44 0.0166
3  3   << ALLELE NUMBERS, NO. OF ALLELES
 0.32 0.16 0.52
 0 0   << SEX DIFFERENCE, INTERFERENCE (IF 1 OR 2)
0.08 0.057
1 0.10000 0.45000 << REC VARIED, INCREMENT, FINISHING VALUE
```

One final input file, called SLINKIN.DAT, is required for the SLINK program, which contains the analysis parameters (note that SLINK does not require the PROBLEM.DAT file of SIMULATE, but rather this SLINKIN.DAT file). The file should consist of four lines as follows:

Line 1–*One* seed for the random number generator between 1 and 30000. As in SIMULATE, numbers over 25000 perform better.

Line 2–The number of replicates to be simulated

Line 3–The locus number of the trait locus (in our example, the trait locus is locus 2. You would input a 0 if there were no trait locus.)

Line 4–The proportion of unlinked families (if you want to allow for heterogeneity, input the value of $(1 - \alpha)$ here, where α is the proportion of linked families as defined in Section 6.3). Typically, this value is set to be 0 and assumes homogeneity in the simulation. (The properties of simulation under heterogeneity are beyond the scope of this book and are not discussed here.)

For our sample data set, let us again simulate 50 replicates of the pedigree set (though in practice, you typically simulate a much larger set of replicates to get more reliable results). The SLINKIN.DAT file should look like the following:

```
28733
50
2
0
```

To perform the simulation, type SLINK at the DOS prompt. Note that SLINK is incredibly slow, taking 33 hours of CPU time on a 486 PC, because each time a new individual is simulated the MLINK program must compute the conditional probability of each possible multilocus genotype for that individual. In fact, the SIMULATE program was developed precisely because incredible amounts of computer time are required for a SLINK analysis. Remember that simulating 50 replicates of the two linked markers (unlinked to the disease) takes a matter of only several seconds, whereas the identical simulation with SLINK takes on the order of 33 hours on a 486 PC. As a tradeoff for the increased computing time, however, much additional flexibility is available, allowing for both simulation conditional on the disease phenotypes and on previously typed marker data. For practice, you may want to try simulating only five replicates for now. We present the analysis results for both 5 and 50 replicates.

The file produced by SLINK is also called PEDFILE.DAT, as was the case with SIMULATE. Again, we have three loci in our simulated data, this time with the disease being locus 2, and the markers being loci 1 and 3. Because we initially want to perform two-point analysis of the data, you should rename the PEDFILE.DAT to SIM.PED. To analyze the data under the model we simulated for the disease and markers, copy the SIMDATA.DAT file to

Table 28–2. Results of MSIM and ISIM Analyses of Disease versus Marker 1 Based on Both 50 and 5 Replicates

θ	$E[Z(\theta)]_{50}$	$StdDev_{50}$	$E[Z(\theta)]_5$	$StdDev_5$
0	0.735496	1.166530	0.414042	1.062897
0.05	0.836342	0.977525	0.622942	0.863761
0.10	0.816879	0.820165	0.655215	0.738885
0.15	0.742267	0.675951	0.617683	0.622972
0.20	0.634117	0.540453	0.540525	0.508303
0.25	0.505767	0.412221	0.439205	0.394128
0.30	0.368617	0.292287	0.324957	0.282457
0.35	0.234871	0.184363	0.208760	0.177726
0.40	0.118823	0.094987	0.103985	0.087554
0.45	0.036177	0.032759	0.028154	0.023666
0.50	0.000000	0.000000	0.000000	0.000000

	$E[maxZ(\theta)]_{50}$	$StdDev_{50}$	$E[maxZ(\theta)]_5$	$StdDev_5$
MSIM	1.045271	0.822056	0.819046	0.582468
ISIM	1.059299	0.808330	0.818405	0.584770

	Observed Lod Scores Greater Than a Given Constant			
Constant	$Number_{50}$	$Percent_{50}$	$Number_5$	$Percent_5$
1	20	40	1	20
2.65	2	4	0	0
3	0	0	0	0

Table 28–3. Results of MSIM and ISIM Analyses of Disease versus Marker 2 Based on Both 50 and 5 Replicates

θ	$E[Z(\theta)]_{50}$	StdDev$_{50}$	$E[Z(\theta)]_5$	StdDev$_5$
0.00	1.344803	1.477235	0.926615	1.352813
0.05	1.578782	1.267425	1.276471	1.165699
0.10	1.555690	1.103191	1.351794	0.985503
0.15	1.428120	0.944638	1.299463	0.822139
0.20	1.236861	0.784552	1.165164	0.670369
0.25	1.004403	0.621787	0.974942	0.525907
0.30	0.749474	0.458352	0.749062	0.386712
0.35	0.493028	0.299932	0.508250	0.253790
0.40	0.261602	0.158164	0.278780	0.133944
0.45	0.087424	0.052783	0.096245	0.044466
0.50	0.000000	0.000000	0.000000	0.000000

	$E[\max Z(\theta)]_{50}$	StdDev$_{50}$	$E[\max Z(\theta)]_5$	StdDev$_5$
MSIM	1.751465	1.171508	1.471560	1.028230
ISIM	1.750680	1.169886	1.467988	1.031358

| | Observed Lod Scores Greater Than a Given Constant | | | |
Constant	Number$_{50}$	Percent$_{50}$	Number$_5$	Percent$_5$
1	36	72	2	40
2.65	11	22	1	20
3	7	14	1	20

SIM.DAT. Then use LSP to extract loci 1 and 2 from these files, setting up the parameter file for MLINK, with θ ranging from 0 through 0.5 in steps of 0.05. Run UNKNOWN, followed by MSIM, as you did in the previous section. Alter the DATAFILE.DAT file to put it in the proper format for ISIM, with a starting value of $\theta = 0.1$. The results should match those found in Table 28–2 (results given for both cases: 5 replicates and 50 replicates). Next, repeat the process for marker 2 (extract loci 2 and 3 from the SIM.PED file with LSP), the results for which are indicated in Table 28–3.

28.10 LSIM

A version of the LINKMAP program is designed to analyze simulated data from SLINK or SIMULATE. In both cases, we simulated multilocus data, so it may be of value to see the properties of the multipoint analysis in terms of expected multipoint lod score, and so on. To do this, use the original SIM.PED file (containing the disease and both markers) by copying it to PEDFILE.DAT. Then modify the SIMDATA.DAT file so it is in LINKMAP format. The file should specify that the locus order is 2 1 3, meaning that the disease starts outside the set of linked marker loci on the right, as is usually the case in a LINKMAP analysis. Then, the recombination fractions are set to 0.5 (because the disease should start out unlinked to the markers) and 0.128 (the recombination fraction between the two markers). Finally, specify that the trait locus is locus 2, with 5 evaluations per interval and a finishing value of 0 (this number is irrelevant to the analysis but is required in the parameter file). The final version of this parameter file should look like this:

```
3 0 0 5 << NO. OF LOCI, RISK LOCUS, SEXLINKED (IF 1) PROGRAM
 0 0.0 0.0 0 << MUT LOCUS, MUT MALE, MUT FEM, HAP FREQ (IF 1)
  2  1  3
3  2  << ALLELE NUMBERS, NO. OF ALLELES
 0.33 0.67
1  2  << AFFECTION, NO. OF ALLELES
 0.010000 0.990000  << GENE FREQUENCIES
 3 << NO. OF LIABILITY CLASSES
0.44 0.44 0.0166
0.44 0.44 0.0166
0.44 0.44 0.0166
 3  3  << ALLELE NUMBERS, NO. OF ALLELES
 0.32 0.16 0.52
 0 0  << SEX DIFFERENCE, INTERFERENCE (IF 1 OR 2)
0.50 0.128
 2  0  5 << LOCUS VARIED, FINISHING VALUE, NU OF EVALUATIONS
```

Save this file as DATAFILE.DAT and run the UNKNOWN program followed by the LSIM program. The resulting expected lod scores are given in Table 28–4. If there is linkage, the multipoint lod scores are typically much higher than the two-point lod scores from the same data set. In this situation our ELOD is 2.25, which is substantially higher than the ELOD from either two-point linkage analysis, because there are many more informative meioses for linkage when both markers are typed. It is perhaps more striking to look at the power of these pedigrees. If we examine the probability of finding a lod score greater than 3, we note that with the more informative marker (marker 2), the probability of exceeding a lod score of 3 in two-point analysis was 0.14, and with marker 1 the probability was approximately 0. However, in the three-point LSIM analysis, the probability of getting a multipoint lod score greater

Table 28–4. Results of LSIM Analysis of Disease versus Fixed Map of Two Linked Markers in Replicates Simulated with SLINK in File SIM.PED

Locus Order	$E[Z(x)]_{50}$	StdDev$_{50}$	$E[Z(x)]_5$	StdDev$_5$
2-0.500-*1*-0.128-*3*	0.000000	0.000000	0.000000	0.000000
2-0.400-*1*-0.128-*3*	0.254666	0.133885	0.236215	0.106462
2-0.300-*1*-0.128-*3*	0.767525	0.405632	0.674440	0.293006
2-0.200-*1*-0.128-*3*	1.330319	0.719721	1.109016	0.484413
2-0.100-*1*-0.128-*3*	1.783796	1.039690	1.378166	0.694069
2-0.000-*1*-0.128-*3*	1.888853	1.399177	1.175593	1.087273
1-0.000-*2*-0.128-*3*	1.888853	1.399177	1.175593	1.087273
1-0.026-*2*-0.108-*3*	2.104250	1.369755	1.422980	0.997804
1-0.051-*2*-0.086-*3*	2.208696	1.376830	1.530529	1.034229
1-0.077-*2*-0.060-*3*	2.249394	1.405504	1.561322	1.107357
1-0.102-*2*-0.032-*3*	2.211023	1.457537	1.502997	1.208236
1-0.128-*2*-0.000-*3*	1.961298	1.549443	1.251705	1.329041
1-0.128-*3*-0.000-*2*	1.961298	1.549443	1.251705	1.329041
1-0.128-*3*-0.100-*2*	2.047632	1.148514	1.630032	1.027003
1-0.128-*3*-0.200-*2*	1.574862	0.817627	1.356377	0.700748
1-0.128-*3*-0.300-*2*	0.932305	0.477947	0.848989	0.405352
1-0.128-*3*-0.400-*2*	0.316440	0.164488	0.305904	0.143177
1-0.128-*3*-0.500-*2*	0.000000	0.000000	0.000000	0.000000

	Observed Lod Scores Greater Than a Given Constant			
Constant	*Number*$_{50}$	*Percent*$_{50}$	*Number*$_5$	*Percent*$_5$
1	46	92	4	80
2.65	21	42	1	20
3	18	36	1	20

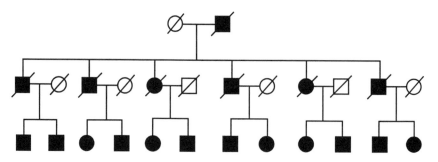

Figure 28–3. Pedigree to be simulated to show the effect of gene frequencies

than 3 was raised to 0.36. Although this is still not enough power to encourage a linkage analysis with these pedigrees and these markers alone, it is substantially better than the power of 0.14 with just marker 2. This increase in information can also be taken advantage of through the polylocus method of Terwilliger and Ott (1993), in the case of complex disease analysis, without the need to rely on the nonrobust and time-consuming process of multipoint analysis.

It is also the case that when there is no linkage in reality, the multipoint lod scores tend to be lower than the two-point lod scores, and the ability to do exclusion mapping is enhanced by multipoint analysis but *only* if the model is known with accuracy. In this case, we did simulation on a data set that is segregating a complex disorder for which the model is not accurately known. We do not consider multipoint results for the simulation with the disease unlinked to the markers, because it is of little meaning with a truly complex disease (cf. Section 25.3).

☐ Exercise 28

Use SLINK to simulate marker 1 from the schizophrenia data set under the recessive model, diagnostic scheme 3, and linked to the disease at $\theta = 0.05$. Then, analyze it under the dominant model for diagnostic scheme 3. Next, simulate the same marker, again at $\theta = 0.05$ from the disease, under the dominant model for diagnostic scheme 3 and analyze the data, assuming the recessive model for the same diagnostic class. Do the results of this experiment confirm what was discussed in Chapter 17 about analysis under the incorrect model?

Finally, to demonstrate the effect of gene frequencies on a linkage analysis, use the SIMULATE program to simulate 100 replicates of an unlinked marker to the fully penetrant dominant disease ($p = 0.00001$) in the family in Figure 28–3. Simulate the marker under the assumption that there are five alleles with gene frequencies 0.05, 0.05, 0.05, 0.05, and 0.80. All symbols with a slash (/) through them represent dead individuals, who therefore should not be simulated (i.e., they should all be assigned genotype *0 0* at the marker locus). Then, analyze the pedigree, assuming equal gene frequencies for all five alleles. Is there false-positive evidence for linkage in this example?

29.□

Solutions to the Exercises in Part III

□ **Exercise 21**

Assuming the disease in the pedigree from Exercise 6 is a fully penetrant, sex-linked, recessive, lethal disorder, the mutation rate must be $p/2 = 0.01/2 = 0.005$ in this example. Reanalyzing this pedigree allowing for $\mu = 0.005$ yields the results shown in Table 29–1. Comparing these results with those obtained when mutation was not allowed for (see Table 12–6) you see that there is negligible difference between the two situations. This is due primarily to the large density of affected individuals in this pedigree, which makes it much more likely that the disease allele is segregating than that a new mutation occurred at some point in the pedigree. Hence, allowing for mutation has little effect on the analysis, as explained in Chapter 21.

In the pedigree from Exercise 7, there is a fully penetrant recessive disease with $p = 0.001$. As explained in that chapter, at equilibrium, $\mu = sp^2$, so in that case, $\mu = sp^2 = (0.5)(0.001)^2 = 0.0000005$. Incorporating this information in the linkage analysis leads to the results shown in Table 29–2. Again, due to the high density of affected persons in this pedigree, allowing for the possibility of mutation has little effect, with extremely slight reductions in lod score. Furthermore, in this case, the mutation rate is 2000 times smaller than the gene frequency, which is minute. This is typically the case with autosomal recessive disorders in contrast to the sex-linked case, in which the mutation rate is as large as half the gene frequency.

To design an experiment to determine the types of mutation allowed for in the LINKAGE programs, we could do the following: Set up a pedigree with an internal inconsistency as shown in Figure 29–1. Now, assume that the disease is autosomal recessive with full penetrance and gene frequency of 0.01; the marker locus has four alleles with equal frequencies. In Figure 29–1, the mother has marker genotype x/x, and her daughter has genotype $1/y$, meaning that she had to have received the y allele from her mother (because her father was homozygous $1/1$. Clearly, whenever $x \neq y$, there is an inconsistency, and our lod scores are all $-\infty$. However, if we allow for mutation rate μ at the **marker** locus, we should get lod scores of 0 everywhere (because there is obviously no information for linkage in this little pedigree, yet the inconsistency is eliminated), whenever allele x is allowed to mutate into allele y with

Table 29–1. Results of Analysis of Sex-linked Recessive Disease Pedigree from Exercise 6, Allowing for $\mu = 0.005$

θ	Lod Score
0.0	-0.234382
0.1	-0.170833
0.2	-0.021145
0.3	0.010842
0.4	-0.019488
0.5	0.000000

ILINK: $\hat{\theta} = 0.862$; $Z(\hat{\theta}) = 0.554451$.

probability μ. If mutation is allowed in all directions, then we always get lod scores of 0 in this pedigree, never lod scores of $-\infty$. To determine which types of mutation are allowed, analyze this pedigree, allowing for mutation rate $\mu = 0.001$ at the marker locus (locus 2 in this example) and assuming all possible combinations of x and $y \in \{1,2,3,4\}$. Then compute the lod score at recombination fraction $\theta = 0.1$ (without loss of generality). The results should match those shown in Table 29–3. This demonstrates that the only types of mutation allowed in the LINKAGE programs are from any allele to the last (i.e., highest numbered) allele at the locus. You can verify this for other locus types and other numbers of alleles, but it is the general solution that mutations to the last (i.e., highest numbered) allele at any locus are the only ones permitted in this implementation of mutation. It is primarily for this reason that we typically specify the second allele to be the disease-predisposing one at an affection status locus, so we could allow for mutations to the disease allele and not away from it.

☐ Exercise 22

In this pedigree, you first need to extract the disease locus and the ABO blood group locus from the files USEREX8.* with LSP. Then, you must modify the DATAFILE.DAT file as explained in Chapter 22 to estimate allele frequencies for the ABO locus. There are two different ways of doing this. The first is to set the recombination fraction between disease and ABO to 0.5 and estimate allele frequencies, in which case you get estimates of 0.288, 0.343, and 0.369 for the *A, B,* and *O* alleles, respectively. The second is to estimate them jointly with the recombination fraction, in which case the estimates are revised slightly to 0.277, 0.341, and 0.382, respectively, with a recombination fraction

Table 29–2. Results of Analysis of Autosomal Recessive Disease Pedigree from Exercise 7, Assuming $\mu = 0.0000005$

θ	Lod Score
0.0	3.130937
0.1	2.336976
0.2	1.535554
0.3	0.794584
0.4	0.270785
0.5	0.000000

ILINK: $\hat{\theta} = 0.001$; $Z(\hat{\theta}) = 3.125540$.

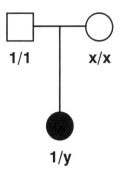

Figure 29–1. Pedigree with internal inconsistency for mutation experiment

$\hat{\theta} = 0.001$. Now, there are three possible ways to compute lod scores, given these gene frequency estimates. The first approach is to consider

$$Z(\hat{\theta}) = \log_{10}\left[\frac{L(\hat{\theta},\hat{p}_i)}{L(\theta = \frac{1}{2},\hat{p}_i)}\right]$$

where the $\hat{p}_i$ are estimated jointly with the recombination fraction in the numerator and kept the same in the denominator. In this case the lod score (at $\theta = 0$) is equal to 3.459960. Another possible approach is to compute lod scores using the gene frequency estimates obtained when the disease was considered to be unlinked to the marker (i.e., do the estimation of allele frequencies in the denominator and use these same estimates in the numerator), in which case the lod score is $Z(\theta = 0) = 3.454484$. The best way to compute this lod score, however, is to treat the gene frequency estimates as nuisance parameters and compute the lod score with separate estimates of the p_i in numerator and denominator as

$$\log_{10}[L(\hat{\theta},\hat{p}_i)] - \log_{10}[L\left(\theta = \frac{1}{2}, \hat{p}_i\right)]$$

where the $\hat{p}_i$ are separately estimated in each term. In this case, the resulting lod score is $(-23.299604) - (-26.756902) = 3.457298$. In this example the lod scores are not greatly affected by the changes in gene frequency estimates at ABO, but in some cases they can be quite significant, so this procedure is usually advisable when accurate allele frequency estimates are unavailable.

Consider the example from Exercise 9 in which a reduced penetrance model is applied to the same pedigree. Reestimate the allele frequencies and

Table 29–3. Lod Scores $Z(\theta = 0.1)$ for Pedigree in Figure 29–1, Assuming that $\mu = 0.001$ at the Marker Locus

	y			
x	1	2	3	4
1	0.0	$-\infty$	$-\infty$	0.0
2	$-\infty$	0.0	$-\infty$	0.0
3	$-\infty$	$-\infty$	0.0	0.0
4	$-\infty$	$-\infty$	$-\infty$	0.0

you obtain identical gene frequency estimates of 0.288, 0.343, and 0.369 for the *A, B,* and *O* alleles, respectively when the disease and marker are assumed to be unlinked. This is true because the estimation of allele frequency is done essentially independently of the disease phenotypes in the pedigree. When we estimate the allele frequencies jointly with recombination fraction, however, we obtain estimates of 0.277, 0.341, and 0.382, which are again identical to those estimated with the full penetrance model. This is not typically the case unless there is little ambiguity as to the disease locus genotypes of the founder individuals, which is clearly the case in this pedigree. The three lod scores, as computed above, are now as follows: using the gene frequency estimates obtained when $\theta = \hat{\theta}$, we get $Z(\theta = 0) = 2.172223$; using the gene frequency estimates obtained under $\theta = \frac{1}{2}$, we get $Z(\theta = 0) = 2.166747$; and finally, separately estimating the gene frequencies in each term, we get $Z(\theta = 0) = (-25.497910) - (-27.667471) = 2.169561$, which is again right between the two lod scores computed with fixed gene frequency estimates.

☐ Exercise 23

First you need to compute the genotype probabilities in terms of haplotype probabilities for use in the EH program, assuming one four-allele locus and one three-allele locus. These frequencies are given in Table 29–4.

The data set from Table 23–10 should yield the following results from the EH program:

Estimates of Gene Frequencies (Assuming Independence)

locus \ allele	1	2	3	4
1	0.2236	0.3650	0.4114	
2	0.3439	0.1857	0.1730	0.2975

# of Typed Individuals: 237

There are 12 Possible Haplotypes of These 2 Loci.
They are Listed Below, with their Estimated Frequencies:

Allele at Locus 1	Allele at Locus 2	Haplotype Frequency Independent	w/Association
1	1	0.076902	0.106861
1	2	0.041518	0.038783
1	3	0.038687	0.045654
1	4	0.066522	0.032331
2	1	0.125510	0.149313
2	2	0.067760	0.077541
2	3	0.063140	0.048721
2	4	0.108570	0.089404
3	1	0.141470	0.087708
3	2	0.076377	0.069330
3	3	0.071169	0.078621
3	4	0.122376	0.175734

# of Iterations = 7

	df	ln(L)	χ^2
H0 : No Association	5	−983.22	0.00
H1 : Allelic Associations Allowed	11	−965.53	35.37

Table 29–4. Table of Genotype Probabilities for One Three-allele Marker and One Four-allele Marker

	1/1	*1/2*	*2/2*	*1/3*	*2/3*	*3/3*
1/1	P_{11}^2	$2P_{11}P_{12}$	P_{12}^2	$2P_{11}P_{13}$	$2P_{12}P_{13}$	P_{13}^2
1/2	$2P_{11}P_{21}$	$2(P_{11}P_{22} + P_{12}P_{21})$	$2P_{12}P_{22}$	$2(P_{11}P_{23} + P_{13}P_{21})$	$2(P_{12}P_{23} + P_{13}P_{22})$	$2P_{13}P_{23}$
2/2	P_{21}^2	$2P_{21}P_{22}$	P_{22}^2	$2P_{21}P_{23}$	$2P_{22}P_{23}$	P_{23}^2
1/3	$2P_{11}P_{31}$	$2(P_{11}P_{32} + P_{12}P_{31})$	$2P_{12}P_{32}$	$2(P_{11}P_{33} + P_{13}P_{31})$	$2(P_{12}P_{33} + P_{13}P_{32})$	$2P_{13}P_{33}$
2/3	$2P_{21}P_{31}$	$2(P_{21}P_{32} + P_{22}P_{31})$	$2P_{22}P_{32}$	$2(P_{21}P_{33} + P_{23}P_{31})$	$2(P_{22}P_{33} + P_{23}P_{32})$	$2P_{23}P_{33}$
3/3	P_{31}^2	$2P_{31}P_{32}$	P_{32}^2	$2P_{31}P_{33}$	$2P_{32}P_{33}$	P_{33}^2
1/4	$2P_{11}P_{41}$	$2(P_{11}P_{42} + P_{12}P_{41})$	$2P_{12}P_{42}$	$2(P_{11}P_{43} + P_{13}P_{41})$	$2(P_{12}P_{43} + P_{13}P_{42})$	$2P_{13}P_{43}$
2/4	$2P_{21}P_{41}$	$2(P_{21}P_{42} + P_{22}P_{41})$	$2P_{22}P_{42}$	$2(P_{21}P_{43} + P_{23}P_{41})$	$2(P_{22}P_{43} + P_{23}P_{42})$	$2P_{23}P_{43}$
3/4	$2P_{31}P_{41}$	$2(P_{31}P_{42} + P_{32}P_{41})$	$2P_{32}P_{42}$	$2(P_{31}P_{43} + P_{33}P_{41})$	$2(P_{32}P_{43} + P_{33}P_{42})$	$2P_{33}P_{43}$
4/4	P_{41}^2	$2P_{41}P_{42}$	P_{42}^2	$2P_{41}P_{43}$	$2P_{42}P_{43}$	P_{43}^2

P_{ij} is the haplotype frequency for allele i at the four-allele marker and allele j at the three-allele marker

In this case, there were 5 free parameters under the assumption of linkage equilibrium and 11 under the assumption of allelic association. Therefore, our chi-square statistic 35.37 has $(11 - 5) = 6$ df and is significant at the 0.000004 level, indicating that some association exists between the alleles of these two loci. If we consider only the unambiguous haplotypes and simply count them up, we fill a 4×3 table like that shown in Table 29–5. A chi-square test of independence on this table produces the chi-square statistic of 30.07 with 6 df corresponding to a *p*-value of 0.000038, which is still highly significant. However, our new haplotype frequency estimates (computed as k_i/n for each cell) are given in Table 29–6. These estimates are somewhat different from those obtained using the EH program but not dramatically so.

In the pedigree from Exercise 8, there are only six founder individuals, three of whom are untyped at the marker locus. Therefore, there is not likely to be much power to estimate haplotype frequencies. For simplicity assume that all 12 haplotype frequencies are 0.08 as starting values (with the last frequency set to 0.12 so they sum to 1). The estimated haplotype frequencies and corresponding lod scores are given in Table 29–7 with lod scores provided, assuming both first that the haplotype frequencies are estimated only in the numerator (then fixed in the denominator) of the likelihood ratio and again with the frequencies are estimated separately in numerator and denominator.

☐ Exercise 24

With the simplifying assumptions that all parents are unaffected and the disease is fully penetrant recessive, we know that every parent is heterozygous for the disease allele, and we can therefore attempt to estimate the haplotype

Table 29–5. Haplotypes Unequivocally Determinable from Genotype Data Given in Table 23–10

	Allele at Locus 2			
Allele at Locus 1	*1*	*2*	*3*	*4*
1	42	14	13	12
2	58	25	16	31
3	37	26	29	63

Table 29–6. Haplotype Frequencies Estimated from Data in Table 29–5

Allele at Locus 1	Allele at Locus 2			
	1	*2*	*3*	*4*
1	0.115	0.038	0.036	0.033
2	0.158	0.068	0.044	0.085
3	0.101	0.071	0.079	0.172

frequencies with the EH program. Do not use the case-control option to make your estimations, but rather enter every parent as if he or she was heterozygous (*1/2*) at the first locus and treat the *H* allele and the $\overline{H}$ allele as alleles *1* and *2*, respectively, at the second locus. Then, we have *A 1/1* haplotypes, (*B* + *C*) *1/2* haplotypes, and *D 2/2* haplotypes in our parental sample. When we run the EH program using the data from Section 24.6, we have *A* = 19, (*B* + *C*) = 52, and *D* = 29. Our output tells us that there is no evidence for any allelic association whatsoever, because everyone is heterozygous *1/2* at the disease locus. It is therefore impossible to discern the phase. However, if we construct pedigrees that match the data and analyze the data with the ILINK program, we might be able to use the offspring genotypes to reconstruct the phases in the parents. Remember in Chapter 24 we showed that nuclear pedigrees with one offspring *do* contain linkage information when there is disequilibrium, but we haven't discussed the reverse situation. Let us do so now. Although we had separate information for the GHRR and HHRR tests collected from the same pedigree set, because the disease is fully penetrant recessive and the parents are unaffected, we only need to match the data in our pedigrees with that provided for the HHRR test. For simplicity's sake, assume there are 9 pedigrees of the structure $HH \times HH \rightarrow HH$, 1 pedigree of the form $HH \times H\overline{H} \rightarrow HH$, 20 of the form $H\overline{H} \times H\overline{H} \rightarrow HH$, 1 of the form $H\overline{H} \times \overline{H}\overline{H} \rightarrow HH$, 5 of the form $H\overline{H} \times H\overline{H} \rightarrow \overline{H}\overline{H}$, and 14 pedigrees of the form $\overline{H}\overline{H} \times \overline{H}\overline{H} \rightarrow \overline{H}\overline{H}$. Then you can run this analysis with ILINK, estimating haplotype frequencies and recombination fraction jointly. First as-

Table 29–7. Haplotype Frequency Estimates from Pedigree in Exercise 8 for Marker 1 versus ABO Blood Group

Haplotype	Haplotype Frequency					
	$\theta = 0.5$	$\theta = 0.4$	$\theta = 0.3$	$\theta = 0.2$	$\theta = 0.1$	$\hat{\theta} = 0.22$
1 A	0.090	0.090	0.090	0.090	0.091	0.090
1 B	0.094	0.094	0.094	0.093	0.092	0.094
1 O	0.095	0.095	0.095	0.095	0.093	0.095
2 A	0.090	0.090	0.088	0.090	0.091	0.090
2 B	0.095	0.095	0.094	0.094	0.093	0.094
2 O	0.082	0.082	0.084	0.082	0.081	0.082
3 A	0.092	0.092	0.094	0.092	0.093	0.092
3 B	0.087	0.087	0.088	0.087	0.088	0.087
3 O	0.102	0.102	0.102	0.101	0.102	0.102
4 A	0.089	0.089	0.087	0.089	0.091	0.089
4 B	0.084	0.084	0.085	0.084	0.084	0.084
4 O	0.000	0.000	0.000	0.002	0.001	0.000
$Z(\theta)$	0.000	0.416	0.760	0.886	0.459	0.898
$-2 \ln L(\theta)$	126.9	125.0	123.3	123.0	125.0	122.8
$Z(\theta, \delta)$	0.000	0.413	0.782	0.848	0.413	0.891

Lod scores are provided both given the estimated haplotype frequencies and given haplotype frequencies are estimated separately in numerator and denominator

sume starting values of 0.4, 0.1, 0.1, and 0.4 for the four haplotype frequencies and 0.1 for the recombination fraction. Use the new estimates as starting values to refine them. Repeat this process two additional times, and the resulting haplotype frequency estimates should be 0.1448, 0.3548, 0.3055, and 0.1949, with $\theta = 0.001$, a lod score of 4.58, and $-2 \ln(\text{Like}) = 531.44$. This lod score, however, is not meaningful to us, because it assumes the same haplotype frequencies under the null hypothesis as well. To be fully accurate reestimate them when $\theta = 0.5$. When this is done, the corresponding haplotype frequency estimates are 0.2807, 0.2192, 0.1692, and 0.3308, with $-2 \ln(\text{Like}) = 552.26$. The overall lod score is therefore

$$\frac{552.26 - 531.44}{4.6} = 4.53$$

which is actually almost the same as with the other haplotype frequency estimates. This similarity occurs because, under the null hypothesis of free recombination, the haplotype frequencies have much less influence on the pedigree likelihood. So far, we have determined a lod score, evaluating our evidence for linkage, but we have yet to test the significance of our disequilibrium. To do this, we need to maximize the likelihood over allele frequencies for each locus, assuming absence of allelic association. The best estimate for the disease allele frequency is 0.5 (which makes sense because we know that every founder is heterozygous for the disease allele), and 0.45 is the best estimate for the *H* allele at the marker locus (coded as the *1* allele in the data files). The likelihood is now going to be independent of the recombination fraction, because phase-unknown pedigrees with only one offspring are uninformative for linkage in the absence of linkage disequilibrium. Therefore, we can calculate the appropriate likelihood with the ILINK program, fixing $\theta = 0.1$, without loss of generality to get $-2 \ln(\text{Like}) = 552.51$. Now, we know that the difference in $-2 \ln(\text{Like})$ is distributed as a chi-square statistic, in this case with 1 df. We have $552.51 - 531.44 = 21.07$, which is significant at the 0.000004 level, so there is very significant evidence for linkage disequilibrium in this parametric analysis. One problem remains, however; we drastically overestimated the disease allele frequency in every case. Consider the haplotype frequencies estimated with ILINK as summarized in Table 29–8. In this table, the "normalized" haplotype frequencies are also provided. These are computed as explained in Section 24.7, given the known disease allele frequency of 0.01. It is always required that you reevaluate the likelihoods and significance level of your test given this constraint, which you applied a posteriori. In this case, reanalyzing the data should have no effect on the significance level of either test, because all genotypes are known with certainty. To demonstrate this note that the lod score at $\theta = 0.001$ is still 4.58, with

Table 29–8. Haplotype Frequency Estimates from HHRR Pedigrees Computed with ILINK and Normalized to Fit the Known Population Gene Frequency of the Disease Allele, $p = 0.01$

Haplotype	$\theta = \hat{\theta}$ Estimated	Normalized	$\theta = 0.5$ Estimated	Normalized
d H	0.3055	0.006105	0.1692	0.003384
d H	0.1949	0.003985	0.3308	0.006616
+ H	0.1448	0.2869	0.2807	0.5558
+ H	0.3548	0.7031	0.2193	0.4342

$-2 \ln(\text{Like}) = 1177.23$. At $\theta = 0.5$, $-2 \ln(\text{Like}) = 1198.04$. The difference is 20.81, corresponding to a lod score of 4.5 as before. The test for linkage disequilibrium as well maintains its significance. To test this compute the likelihood, assuming the disease allele frequency to be 0.01 and the H allele frequency to be 0.45, again at $\theta = 0.1$, without loss of generality. In this case $-2 \ln(\text{Like}) = 1198.30$, for a chi-square statistic of $1198.30 - 1177.23 = 21.07$, exactly as before. In general pedigrees, however, the significance of your statistics may change dramatically after normalization of the haplotype frequencies, and they may no longer be optimal either, given the additional constraint on the disease allele frequency.

☐ Exercise 25

The analysis parameters for the six models to be considered are computed as shown in Table 29–9. The results of the linkage analysis of the schizophrenia pedigrees under these six models are shown in Table 29–10. As you can see, the maximized–over–models maximum lod score is quite a lot larger (2.937), which would be almost significant in a single-model analysis with a simple mendelian disorder, but we should use a cutoff point of $5 + \log_{10}(m)$, where m is the number of models tested. Here, again $m = 6$, so our cutoff point is 5.78, and we are only halfway to a significant lod score in this analysis.

The affecteds-only analysis was done assuming the penetrances $P(\text{Aff}|\text{Genotype})$ were all divided by 1000, making "unaffected" individuals essentially unknown in the analysis, because the penetrance ratio for unaffected persons f_p/f is approximately equal to 1. The results of this analysis are shown in Table 29–11 and are typically less significant than the regular analysis done before (Table 29–10). The most striking change occurs under the recessive model with marker 2, in which highly negative lod scores and estimates of $\hat{\theta} = 0.5$ were changed to slightly positive lod scores in the affecteds-only analysis, with corresponding reductions in the estimate of $\hat{\theta}$. This is especially noticeable under the broad diagnostic class, which had a penetrance of 0.96 for susceptible genotypes in the regular analysis. This translated into a penetrance ratio in unaffected individuals of $k = 24.5$, which made unaffected persons particularly informative for linkage. Eliminating this information led to slightly positive lod scores and $\hat{\theta} = 0.05$. Thus, you can see the potential perils of putting too much emphasis on unaffected individuals when you are dealing with a disease of uncertain diagnosis and mode of inheritance.

The analysis parameters for the diagnostic uncertainty model are presented in Table 29–12, and the output from that linkage analysis is given in Table 29–13. In this case our maximum lod score dropped to 2.054 (a loss of 0.883), whereas the number of models was reduced by two, causing our critical value to drop to $5 + \log_{10}(2) = 5.3$, a drop of 0.4 units. Although more

Table 29–9. Penetrance Models Used in Exercise 25

Model	Diagnosis	φ	R	p	f	f_P	k
Dominant	Narrow	0.005	0.1	0.01	0.23	0.0005	0.0023
	Medium	0.01	0.35	0.01	0.33	0.0036	0.0109
	Broad	0.03	0.50	0.01	0.75	0.015	0.0203
Recessive	Narrow	0.005	0.1	0.125	0.288	0.0005	0.0018
	Medium	0.01	0.35	0.125	0.416	0.0036	0.0085
	Broad	0.03	0.50	0.125	0.96	0.0152	0.0158

Table 29–10. Results of Linkage Analysis of Schizophrenia Pedigrees Using the Penetrance Models in Table 29–9

Diagnosis	θ	Dominant Lod Scores				Recessive Lod Scores			
		Marker 1		*Marker 2*		*Marker 1*		*Marker 2*	
Narrow	0	1.649		−0.580		0.584		−1.503	
	0.1	1.266		0.630		0.751		−0.639	
	0.2	0.819		0.720		0.546		−0.269	
	0.3	0.395		0.469		0.275		−0.093	
	0.4	0.098		0.147		0.072		−0.020	
ILINK:	0.001	1.646	0.164	0.743	0.071	0.765	0.500	0.000	
Medium	0	2.239		0.770		0.945		−0.993	
	0.1	1.818		1.613		1.200		−0.351	
	0.2	1.206		1.389		0.874		−0.117	
	0.3	0.603		0.835		0.447		−0.034	
	0.4	0.158		0.249		0.119		−0.008	
ILINK:	0.001	2.238	0.109	1.615	0.072	1.227	0.500	0.000	
Broad	0	2.937		1.143		0.970		−5.767	
	0.1	2.518		2.584		2.066		−1.800	
	0.2	1.776		2.234		1.746		−0.666	
	0.3	0.963		1.406		1.016		−0.222	
	0.4	0.276		0.462		0.301		−0.048	
ILINK:	0.003	2.937	0.107	2.586	0.108	2.069	0.500	0.000	

Table 29–11. Results of Affecteds-only Linkage Analysis of Schizophrenia Pedigrees Based on the Penetrance Models in Table 29–9

Diagnosis	θ	Dominant Lod Scores				Recessive Lod Scores			
		Marker 1		*Marker 2*		*Marker 1*		*Marker 2*	
Narrow	0	1.625		0.095		0.675		−0.651	
	0.1	1.231		0.693		0.625		−0.280	
	0.2	0.782		0.632		0.421		−0.119	
	0.3	0.372		0.377		0.208		−0.041	
	0.4	0.092		0.112		0.055		−0.009	
ILINK:	0.001	1.623	0.127	0.709	0.029	0.693	0.500	0.000	
Medium	0	2.003		0.951		0.909		−0.168	
	0.1	1.530		1.212		0.763		−0.017	
	0.2	0.982		0.954		0.494		0.016	
	0.3	0.476		0.529		0.239		0.013	
	0.4	0.121		0.146		0.062		0.003	
ILINK:	0.001	2.000	0.079	1.118	0.003	0.909	0.238	0.017	
Broad	0	2.249		1.335		0.996		0.268	
	0.1	1.721		1.360		0.924		0.279	
	0.2	1.124		1.025		0.625		0.195	
	0.3	0.563		0.564		0.312		0.099	
	0.4	0.150		0.162		0.083		0.026	
ILINK:	0.003	2.246	0.050	1.415	0.030	1.025	0.050	0.297	

Table 29–12. Penetrance Models for Dominant and Recessive Analysis with Certainty of Diagnosis Parameters p_i from Exercise 25

Diagnostic Class	p_i	Dominant			Recessive		
		f	f_P	*k*	*f*	f_P	*k*
1	0.99	.333	.0135	.0405	.418	.0135	.0323
2	0.80	.398	.2022	.5080	.450	.2022	.4493
3	0.65	.449	.3511	.7820	.475	.3511	.7392

Table 29–13. Results of Linkage Analysis of Schizophrenia Pedigrees with Penetrance Models Outlined in Table 29–12

	θ	Dominant Lod Scores				Recessive Lod Scores			
		Marker 1		*Marker 2*		*Marker 1*		*Marker 2*
	0	2.057		0.948		1.338		−0.950
	0.1	1.606		1.327		1.217		−0.433
	0.2	1.051		1.088		0.823		−0.185
	0.3	0.518		0.629		0.406		−0.068
	0.4	0.133		0.185		0.106		−0.015
ILINK:	0.001	2.054	0.093	1.328	0.025	1.360	0.500	0.000

information was lost in this example from the combining of the diagnostic criteria, there is still a great reduction in computing time and roughly the same degree of significance in the results.

☐ Exercise 26

Analysis with the ESPA program is very straightforward. The results are shown in Table 29–14 for marker locus 1 and in Table 29–15 for marker locus 2. Clearly, the broad diagnostic scheme provides the most significant result, whereas the narrowest diagnostic class shows almost no evidence for linkage. The total *p*-value under the broad diagnostic class with marker 1 is 0.0002, which looks very significant. However, if we assume a *p*-value of 0.00001 is required to declare a linkage significant, and we try three models, we need to divide that *p*-value by 3 to find the critical limit of 0.0000033. In this example, however, we also considered two separate loci as well, so we divide the critical *p*-value by 2 again (for the two loci tested) to get an overall critical value of 0.0000017. By this criterion, we are not even close to getting a significant result, but this is still an interesting finding that corroborates our highest lod score (which also occurred in the broad diagnostic class). If we consider only the fully known sibships (i.e., all parents and sibs typed, so IBD status can be uniquely determined), then under the broad criterion we have *p*-values of around 0.001 for each marker. Similarly for all three diagnostic schemes, the *p*-values are always less than 0.05 with each marker when only completely known sibships were used. This is the most robust portion of the analysis and

Table 29–14. ESPA Results for Schizophrenia Pedigrees with Disease versus Marker 1

Diagnosis	Analyzed Sibships	Not Shared	Shared	CHI	*p*
BROAD	Completely known	4.00	19.00	9.78	0.0009
	Unknown parents	8.00	16.82	3.14	0.0383
	Unknown sib	0.00	0.88	0.88	0.1744
	TOTAL	12.00	36.70	12.53	0.0002
MEDIUM	Completely known	3.00	9.00	3.00	0.0416
	Unknown parents	7.00	16.53	3.86	0.0248
	Unknown sib	0.00	0.88	0.88	0.1744
	TOTAL	10.00	26.41	7.39	0.0036
NARROW	Completely known	3.00	9.00	3.00	0.0416
	Unknown parents	5.00	8.71	1.01	0.1580
	Unknown sib	0.00	0.88	0.88	0.1744
	TOTAL	8.00	18.59	4.22	0.0200

Table 29–15. ESPA Results for Schizophrenia Pedigrees with Disease versus Marker 2

Diagnosis	Analyzed Sibships	Not Shared	Shared	CHI	*p*
BROAD	Completely known	6.00	22.00	9.14	0.0013
	Unknown parents	20.00	18.06	0.10	0.6239
	Unknown sib	0.00	0.56	0.56	0.2269
	TOTAL	26.00	40.62	3.21	0.0367
MEDIUM	Completely known	4.00	12.00	4.00	0.0228
	Unknown parents	18.00	15.44	0.20	0.6714
	Unknown sib	0.00	0.56	0.56	0.2269
	TOTAL	22.00	28.00	0.72	0.1983
NARROW	Completely known	3.00	9.00	3.00	0.0416
	Unknown parents	12.00	10.22	0.14	0.6476
	Unknown sib	0.00	0.56	0.56	0.2269
	TOTAL	15.00	19.78	0.66	0.2091

supports the idea that there may be linkage in these pedigrees. The cases in which we included sibships with unknown parents or sibs are more dependent on the allele frequencies of the marker alleles, a dependency that can strongly affect the significance of the analysis. For example, try repeating the analysis of marker 1 under the broad diagnostic scheme, assuming allele frequencies of 0.01 and 0.99 for the two marker alleles. The results now show that in the sibships with one or more parents unknown, 37.17 alleles are now shared and 8 not shared. Similarly, in the sibship with one or more sibs untyped, 1.31 alleles are shared IBD and 0 are not shared. The overall chi-square statistic is also increased to 29.77, which is highly significant. Thus, you can see the major effect the allele frequencies could play in such an analysis.

☐ Exercise 27

Running the linkage analysis on these fully penetrant dominant disease pedigrees produces the lod scores shown in Table 29–16. The best estimate of θ in the entire family set together is obviously $\hat{\theta} = 0.5$, yet it appears that in families 1 and 3 there are no recombinants, which might be indicative of some heterogeneity. There is the problem, however, that we have no evidence for linkage, so we must use the techniques outlined in Section 27.3 to test for linkage and heterogeneity jointly (because proving one exists obligates the other to exist).

Table 29–16. Results, by Family, of Linkage Analysis with Pedigrees in Figure 27–1

θ	Family 1	Family 2	Family 3	Family 4	Total
0	2.41	−∞	3.01	−∞	−∞
0.05	2.23	−8.00	2.79	−10.00	−12.98
0.1	2.04	−5.59	2.55	−6.99	−7.99
0.15	1.84	−4.18	2.30	−5.23	−5.26
0.2	1.63	−3.18	2.04	−3.98	−3.49
0.25	1.41	−2.41	1.76	−3.01	−2.25
0.3	1.17	−1.77	1.46	−2.22	−1.36
0.35	0.91	−1.24	1.14	−1.55	−0.74
0.4	0.63	−0.78	0.79	−0.97	−0.32
0.45	0.33	−0.37	0.41	−0.46	−0.08

After running these lod scores through the HOMOG program (assuming STEPSIZE = 0.05 and ALOW = 0), the output should resemble the following:

```
                                   Estimates of
Hypotheses                    Max.ln L    Alpha     Theta
H2: Linkage, heterogeneity     9.7123     0.5000    0.0000
H1: Linkage, homogeneity       0.0000      (1)     99.0000
H0: No linkage                  (0)        (0)       (0.5)

Source                   df   Chi-square   L Ratio
H2 vs. H1 Heterogeneity   1     9.712       16520
H1 vs. H0 Linkage         1     0.000           1
H2 vs. H0 Total           2     9.712       16520
```

Since there is absolutely no evidence for linkage (H_1), the test of H_2 versus H_1 is not meaningful, because the null hypothesis is not a valid null hypothesis. Instead, we must consider the comparison of H_2 versus H_0 (the correct null hypothesis of no linkage). Remember that this likelihood ratio test must exceed 2000 for there to be significant evidence for linkage and heterogeneity. In this case, we have a likelihood ratio of 16,520, which is highly significant evidence for linkage and heterogeneity. In this case therefore although there is no evidence for linkage whatsoever under the assumption of locus homogeneity, as soon as we allow for heterogeneity, we have significant evidence for linkage (in at least some of the families) with $Z(\hat{\theta}, \hat{\alpha}) > 4$.

☐ Exercise 28

For the first problem, we simulated 50 replicates of the pedigree set using a seed of 27,801 for the random number generator. If you use a different seed or a different number of replicates, your results will be somewhat different but similar in their interpretation if everything was done correctly. The results of the analyses are presented in Table 29–17. As we explained in Part I, when analyzing something as a dominant disease when it is truly recessive, you are throwing away information, yet you should still see positive lod scores. We demonstrate this result in this exercise. The EMLOD is about 0.74, and the probability of getting a lod score over 3 is about 0.02—not bad, considering the model is wrong, and roughly half of the meioses are being thrown away by treating the recessive condition as if it were dominant. On the other hand, when something is really dominant and misanalyzed as a recessive condition, the recombination fraction estimates are biased dramatically upward. In this

Table 29–17. Expected Lod Scores in the Schizophrenia Pedigrees When Simulated under One Model and Analyzed under the Wrong Model

	Expected Lod Scores	
θ	*Simulated Recessive Analyzed Dominant*	*Simulated Dominant Analyzed Recessive*
0	0.172	−1.704
0.1	0.436	−0.119
0.2	0.374	0.245
0.3	0.220	0.239
0.4	0.066	0.092
EMLOD	0.740	0.466
$P(Z_{max} > 3)$	0.02	0.000

Table 29–18. Expected Lod Scores for the Pedigree in Figure 28–3 When Simulated, Assuming a Marker with One Common Allele and Four Rare Ones, and Analyzed under the Assumption of Five Equally Frequent Alleles, Simulated Both under Absence of Linkage ($\theta_0 = 0.5$) and under Tight Linkage ($\theta_0 = 0.05$)

θ	$\theta_0 = 0.5$	$\theta_0 = 0.05$
0	$-\infty$	$-\infty$
0.1	0.894	1.013
0.2	0.541	0.594
0.3	0.246	0.265
0.4	0.061	0.065
EMLOD	1.370	1.517
$P(Z_{max} > 1)$	0.800	0.900

case, although one meiosis to each affected offspring truly does contain the disease allele, the other one doesn't, so from one parent the disease and marker appear to be linked (in this case, at $\theta = 0.05$), and from the other parent they appear to segregate independently (since there really is no disease allele there). The overall recombination fraction estimate should therefore be somewhere around the average of 0.05 and 0.5, which is 0.275. In this example the MELOD occurs somewhere between 0.2 and 0.3, consistent with this theoretical prediction. Thus, you can see not only the importance of having an accurate model but also why analyzing under a dominant model is typically more robust than under a recessive model, when it is actually an incorrect model.

The results for the example with the SIMULATE program are presented in Table 29–18, given seeds for the random number generator of 27801, 29721, and 24562. In this case, even though the disease and marker are truly unlinked, by using equal gene frequencies for the marker alleles when this is not the true state of nature, you get positive *expected* lod scores, with an EMLOD of 1.37! Remember, this is in a pedigree in which the marker is actually *unlinked* to the disease. In this example, you can see how important good gene frequency estimates are for your markers, becuase the false-positive rate can easily lead you on a wild goose chase. Some investigators have remarked that they don't mind a few false-positives, if it means they have increased power to detect a true linkage, but the problem is that in these situations the expected lod scores are not much different with or without linkage. To illustrate this, simulate 50 replicates of this pedigree with the SLINK program at $\theta = 0.05$ between disease and marker (again with frequencies 0.05, 0.05, 0.05, 0.05, and 0.80 for the five marker alleles) and analyze them, assuming equal gene frequencies at the marker locus. The results of this should be approximately the same as those shown in Table 29–18 in the right-hand column. The expected lod scores are almost identical, whether or not there really is linkage, when the analysis is done under such an incorrect model for the marker allele frequencies. The expected lod scores are thus essentially independent of the true recombination fraction when these data are analyzed assuming equal gene frequencies. Further, if the simulated replicates are analyzed under the correct model, the expected lod scores are naturally lower (the MELOD for the unlinked replicates is 0.00), yet the power is somewhat increased because now there is a 6% chance that $Z_{max} > 2$. It was 0 when the data were analyzed under the equal gene frequencies model. All of this together should dissuade you from using erroneous gene frequency information and emphasize the importance of getting accurate estimates of the gene frequencies.

Appendix A □

The Linkage Utility Programs

The linkage utility programs are a collection of small programs that prove useful in everyday linkage analysis. For example, the program CHIPROB computes the p-value associated with an observed chi-square with n degrees of freedom, NORPROB carries out analogous calculations for the standard normal distribution, and NORINV does the reverse—computing standard normal deviates from given p-values. Some of these programs were used in this book. Read through the documentation of these programs to find useful hints. A few selected programs are applied below to examples found in practical applications.

A.1 The BINOM Program

Conventionally, linkage is declared significant when the lod score attains or exceeds the value 3, which is associated with a p-value of at most 0.001. If your data consist of counts of recombinants and nonrecombinants you can compute the p-value directly and declare linkage significant if $p \leq 0.001$. The p-value is defined as the probability, given the null hypothesis (of no linkage, in this case), of finding a maximum lod score as large or larger than the one actually observed.

Assume that in an experiment $k = 4$ recombinants are observed in a total of $n = 20$ opportunities for recombination (phase-known meioses). Does this result represent significant evidence for linkage? What about $k = 2$ recombinants in $n = 20$ meioses? To find out, compute the p-value as the probability, given a (true) recombination fraction of $r = \frac{1}{2}$ of observing $k = 4$ or fewer recombinants because decreasing the number of recombinants leads to an increase in the maximum lod score. Call up the BINOM program and choose the binomial probabilities option. Then, select $n = 20$ and $p = 0.5$ and have the program calculate the binomial probabilities of $k = 0 \cdots 4$ (choose $k_1 = 0$ and $k_2 = 4$). What do you get? Repeat this analysis assuming $k = 2$ recombinants are observed. Which of the two outcomes is significant? You should find that for $k = 4$, the p-value is equal to 0.006 (not significant), and for $k = 2$ it is 0.0002 (significant).

A result of $k = 4$ or $k = 2$ recombinants in 20 phase-known meioses leads to recombination fraction estimates of $\hat{\theta} = 0.20$ and $\hat{\theta} = 0.10$, respectively. To assess the accuracy of such point estimates construct support intervals or confidence intervals for the (true) parameter for which an estimate was obtained. Support intervals are generally easy to obtain (see below for an example); however, calculating a confidence interval can be difficult. Usually we work with the normal approximation to the binomial distribution, but this has the disadvantage that the confidence intervals are forced to be symmetric about the estimate of the recombination fraction (the lower bound may become negative). Using the BINOM program we can calculate proper confidence intervals (it does the calculations numerically using an interactive procedure to solve the relevant equations). For further explanations on confidence intervals, consult Section 3.6 in Ott (1991). Before proceeding, take a guess at the 95% confidence intervals for r based on $k = 4$ and $k = 2$. What are its lower and upper bounds?

For each of the two observations $k = 4$ and $k = 2$, calculate the 95% confidence interval for r. Call up the BINOM program, choose the confidence interval option, and for each of $k = 4$ and $k = 2$ compute the two-sided confidence interval using 0.025 each for the lower and upper error probabilities. Write down the resulting 95% confidence intervals with three decimal places. You should find [0.057, 0.437] for $k = 4$ and [0.012, 0.317] for $k = 2$. Note, however, that in linkage analysis a confidence coefficient of 95% is insufficient. For consistency with the lod score criterion of 3, a confidence coefficient of at least 99.9% should be chosen. With our two observations of $k = 4$ and $k = 2$, using a lower and upper error probability of 0.0005 each, we find confidence intervals of [0.019, 0.586] for $k = 4$ and [0.002, 0.471] for $k = 2$. The first includes the value $r = 0.5$, which agrees with the verdict we found above of not significant.

It is unclear which is more appropriate, support or confidence intervals. Statisticians are divided about this issue, and different schools of thought have different preferences. In linkage analysis, it is customary to compute support intervals rather than confidence intervals for r. The support interval often applied is the 1-lod-unit support interval, which is constructed by finding the maximum lod score, Z_{max}, and determining those points of θ for which the lod score is at least $Z_{max} - 1$; these θ points form the desired support interval. As outlined in Section 1.3.5, however, 3-lod-unit support intervals are more appropriate in linkage analysis. One way to compute the 3-lod-unit support interval for the observation $k = 2$ recombinants in $n = 20$ meioses is to use a spreadsheet program, fill one column with values of θ from 0.001 through 0.5 in steps of 0.001 and fill another column with the formula for the lod score corresponding to $k = 2$ and $n = 20$. Then find the maximum lod score, subtract 3 from it, and find the θ values with associated lod scores closest to $Z_{max} - 3$. You may also proceed as follows. Create a family with 20 offspring, two parents, and the parents of one of the parents. Of the grandparents, one has genotype *1/1* at each of two loci, and the other is *2/2* at each locus. Their offspring (a parent) is *1/2* at each locus, and this parent's mate is *1/1* at each locus. Then, assume two types of offspring. *1 2/1 1* (recombinants) and *1 1/1 1* (nonrecombinants). This way a family can be created with exactly two recombinants and 18 nonrecombinants. Now, run the MLINK program and have it compute lod scores at θ between 0 and 0.40 in steps of 0.001. You should find a 3-lod-unit support interval of [0.002, 0.485], which is similar to the 99.9% confidence interval found above.

A.2 The PIC and HET Programs

Genetic marker loci may be more or less polymorphic depending on the number of alleles and their population frequencies. The degree of polymorphism of a marker may be assessed by the proportion of individuals in the population who are heterozygous for that marker. In other words, the probability that a random individual is heterozygous is used as a measure of the degree of polymorphism. This probability may be estimated in two principal ways, each based on a random sample of unrelated individuals.

The first measure is the amount of heterozygosity observed $\hat{h}$ and is simply the proportion of heterozygous individuals observed in the sample (Weir, 1990). It is an unbiased estimate of the proportion h of heterozygous individuals in the population.

In human genetics, a more precise estimate is usually used. It rests on the assumption that the genotypes are in Hardy-Weinberg equilibrium (HWE), which is the reason for its increased precision. This expected heterozygosity (or, in human genetics, just heterozygosity) is defined as $H = 1 - \Sigma p_i^2$, where the sum is taken over all alleles, with p_i denoting the frequency of the i-th allele. The maximum likelihood estimate of h is given by $\hat{H}_M = 1 - \Sigma(\hat{p}_i)^2$ and is slightly biased. An unbiased estimate is $\hat{H}_U = \hat{H}_M n/(n - 1)$, where n is the number of alleles observed in a sample (Ott, 1992). The estimate $\hat{H}_U$ is preferable over $\hat{H}_M$ because it is unbiased and has a smaller mean squared error than $\hat{H}_M$.

An older measure of heterozygosity is the Polymorphism Information Content (PIC) value (Botstein et al., 1980), which is defined as

$$PIC = 1 - \sum_{i=1}^{n} p_i^2 - \sum_{i=1}^{n-1} \sum_{j=i+1}^{n} 2p_i^2 p_j^2$$

where a is the number of alleles at the given locus. In the PIC value a quantity is subtracted from the heterozygosity that corresponds to the probability that offspring are uninformative, because if both parents are identically heterozygous, on average half of their children (the homozygotes) are informative and half (the heterozygotes) are uninformative. For family data PIC may be somewhat more appropriate, whereas the heterozygosity is more general. The maximum likelihood estimate of the PIC value is obtained by replacing the gene frequencies by their estimates.

Genotype	*1/1*	*1/2*	*1/3*	*2/2*	*2/3*	*3/3*
Number of Individuals	2	23	2	13	9	1

As an application, assume you find a new DNA polymorphism. You type 50 unrelated individuals to estimate the number of alleles, their population frequencies, and the heterozygosity of the system. The genotyping results are summarized in the preceding table. We easily estimate the observed heterozygosity *(h)* by the proportion of heterozygous individuals, that is, as $\hat{h} = (23 + 2 + 9)/50 = 0.68$. Also, we easily find the 95% confidence interval for the proportion of heterozygous individuals in the population. Call up the BINOM program and select the confidence intervals option. Enter 34 (for k) and 50 (for n) and choose 0.025 each for the lower and upper error probabilities. You should find a confidence interval of [0.533, 0.805].

The expected heterozygosity *(H)* is more difficult to calculate by hand, so we make use of the PIC program to compute it. In addition to the biased (maximum likelihood) estimate, it also furnishes the unbiased heterozygosity estimate and the PIC value. Because these quantities are based on allele counts rather than genotype counts, we first make a list of the different alleles and how often they occur. For our alleles *1, 2,* and *3,* we find 29, 58, and 13 copies in the 50 individuals, respectively (the number of alleles must sum to $2 \times 50 = 100$). Now call up the PIC program and choose the *Count alleles* option. You should find the following estimates: $\hat{H}_M = 0.5626$ (maximum likelihood, biased), $\hat{H}_U = 0.5683$ (unbiased), and PIC = 0.4918. These values happen to be quite a bit lower than $\hat{h} = 0.68$.

As the observed proportion of heterozygous individuals is an estimate for the corresponding proportion in the total population, so are the expected heterozygosities $\hat{H}_U$ and $\hat{H}_M$ estimates for the population value *H.* A support interval for *H* can be found with the help of the HET program (Shugart and Ott, 1992). HET works in terms of *m*-unit support intervals, where *m* refers to the number of units and natural log likelihood. Thus, $m = 2$ corresponds to a likelihood ratio of 7.4. Asymptotically, it is equivalent to a 95% confidence interval.

Call up the HET program and follow the directions to calculate a 2-unit support interval for *H.* You should find [0.492, 0.622], which is less than half as long as the 95% confidence interval for *h* computed above. This difference clearly demonstrates the gain in precision when we can rely on HWE, which is generally reliable for a stable population.

A.3 The CHIPROB Program and Testing HWE

In the previous section, the observed heterozygosity of 0.68 deviates quite a bit from the value of 0.57 expected under HWE, and we wonder whether the assumption of HWE might not be violated here. To investigate this, we carry out a test of HWE, that is, we test whether the genotype frequencies are compatible with HWE. Before proceeding, we take a hint from the confidence interval for the population heterozygosity—it includes the point estimate under the assumption of HWE, $\hat{H}_U = 0.57$, so we suspect that the genotype frequencies are compatible with HWE.

We test the assumption of HWE for the observed genotype frequencies given in Section A.2 using a chi-square test. We first calculate expected genotype frequencies assuming HWE and do this on the basis of the allele frequencies already obtained, that is, with $\hat{p}_1 = 0.29$, $\hat{p}_2 = 0.58$, and $\hat{p}_3 = 0.13$. Our expected genotype frequencies are then estimated, for example, as $P(1/1) = (\hat{p}_1)^2$ and $P(1/2) = 2\hat{p}_1\hat{p}_2$. These estimates are biased; unbiased or less biased genotype frequency estimates have been derived but are not generally used in practice. For our chi-square test, we use the (biased) maximum likelihood estimates. We multiply each of the expected genotype frequencies by 50 to obtain the expected number of individuals with the respective genotypes. Carry out these calculations for all genotypes. You should find, in the order of genotypes given in the table in Section A.2, 4.205, 16.82, 3.77, 16.82, 7.54, and 0.845. As a check, the sum of these figures should equal 50. Then, for each of the genotypes we calculate its contribution to chi-square in the usual manner as $(O - E)^2/E$ where *O* stands for the observed number and *E* for the expected number of individuals. For example, the contribution from the *1/1* genotype is $(2 - 4.205)^2/4.205 = 1.156$. Calculate all six contributions and sum them. You should obtain a chi-square value of 5.44. The number of degrees of freedom associated with this chi-square is given by $6 - 1 - 2 = 3$, where 6 is the number of classes in which the observed and expected number of observations are contrasted. We subtract 1 from the number of classes because the total number of observations is fixed, and the numbers in the sixth class are given once we know the numbers in the first five classes. We estimated three gene frequencies, but only two of them represent independent estimates; the third is again given once we know the first two. Thus, we subtract 2 to arrive at a number of 3 df.

Is the chi-square of 5.44 on 3 df significant? Instead of looking up critical values for chi-square in a table, we calculate the empirical significance level p associated with this result, that is, the probability that, under the null hypothesis (HWE in this case), the observed chi-square value is exceeded by chance. We declare the result significant if $p \leq 0.05$ and highly significant if $p \leq 0.01$. Call up the CHIPROB program and enter the two values 5.44 and 3. You quickly find that $p = 0.14$, which is larger than 0.05, so there is no significant evidence for a deviation from HWE.

In addition to the application of CHIPROB shown above, this program also allows combining p-values from different independent investigations into one overall p-value, in which the individual p-values may result from any statistical test furnishing a p-value. The approach, based on a method by R. A. Fisher, specifies that each value of p, which has a uniform distribution under the null hypothesis should be transformed into $c = -2 \ln(p)$, which has a chi-square distribution on 2 df. Assume that n independent p-values should be combined. The corresponding n c-values are then added. Their sum $\Sigma(c)$ represents a chi-square variable with $2n$ df. So, if $\Sigma(c)$ is entered in the CHIPROB program with $2n$ df, the p-value returned is the desired overall empirical significance level. As an example, assume that three independent tests (not necessarily chi-square tests) have furnished the respective p-values 0.011, 0.047 and 0.35. The corresponding c-values are 9.02, 6.12, and 2.10. Their sum, 17.24 with 6 df, yields a combined p-value of 0.008.

Appendix B □

Practical Considerations

B.1 Overview of Linkage Programs

Linkage programs can be divided into two groups. The major programs belonging to the first group are LIPED (Ott, 1974), PAP (Hasstedt and Cartwright, 1981), LINKAGE (MLINK, LINKMAP, ILINK, etc.) (Lathrop et al., 1984), MENDEL (Lange et al., 1988), and GRONLOD (te Meerman, 1991) (see Section B.4 and Appendix C for ordering information). These programs are able to carry out linkage analyses for families of an arbitrary structure, with possibly incomplete penetrance, and other complicating factors. The second group of programs comprising MAPMAKER (Lander et al., 1987), CRI-MAP (P. Green, personal communication) and the CEPH version of LINKAGE (CLINKAGE), is applicable only to special loci or pedigree types. For example, a version of MAPMAKER and the CEPH version of LINKAGE work with codominant markers in three-generation pedigrees with a nuclear family and up to four grandparents (Figure 13-1). The CRI-MAP program was originally written for this type of application also but has been extended to some other pedigree structures and loci. Also, other programs (for example, special versions of MAPMAKER and LINKAGE) work with quantitative traits observed on experimental crosses. MAPMAKER is very user-friendly and has many options for automated linkage analysis and map building.

The LINKAGE package, like most of the other linkage analysis programs, is available for a variety of computer systems. Its programs were developed by Mark Lathrop with contributions by Jean-Marc Lalouel, Cécile Julier, and Jurg Ott. Peter Cartwright made major contributions to the development of the shell programs, which greatly increased the usefulness of LINKAGE. Mark Lathrop regularly updates these programs.

The LINKAGE and MENDEL programs are very similar in their focus. They both handle pedigrees of arbitrary structure and various phenotypes, but MENDEL is more flexible in the problems it can address. For example, the user can impose linear constraints on the parameters to be estimated, which is not possible in ILINK. On the other hand, MENDEL is more demanding both of the user (it requires fluency in FORTRAN) and of computer resources (it requires more memory than LINKAGE for the same problem). On a PC many linkage problems that cannot be handled by MENDEL can be carried out successfully by the LINKAGE programs.

A special version of the LINKAGE programs, TLINKAGE, allows for two loci jointly leading to disease (Lathrop and Ott, 1990). This possibility has also been incorporated in the MENDEL program (Schork et al., 1993).

GRONLOD is the newest member of these programs. It is written in PROLOG and takes advantage of PROLOG's capacity to represent abstract objects and work with dependencies among those objects.

B.2 Data Base and Pedigree-drawing Programs

How should pedigree data be stored in a computer? Many people simply keep it in files (in ASCII or another format) with rows corresponding to individuals and columns corresponding to phenotypes at different loci. In addition to the phenotypes, there are columns containing the sex of an individual and pointers to the two parents (analogous to a LINKAGE pedigree file). This approach is probably easiest and sufficient if the amount of data is small enough to be manageable in this form.

Another method is to enter the data into a data base using one of the commercially available data base programs, such as dBASE, Foxbase, or Paradox. Data bases have various advantages: some columns can be singled out for special consideration, or a printout of that data base can be made that suppresses some columns containing sensitive data. On the other hand, the user must learn commands specific for that data base. Specialized data bases have been developed for family pedigree data. They are typically capable of writing output in a format suitable for analysis by a linkage program or of graphically displaying the pedigree.

B.3 Sources of Information

To carry out a linkage analysis, a variety of information is needed. This section is intended to guide you in your search for the required information. We tried to provide as much useful material as possible, but the list given below is by no means exhaustive.

Programs and other files can be down-loaded from a data base with the use of the FTP (file transfer protocol) program, which is generally available to computers that have access to the INTERNET. Typically a so-called anonymous FTP site is accessed by logging in as "anonymous," and leaving his E-MAIL address as the password.

A data base called ARCHIE, which is accessible via TELNET (on the INTERNET), is a searchable list of all programs and files available at a large number of FTP sites around the world. To connect to the ARCHIE site at Rutgers University, for example, you type TELNET ARCHIE. RUTGERS.EDU, and login as ARCHIE. Then, you search the data base for the LINKAGE programs by typing prog linkage at the Archie prompt, for example. This returns a listing of all files available with the word *linkage* in their program name, and the anonymous FTP site (and directory) from which the file can be obtained.

Information on locus parameters, such as gene frequencies and mode of inheritance, can be found in review articles or regular scientific articles in human genetics journals (listed at the end of this section). The "McKusick catalog," or *Medelian Inheritance of Man* (McKusick, 1990) contains information on loci with an established mode of inheritance, for which each locus carries a unique number—the MIM (from the book title) number. Its contents are also available electronically. To access OMIM (On-line Mendelian Inheritance of Man), or its companion data base of locus data, the GDB (genetic data base), which grew out of the International Human Gene Mapping Workshops, you can register them free of charge by writing to

GDB/OMIM User Support
William H. Welch Medical Library
1830 Monument Street, Third Floor
Baltimore, MD 21205
E-MAIL: help@gdb.org

Numerous good textbooks in human genetics contain a wealth of information. Some of them are not very accurate in terms of background for linkage analysis, but they provide general genetics background and details on specific topics. Only a brief list can be given here. A well-known compendium in medical genetics is the textbook by Vogel and Motulsky (1986), a new edition of which is being written in 1993–1994. This text also contains valuable sections on population genetics. Another similar book is *Thompson and Thompson: Genetics in Medicine* (Thompson et al., 1991), which covers a wide range of topics in medical genetics.

An older book, which is unfortunately out of print but treasured by many geneticists, is Cavalli-Sforza and Bodmer's *The Genetics of Human Population* (1971). It focuses on the population genetic aspects of human genetics, provides locus information for many classical genetic markers, and presents a very readable and lucid discussion of population genetic phenomena. Other useful population genetics textbooks include works by Hartl (1988), Weir (1990), and a classic four-volume population text by Wright (1968).

Issues in segregation analysis and some population genetics issues are discussed in Elandt-Johnson (1971), but this book is also quite old although still a useful reference source. As far as linkage analysis textbooks are concerned, Ott (1991), the companion book to this volume, is the most complete modern source. However, there is much useful information in older sources, such as Bailey (1961).

Among the journals specializing in human genetics, the *American Journal of Human Genetics* is probably the most widely known worldwide. Other general journals are the *American Journal of Medical Genetics* and *Human Genetics*. Smaller journals that emphasize methodology, linkage analysis, and pedigree analysis are the *Annals of Human Genetics* (formerly *Annals of Eugenics*), *Human Heredity* (formerly *Acta Genetica* and *Statistica Medica*), and *Genetic Epidemiology*. Other journals in human genetics include *Clinical Genetics,* the *Journal of Medical Genetics,* and *Genomics.* Several new journals have appeared in recent years, for example, *Human Molecular Genetics* and the *European Journal of Human Genetics.*

B.4 How to Order the LINKAGE Programs

The LINKAGE programs, LIPED, HOMOG, and other programs for PCs running under DOS and OS/2 can be obtained from:

Katherine Montague/Jurg Ott
Columbia University, Unit 58
722 West 168th Street
New York, NY 10032, USA
Fax: (212) 568-2750 Tel: (212) 960-2507
E-MAIL: `ott@nyspi.bitnet` or `jurg.ott@columbia.edu`

In the near future, we will provide programs also for Sparcstations (UNIX) and Vax computers (VMS). Our program list (to be made available on line) describes the current status of programs. The *Linkage Newsletter* is sent free of charge (by E-MAIL or postal mail) to anyone requesting it or who has obtained programs from us.

An anonymous FTP site has recently been installed in our department at internet address YORK.CPMC.COLUMBIA.EDU (128.59.101.161). The LINKAGE programs, as well as most of the companion programs used in this book, can be obtained from this anonymous FTP site. To access our site, type

`FTP YORK.CPMC.COLUMBIA.EDU` or `FTP 128.59.101.161`

When asked for a login name, type ANONYMOUS (no password is required). You may then proceed to download whatever files you require from the site. The host computer is running Desktop-VMS version 1.2, so directory syntax must be given in VMS format, which is different from UNIX-based FTP sites. When you login to the computer, you are in directory [ANONYMOUS], which is the root directory for the FTP site. All higher directories are off limits, and any attempt to access such directories blocks any further activity for you. A file called README.TXT is available in directory [ANONY-MOUS.PUB] and contains a list of all files available from the FTP site and their location.

When you log on, notice that there are some files in the root directory. These are all account-specific files, which are read/write protected. You must go to the subdirectory PUB.DIR with VMS syntax [ANONYMOUS.PUB] by typing CD [.PUB], for example, if your computer is running UNIX FTP software. A directory name preceded by a period (.) means a subdirectory. If the period is not given, the computer thinks you are trying to access a higher-level directory and blocks further access to the system. If, for example, you are in the directory [ANONYMOUS.PUB.LINKAGE.DOS] and you want to move to the directory [ANONYMOUS.PUB.LINKAGE], enter CD [−], where the minus (−) sign means to go back one directory level. To move to the directory [ANONYMOUS.PUB.TLINKAGE.DOS], you could enter CD [− − .TLINK-AGE.DOS], meaning back up two levels, and then move forward to subdirectory [.TLINKAGE.DOS]. If you have any further questions about VMS directory syntax or are having difficulty navigating around the FTP site, send E-MAIL to Joseph Terwilliger (JOE@YORK.CPMC.COLUMBIA.EDU) (or JDT3@COLUMBIA.EDU).

To get any files other than ASCII files (*.ZIP or *.W51 files, for example), please make sure you do this in binary mode. Typically, type SET TYPE BINARY at the FTP prompt, though the exact syntax may vary from system to system. If you must use communications software such as KERMIT to get the binary files from a UNIX or VMS machine to your PC, be sure to do those transfers in BINARY format as well.

Many of the programs and data files are in compressed form and must be decompressed after down-loading. Compressed files are compressed with either PKZIP V2.04g or ZIP V1.9. These formats are cross-compatible, and the compressed files can be decompressed with either PKUNZIP V2.04 (or a later version) or UNZIP V5.0 (or a later version). We have made available the UNZIP V5.0 executable program for DOS, OS2, VMS, and UNIX. You can UNZIP any of our files on any computer, as long as the UNZIP program is correct for your machine (i.e., you can UNZIP the DOS version of LINKAGE on a VMS machine, using the VMS version of UNZIP.EXE).

The LINKAGE programs for Sparcstations (UNIX) and other machines may be obtained from the following anonymous FTP site. To access it, issue the following command (directions taken from a document obtained from that site):

```
ftp corona.med.utah.edu    or    ftp 128.110.231.1
```

When prompted to provide a user name, enter "anonymous." As the password, give your last name. Then, issue the commands

```
cd pub/linkage/sun
binary
get linkage.tar.Z
quit
```

This ends your FTP session. On your Sun machine, issue the commands

```
uncompress linkage.tar.Z
tar xvf linkage.tar
rm linkage.tar
```

A new, faster version of some of the LINKAGE programs for large Sun machines written in the C language (Cottingham et al., 1993), is available from Robert Cottingham at the Baylor College of Medicine via anonymous FTP. The address of the FTP site is GC.BCM.TMC.EDU, and he can be contacted via E-MAIL at BWC@BCM.TMC.EDU if further information about this implementation is required.

A list of other programs and the addresses of contact people for ordering these programs is given in Appendix C.

B.5 PC Hardware and Operating Systems

The IBM PC/AT and other machines containing an Intel microprocessor have long been dominated by Microsoft DOS (Disk Operating System), the latest version of which is 6.0. Current Intel microprocessors, such as the 80486 and Pentium, are very powerful, but DOS makes only little use of this power. In this respect, Microsoft Windows does a better job because programs specifically developed to run under Windows can address much more memory than the maximum of 640K bytes allowed under DOS (the LINKAGE programs are not yet available for Windows, but we are working on making them Windows-compatible). IBM's OS/2 version 2 exploits much (but not all) of the power of the 80486; it is a powerful and inexpensive operating system for Intel-based machines. For good performance, a minimum of 16 megabytes of RAM is recommended. Presently, one of the shortcomings of OS/2 is the relative lack of software developed to run under it. Of course, DOS-based software runs under the DOS emulator within OS/2. Several programs can run concurrently in different DOS windows, each window with its own 640 kilobytes of RAM, environment, and expanded and extended memory. Examples of compilers capable of producing programs running under OS/2 are Microsoft Pascal and FORTRAN, Prospero Pascal, and NDP Pascal.

Several UNIX operating systems are available for PCs, but we have no experience with these systems. They are generally much more expensive than

OS/2. Also, UNIX (a multi-user system) is more complex than OS/2 (a single-user multitasking system) and requires careful maintenance, whereas for DOS users the transition to OS/2 is essentially effortless. On the other hand, much software is available for UNIX, including compilers. Currently, many linkage analysts running UNIX do so on one of the Sparcstations from Sun Microsystems. Other machines that run under UNIX are the IBM R6000 and Vax computers, but their UNIX versions and corresponding Pascal compilers are sufficiently different from Sun Pascal that the LINKAGE programs cannot easily be adapted to them.

B.6 Program Constants and Recompiling the LINKAGE Programs

In the Pascal version of LINKAGE (a C version is in preparation), array bounds, such as maximum number of alleles, are given as program constants. They may be changed and set to a user's needs. Once such constants are changed, the programs need to be recompiled for the new constant values to take effect. We first discuss the most important constants for the general analysis programs. Deviating constant definitions for CEPH and other programs are noted. Then we outline the steps necessary to recompile the programs. The *Users' Guide to Analysis Programs,* which comes with the LINKAGE programs, also contains explanations of these constants. Ideally, all constants are set to high values so no recompiling of the programs is required. However, to keep the size of the program to a manageable level, the program constants should be set to small values whenever possible. Also, in Turbo Pascal, the total of all arrays cannot exceed more than 64 kilobytes of memory.

MAXNEED sets the upper bound to an array containing various recombination probabilities. Its value depends only on the number of loci. For locus numbers from 2 through 8, the minimum values of MAXNEED are 7, 32, 157, 782, 3907, 19532, and 97657, respectively. If the array size required by the program is larger than MAXNEED, the program terminates with an error. If MAXNEED is larger than necessary, the program writes on the screen the minimum value of MAXNEED it requires in this run.

MAXCENSOR determines the length of an array that holds intermediate results for pedigree members. In a given run, there is an optimal value for MAXCENSOR. If MAXCENSOR is smaller than this optimal value, the program runs less efficiently and prints on the screen that it would benefit from an increase in MAXCENSOR. If MAXCENSOR is larger than the optimal value, the program does not run faster than with the optimal value and prints on the screen the optimal value for MAXCENSOR.

MAXLOCUS determines the maximum number of loci allowed. This and all of the constants described below represent upper limits. If these upper limits are insufficient for a particular run, the program stops with an error message.

MAXSEG should be set equal to 2 to the power of (maxlocus-1). For example, MAXLOCUS = 5 calls for MAXSEG = 16.

MAXALL specifies the maximum number of alleles at a single locus.

MAXHAP is the maximum number of multilocus haplotypes the program can handle. To be safe, set MAXHAP to a value as large as the product of the number of alleles at all loci used in a particular run. In Turbo Pascal, MAXHAP must not be larger than 126 or the program cannot be compiled.

MAXFEM is the maximum number of female multilocus genotypes the program can handle, and MAXMAL is the analogous quantity for males. These two values should be set to a value at least as large as MAXHAP·(MAXHAP + 1)/2; larger values are wasteful of memory space. Some versions of Pascal allow setting constants as simple functions of other constants. In Turbo Pascal, for example, the user need not set MAXFEM and MAXMAL because they are determined by the constant MAXHAP as given above. Note that in Turbo Pascal, the product MAXFEM·MAXPED must not be larger than 65,536, where MAXPED = maximum number of pedigrees. For example, with MAXHAP = 64 (MAXFEM = 2080), no more than MAXPED = 31 pedigrees can be analyzed in a single run.

MAXIND is the maximum number of individuals in all pedigrees combined.

AFFALL is an integer number indicating which allele is the disease allele. In most applications, a low allele frequency together with the penetrances imply which allele is the disease allele. In these cases the value of AFFALL is irrelevant. At sex-linked quantitative trait loci, the phenotype in males is assumed to be of a fully penetrant affection status type, and no penetrances must be specified. In this case AFFALL is used to identify the disease allele. Also, for rare dominant diseases, homozygotes may be disregarded in the analysis (see MINFREQ below). In this case, too, AFFALL is used to identify the disease allele.

MINFREQ represents a gene frequency limit for the AFFALL allele in the following sense: If the specified frequency of the AFFALL allele is smaller than MINFREQ, homozygotes for the AFFALL allele are not considered. This is only meaningful for rare dominant diseases for which AFFALL is the disease allele. In practice, one usually has MINFREQ = 0. Homozygotes may be eliminated from consideration with the use of liability classes.

MAXTRAIT is the maximum number of (quantitative) variables at a quantitative trait locus type. In most applications this is equal to 1 (univariate phenotype). Some compilers require MAXTRAIT to be at least 2.

MAXFACT is the maximum number of binary codes at a locus. MAXFACT must be at least as large as MAXALL.

SCALE and SCALEMULT are used to increase the likelihood so it does not grow to too small a number, thereby causing an underflow. If problems with underflow or overflow occur, SCALE and SCALEMULT should be changed. The best protection against underflow and overflow, however, is to work with double-precision instead of single-precision variables.

FITMODEL is either true or false. If true, the program calculates likelihoods whether or not a family is informative. If FITMODEL = false, uninformative families are skipped.

DOSTREAM should be set to true if the locus report program, LRP, is to be used to interpret program output.

BYFAMILY is either true or false. If set to true, likelihoods (not lod scores) are output for each family, otherwise no individual family results are provided.

NBIT indicates the precision of real variables and should be set to a value as large as the mantissa length of real variables. For example, it is equal to 23 for single-precision and 52 for double-precision variables. In some versions of LINKAGE, a procedure called precision is furnished, which calculates NBIT as a variable obviating the need for the user to set it as a constant.

MAXN is the maximum number of parameters that ILINK can iteratively estimate for that locus identified at the bottom of the data file by this locus may have iterated parameters. This number of parameters includes the penetrances in all liability classes.

In the CEPH programs, MAXSYSTEM, MAXIND, and MAXPED refer to the respective maximum number of loci, individuals, and pedigrees after the transformation step. These values may be considerably larger than the corresponding values in the pedigree data and cannot be determined before the CFACTOR program has completed. CFACTOR produces two output files—TEMPDAT.DAT and TEMPPED.DAT—which contain the numbers of loci, individuals, and pedigrees to which the three constants above refer.

In the Turbo Pascal version of LINKAGE, the constants reside in the file GENC.PAS (THGC.PAS for the CEPH programs). We also use the Prospero Pascal compiler for the LINKAGE programs. It has the advantage that arrays in the main program body can occupy more than 64 kilobytes of storage area if programs are compiled with the /H2 compiler switch (see file PROSPERO.TXT that comes with the Prospero version of LINKAGE). Also, Prospero Pascal can produce programs running under OS/2 so much more memory than the 640 kilobytes under DOS can be addressed (the maximum is currently 4 megabytes). We are currently evaluating a third compiler, NDP Pascal. It is the most general of the compilers we have found for PCs and produces code for OS/2. Programs typically run twice as fast when compiled with NDP than when compiled with Turbo or Prospero Pascal. Below, the discussion on compiling refers to Turbo Pascal under DOS.

Various compiler switches allow for the production of executable programs suitable for your particular needs. They reside in an include file, SWGEN.PAS (SWTHG.PAS), that is furnished with the source code and is read by each of the LINKAGE programs and each of the units. Part of it looks as follows:

{$DEFINE mlink}	{Program name; MLINK or LINKMAP or ILINK}
{$DEFINE double}	{Precision; single or . . . or turbo}
{$O −}	{Overlays; + or −}
{$N +}	{Use numeric coprocessor; + or −}
{$E +}	{Emulate coprocessor}

The first switch, on the second line in the file, defines the program name. It is automatically set when you use the COMPILE batch program to recompile the programs. The precision switch determines the number of bytes used for a real variable. It is recommended to use "double" whenever possible. This setting requires 8 bytes of memory per real variable but allows numbers to be as small as 10^{-308}, which largely avoids problems with underflows. On the other hand, "single" variables require only 4 bytes each but can be only as small as 10^{-38}. Further details on the switches are given in the LINKAGE.TXT file, which comes with the programs.

We highly recommend that you use the LINKAGE programs on a machine with a numerical coprocessor (e.g., Intel 8087, 80287, 80387) or with a processor such as the 80486, which contains an integrated coprocessor. If a program is compiled with the N+ and E+ compiler switches, it senses the presence of a coprocessor and uses it. On some non–IBM-compatible machines, the signals received by the program may be wrong, so that, for example, a coprocessor is assumed present when in reality it is absent. Such a situation crashes the program and probably freezes the machine (an analogous situation occurs when a coprocessor is installed but no longer functions properly). To prevent this from happening, type SET 87 = N once before using the programs if no coprocessor is present or the installed coprocessor fails to work properly, and type SET 87 = Y if a good coprocessor is installed. This SET command is profitably made part of the AUTOEXEC.BAT file, which is executed automatically at start-up.

B.7 How to Set Up a Linkage Study

Assume that you want to investigate the genetics of a particular disease. One of the first questions is how much of the variability of the phenotype is due to genes as opposed to effects of common family environment or random environment. Generally, the fact that a disease "runs in families" is taken as evidence for a genetic component, and it usually is. But well-known exceptions exist. For example, kuru (a disease previously quite prevalent in Papua-New Guinea) was once thought to be due to a dominant gene but was later found to be transmitted by a virus through cannibalism (Lindenbaum, 1979).

Classical methods of addressing the question of genetic involvement compare the concordance rate among monozygotic siblings (who share 100% of their genes) with the concordance rate among dizygotic twins (who on average share 50% of their genes). To avoid the confounding effects of common family environment, siblings reared apart are often also investigated. Such analyses only show genetic effects, but these may be due to one or several genes. Specialized analyses can help discriminate between these possibilities. For example, the major gene statistic designed by Jayakar and associates (1984) is sensitive to the presence of single major genes influencing quantitative characters. It has been applied to obesity and gave weak evidence for the presence of a major gene influencing body weight (Zonta et al., 1987).

A method often used to dissect effects of major genes from other effects is complex segregation analysis (Morton and MacLean 1974; Bonney et al., 1988). Also, the comparison of recurrence risks among different types of relatives (Risch, 1990b) appears to be a powerful tool for detecting major genes.

Segregation analysis typically is very sensitive to ascertainment, and false assumptions on ascertainment may easily invalidate a segregation analysis (Greenberg, 1986). Linkage analysis, on the other hand, does not suffer from this problem, meaning that family members can be selected by any method on the basis of the phenotypes at one locus and the linkage analysis is still valid and furnishes unbiased estimates of the recombination fraction. For this reason, many investigators skip formal segregation analysis and make a small number of "reasonable" assumptions on the mode of inheritance of the disease to be investigated. The problems addressed here are beyond the scope of this book, so we only make a few additional comments on the treatment of "complex" diseases. You may also want to consult Section 11.9 in Ott (1991).

If multiple genes jointly have an effect on a disease, several investigations have shown that in many cases analysis under a single-gene model retains much of the linkage information of the multilocus situation, but the recombination fraction tends to be biased upwards. This implies that in testing a disease versus a map of markers, a complex trait tends to be localized outside of the map even if in reality a gene exists inside the map. Therefore, for complex traits, use two-point analysis as long as possible. Below, we focus on analyses under a single-gene model.

If it is unclear how to define the genetically relevant affectation status, investigators often use several different diagnostic schemes and carry out a linkage analysis under each one. This represents a case of multiple testing, which tends to inflate the maximum lod score. This problem may be addressed by computer simulation (Weeks et al., 1990b) or by the formula shown below.

Testing for linkage between disease and many markers also represents a case of multiple comparisons. For monogenic diseases, the critical lod score of 3 is then still appropriate because the increased Type I error (false-positive rate) is counterbalanced by an increased prior probability of linkage as more and more of the genome is excluded with the testing of multiple markers. If, however, the presence of major genes is unknown and linkage analysis is undertaken as a means of showing the existence of single genes, the arguments for an increased prior probability of linkage do not apply and multiple testing must be allowed for. This may be done by a formula due to Kidd and Ott (1984), which states that the relevant critical lod score for significant linkage is

$$Z_{crit} = 3 + \log_{10}(m)$$

where m is the number of multiple comparisons. If m refers to multiple marker loci, only "independent" comparisons should be considered, that is, markers 30 cM or 40 cM apart. Therefore, with a genome length of roughly 3000 cM, there are about $m = 100$ "independent" tests with multiple markers throughout the genome such that $Z_{crit} = 5$ is an adequate critical limit for a genome-wide screen of a complex disease. However, multiple tests resulting from multiple disease classification schemes must additionally be allowed for.

Now, we assume the presence of a single gene responsible for a disease. The first task is to find a number of suitable families willing to collaborate and donate small amounts of blood for marker typing. Ideally, there should be several affected individuals in one sibship. For dominant diseases, extended families are more useful than nuclear families. Also, parents should be available for marker typing whenever possible. Once a set of families has been ascertained and affection status has been established at least in a preliminary manner, before marker typing has even begun, you may want to estimate the expected lod score or the power for detecting linkage with the given family data. This is usually done by computer simulation under the assumption that it is possible to find a marker close to the disease gene, say, at a distance of 2–5 cM. The simulation may also be carried out with two flanking markers but that takes much more computer time. Therefore, we usually work with a single "virtual" marker tightly linked (1 cM) with the disease gene.

At the true (simulated) recombination fraction r an expected lod score of, say, 3 means that on average the lod score you find at $\theta = r$ is equal to 3. There is, approximately, a 50% chance that the lod score in your study is equal to 3 or higher. Usually, a power larger than 50% is desired. Of course, these simulations are reliable only when carried out with reasonable parameter values. For example, if penetrance for the disease at high age is 50% but you assume 80% in the simulation, the simulation indicates more power than is available in the data, and the results of the linkage analysis tend to be disappointing. Also, at least in complex traits, be sure to allow for phenocopies (nongenetic cases), and make their penetrance age-dependent if the penetrance of genetic cases is also age-dependent.

Once you have recruited a sufficient number of families or are certain that a sufficient number can be obtained, several tasks need to be carried out. Depending on your background, you need to secure the collaboration of different specialists. A medical person is often responsible for seeing the family members and determining who among them is affected and unaffected, and these decisions should be made blindly with regard to genetic marker determinations. For maximum efficiency, a linkage analyst can determine who should be typed for genetic markers. Blood must then be obtained from these individuals. A molecular geneticist (or a laboratory) is required to carry out the marker typing. Linkage analysts and molecular geneticists interact to determine which markers should be typed. Initially, markers should be relatively far apart from each other, and "promising" lod scores should be followed up by typing additional markers or making markers more informative in the vicinity of a promising lod score. Such two-stage procedures have been proposed by Elston (1993). Assuming homogeneity, he recommends an initial marker spacing of 28 cM for sib-pair linkage tests (corresponding to a set of 117 equally spaced markers throughout the genome) and an initial critical "promising" lod score of 0.23. Until recently, researchers had no theoretical basis for choosing these parameters. In practice, they used to choose markers 10–20 cM apart and considered maximum lod scores between 0.5 and 1 as interesting.

In addition to incomplete penetrance, you must often allow for genetic heterogeneity, that is, that the disease might be caused by different genes in different families. With respect to a particular marker, you then have two family types: those with linkage between disease and marker and those without linkage. If heterogeneity is suspected, it should be allowed for already at the planning stage, that is, in the computer simulation.

Appendix C □

List of Programs, and Where to Obtain Them

The following list is not intended to be exhaustive but rather to provide an overview of some of the programs available for human genetic analysis. The programs are listed alphabetically by name under each heading, and the name of a contact person from whom you can order the programs or obtain further details about the programs is given. Finally, a list of addresses of those individuals is provided, again in alphabetical order. This information is provided as a source of information for the reader, and it is requested that only serious inquiries and program requests be made. By listing these programs, the authors do not wish to imply any endorsement of them but merely provide this list as a service to the readers.

Segregation Analysis

PAP (Hasstedt and Cartwright, 1981)—Sandra Hasstedt

POINTER (Lalouel and Yee, 1980)—Newton Morton, or Jurg Ott's FTP site

REGRESS (Bonney et al., 1988)—George Bonney

SAGE (Elston et al., 1986)—Robert Elston

Database Programs

CYRLLIC (Chapman, 1990)—Cherwell Scientific Publishing Limited

dbLINK (Sarfarazi, 1990)—Mansoor Sarfarazi

dGENE (Lange et al., 1988)—Daniel E. Weeks, Kenneth Lange

KINDRED—Epicenter Software

LABMAN/LINKMAN (Adams et al., 1990)—Phil Adams, Jurg Ott's FTP site

Linksys (Attwood and Bryant, 1988)—John Attwood

LIPIN (Trofatter et al., 1986)—James Trofatter

Megabase (Fenton et al., 1990)—Iain Fenton

MEGADATS (Gersting, 1987)—John Gersting

PEDSYS (Dyke and Mamelka, 1987)—Bennett Dyke

Pedigree-Drawing Programs

CYRILLIC (Chapman, 1990)—Cherwell Scientific Publishing Limited

FTREE—Rodney Go

GENETREE—Ellen Wijsman

KINDRED—Epicenter Software

PEDIGREE/DRAW (Dyke and Mamelka, 1987)—Bennett Dyke

PEDRAW (Curtis, 1990)—Dave Curtis

PLOT2000 (Wolak and Sarfarazi, 1987)—Iain Fenton

SCHESIS (Round, 1990)—Anthony Round

Linkage Analysis

CINTMAX (Weeks et al., 1991)—Daniel Weeks

CRI-MAP (Lander and Green, 1987)—Phillip Green

EXCLUDE (Edwards, 1987)—John Edwards

GRONLOD (te Meerman, 1993)—Gerard te Meerman

LINKAGE (Lathrop et al., 1984)—(See Section B.4)

LIPED (Ott, 1974)—Jurg Ott

MAPMAKER (Lander et al., 1987)—Eric Lander

MAP90 (Morton and Andrews, 1989)—Newton Morton, Jurg Ott's FTP site

MDMAP (Falk, 1991)—Catherine Falk

PAP (Hasstedt and Cartwright, 1981)—Sandra Hasstedt

PROGRAMS FOR PEDIGREE ANALYSIS (MENDEL/FISHER/ SEARCH) (Lange et al., 1988)—Kenneth Lange

RHMAP (Boehnke, 1992)—Michael Boehnke

SAGE (Elston et al., 1986)—Robert Elston

SCHESIS (Round, 1990)—Anthony Round

Simulation Programs

CHRSIM (Speer et al., 1992)—Jurg Ott

MOM (Ott and Terwilliger, 1992)—Jurg Ott

SIMLINK (Boehnke, 1986)—Michael Boehnke

SIMULATE (Ott and Terwilliger, 1992)—Jurg Ott

SLINK (Including **MSIM/ISIM/LSIM**) (Weeks et al., 1990b)—Jurg Ott

TYPENEXT (Ott et al., 1992)—Jurg Ott

Nonparametric Analysis Programs

APM (Weeks and Lange, 1988)—Daniel Weeks, Kenneth Lange

ESPA (Sandkuyl, 1989)—Lodewijk Sandkuyl

SAGE (Elston et al., 1986)—Robert Elston

Heterogeneity Testing

B-TEST (Risch, 1988)—Neil Risch

HOMOG (Ott, 1991)—Jurg Ott

MTEST (Ott, 1991)—Jurg Ott

C-GEN (MacLean et al., 1992)—Charles MacLean

Miscellaneous Programs

CHROMLOOK (Haines, 1992)—Jonathan Haines

EH—Jurg Ott

LINKAGE UTILITY PROGRAMS (Ott, 1991)—Jurg Ott

Miscellaneous Population Genetics Programs (Weir, 1993)—(Source Code given in Weir, 1993)

MULTIMAP (Cox et al., 1992)—Tara Cox

SENSEN—Sensitivity Analysis (Hodge and Greenberg, 1992)—David Greenberg

VARYPHEN (Xie et al., 1991)—Jurg Ott

Addresses

Phil Adams
New York State Psychiatric Institute
722 West 168th Street, Unit 14
New York, NY 10032

John Attwood
Genetic and Biometry Department
U.C.L.
Wolfson House
4 Stephenson Way
London NW1 2HE
UNITED KINGDOM

Michael Boehnke
Department of Biostatistics
School of Public Health
109 South Observatory
University of Michigan
Ann Arbor, MI 48109

George Bonney
Department of Biostatistics
Fox Chase Cancer Center
Philadelphia, PA 19111

Cherwell Scientific Publishing, Inc.
The Magdalen Centre
Oxford Science Park
Oxford OX4 4GA
UNITED KINGDOM

Tara Cox
The MULTIMAP program is distributed via FTP at site
CHIMERA.HGEN.PITT.EDU (Directory: /dist/multimap)

David Curtis
Academic Department of Psychiatry
St. Mary's Hospital Medical School
Praed Street
London W2 1NY
UNITED KINGDOM

Bennett Dyke
Department of Genetics
Southwest Foundation
P.O. Box 28147
San Antonio, TX 78274

John Edwards
Genetics Lab
Department of Biochemistry
Oxford University
S Parks Road
Oxford OX1 3QU
UNITED KINGDOM

Robert Elston
Department of Biometry and Genetics
Louisiana State University Medical Center
1901 Perdido Street
New Orleans, LA 70112

Catherine Falk
New York Blood Center
310 E. 67th Street
New York, NY 10021

Epicenter Software
P.O. Box 990073
Pasadena, CA 91109

Iain Fenton
Institute of Medical Genetics
University of Wales College of Medicine
Heath Park
Cardiff CF4 4XN
UNITED KINGDOM

John Gersting
Helios Software Works
P.O. Box 40068
Indianapolis, IN

Rodney Go
Department of Epidemiology
School of Public Health
University of Alabama
Birmingham, AL 35294

Philip R. Green
Genetics Department
Washington University School of Medicine
Box 8232
St. Louis, MO 63110

David Greenberg
Box 1229
Mount Sinai Medical Center
New York, NY 10024

Jonathan Haines
Department of Molecular Neurogenetics
Massachusetts General Hospital E
13th Street, Building 149 6th
Charlestown, MA 02129

Sandra Hasstedt
Department of Human Genetics
University of Utah
2100 Eccles Genetics Institute
Salt Lake City, UT 84112

Eric Lander
Whitehead Institute for Biomedical Research
9 Cambridge Center
Cambridge, MA 02142

Kenneth Lange
Department of Biomathematics
University of California, Los Angeles
Los Angeles, CA 90024

Charles MacLean
Department of Psychiatry and Human Genetics
Medical College of Virginia, Box 710
Richmond, VA 23298

Newton Morton
CRC Genetic Epidemiology Research Group
Department of Community Medicine
Southampton General Hospital
Southampton, SO9 4XY
UNITED KINGDOM

Neil Risch
Department Epidemiology/Public Health
Yale University School of Medicine
60 College Street
P.O. Box 3333
New Haven, CT 06510

Anthony P. Round
192, Wingrove Avenue
Newcastle upon Tyne NE4 9AD
UNITED KINGDOM

Lodewijk Sandkuijl
Voorstraat 27
Delft 2611 JK
THE NETHERLANDS

Mansoor Sarfarazi
Department of Pediatrics
University of Connecticut Health Center
263 Farmington Ave
Farmington, CT 06032

Mark Skolnick
Genetic Epidemiology, Research Park
University of Utah
420 Chipeta Way, 180
Salt Lake City, UT 84108

Gerard J. te Meerman
Dept. of Medical Genetics
A. Deusinglaan 4
9713 AW Groningen
THE NETHERLANDS

James Trofatter
Department of Molecular Neurogenetics
Massachusetts General Hospital E
13th Street, Building 149 6th
Charlestown, MA 02129

Daniel E. Weeks
Department of Human Genetics
University of Pittsburgh
Pittsburgh, PA 15261

Ellen Wijsman
Dept. of Medical Genetics
School of Medicine
University of Washington
RG-25
Seattle, WA 98195

References

Adams, P. B., J. D. Lish, N. Freimer, et al. 1990. Pedigree and DNA Marker management: integrated system for molecular and family-genetic studies. *Am J Med Genet* 46:A171.

Anderson, T. W., and S. L. Sclove. 1986. *The statistical analysis of data*. 2nd ed. Palo Alto, Calif.: Scientific Press.

Attwood, J., and S. Bryant. 1988. A computer program to make linkage analysis with LIPED and LINKAGE easier to perform and less prone to input errors. *Ann Hum Genet* 52:259.

Ayala, F. J., and J. A. Kiger. 1984. *Modern genetics*. Menlo Park, Calif.: Benjamin/Cummings.

Bailey, N. T. J. 1961. *Introduction to the mathematical theory of genetic linkage*. Oxford: Clarendon Press.

Blackwelder, W. C., and R. C. Elston. 1985. A comparison of sib-pair linkage tests for disease susceptibility loci. *Genet Epidemiol* 2:85–97.

Boehnke, M. 1986. Estimating the power of a proposed linkage study: a practical computer simulation approach. *Am J Hum Genet* 39:513–527.

Boehnke, M. 1991. Allele frequency estimation from data on relatives. *Am J Hum Genet* 48:22–25.

Boehnke, M. 1992. Radiation hybrid mapping by minimization of the number of obligate chromosome breaks. *Cytogenet Cell Genet* 59:119–121.

Bonney, G. E., G. M. Lathrop, and J. -M. Lalouel. 1988. Combined linkage and segregation analysis using regressive models. *Am J Hum Genet* 43:29–37.

Botstein, D., R. L. White, M. H. Skolnick, et al. 1980. Construction of a genetic linkage map in man using restriction fragment length polymorphisms. *Am J Hum Genet* 32:314–331.

Brzustowicz, L. M., C. Mérette, X. Xie, et al. 1993. Detecting marker inconsistencies in human gene mapping. *Hum Hered* 43:25–30.

Cavalli-Sforza, L. L., and W. F. Bodmer. 1971. *The genetics of human populations*. Paperback reprint 1977. San Francisco: Freeman.

Chakravarti, A., C. C. Li, and K. H. Buetow. 1984. Estimation of the marker gene frequency and linkage disequilibrium from conditional marker data. *Am J Hum Genet* 36:177–186.

Chance, P. F., T. D. Bird, P. O'Connell, et al. 1990. Genetic linkage and heterogeneity in type I Charcot-Marie-Tooth disease (hereditary motor and sensory neuropathy type I). *Am J Hum Genet* 47:915–925.

Chapman, C. J. 1990. A visual interface to computer programs for linkage analysis. *Am J Med Genet* 36:155–160.

Chotai, J. 1984. On the lod score method in linkage analysis. *Ann Hum Genet* 48:359–378.

Clerget-Darpoux, F., C. Bonaïti-Pellié, and J. Hochez. 1986. Effects of misspecifying genetic parameters in lod score analysis. *Biometrics* 42:393–399.

Conneally, P. M., J. H. Edwards, K. K. Kidd, et al. 1985. Report of the committee on methods of linkage analysis and reporting. *Cytogenet Cell Genet* 40:356–359.

Cottingham, R. W., R. M. Idury, A. A. Schaeffer. 1993. Faster sequential genetic linkage computations. *Am J Hum Genet* 53:252–263.

Cox, T. K., M. Perlin, A. Chakravarti. 1992. Multimap: automatic construction of linkage maps. *Am J Hum Genet* 51:A33.

Crow, J. F. 1966. The quality of people: human evolutionary changes. *Bioscience* 16:863–867.

Curtis, D. 1990. A program to draw pedigrees using LINKAGE or LINKSYS data files. *Ann Hum Genet* 54:365–367.

Dausset, J., H. Cann, D. Cohen, et al. 1990. Centre d'Étude du Polymorphisme Humain (CEPH): collaborative genetic mapping of the human genome. *Genomics* 6:575–577.

Davies, R. B. 1977. Hypothesis testing when a nuisance parameter is present only under the alternative. *Biometrika* 64:247–254.

Dyke, B., and P. Mamelka. 1987. A computer program that draws pedigrees. *Am J Hum Genet* 41:A253.

Edwards, A. W. F. 1992. *Likelihood,* expanded edition. Baltimore, Maryland: Johns Hopkins University Press.

Edwards, J. H. 1987. Exclusion mapping. *J Med Genet* 24:539–543.

Elandt-Johnson, R. C. 1971. *Probability models and statistical methods in genetics.* New York: Wiley.

Elston, R. C. P-values, power and pitfalls in the linkage analysis of psychiatric disorders. In: *Genetic approaches to mental disorders,* edited by E. S. Gershon and C. R. Cloninger. Washington, D.C.: American Psychiatric Press, (in press).

Elston, R. C., J. E. Bailey-Watson, G. E. Bonney, et al. 1986. *A package of computer programs to perform statistical analysis for genetic epidemiology.* Presented at the Seventh International Congress of Human Genetics, Berlin.

Falk, C. T. 1991. A simple method for ordering loci using data from radiation hybrids. *Genomics* 9:120–123.

Falk, C. T., and P. Rubinstein, 1987. Haplotype relative risks: an easy reliable way to construct a proper control sample for risk calculations. *Ann Hum Genet* 51:227–233.

Faraway, J. J. 1993. Distribution of the admixture test for the detection of linkage under heterogeneity. *Genet Epidemiol* 10:75–83.

Fenton, I., L. A. Sandkuijl, J. R. Sampson, et al. 1990. MEGABASE: A pedigree-based computer program for genetic data management which facilitates risk assessment. *Proc Clin Genet Soc,* Newcastle, England.

Gersting, J. M. 1987. Rapid prototyping of database systems in human genetics data collection. *J Med Syst* 11:177–189.

Greenberg, D. A. 1986. The effect of proband designation on segregation analysis. *Am J Hum Genet* 39:329–339.

Greenberg, D. 1993. Linkage analysis of "necessary" disease loci versus "susceptibility" loci. *Am J Hum Genet* 52:135–143.

Haines, J. L. 1992. CHROMLOOK: an interactive program for error detection and mapping in reference linkage data. *Genomics* 14:517–519.

Haldane, J. B. S. 1935. Spontaneous mutation of a human genome. *J Genet* 31:317–326.

Hartl, D. L. 1988. *A primer of population genetics.* Sunderland, Mass.: Sinauer Associates, Inc.

Hasstedt, S. J., and P. E. Cartwright. 1981. *PAP—pedigree analysis package,* University of Utah, Department of Medical Biophysics and Computing, Technical Report No. 13. Salt Lake City, Utah.

Hodge, S. E., and D. A. Greenberg. 1992. Sensitivity of lod scores to changes in diagnostic status. *Am J Hum Genet* 50:1053–1066.

Hsiao, K., H. F. Baker, T. J. Crow, et al. 1989. Linkage of a prion protein missense variant to Gerstmann-Straussler syndrome. *Nature* 338:342–344.

Jayakar, S. D., J. A. Williamson, and L. Zonta-Sgaramella. 1984. A nonparametric and parametric version of a test for the detection of the presence of a major gene applicable on data for the complete nuclear family. *Hum Genet* 67:143–150.

Karlin, S., and U. Liberman. 1978. Classifications and comparisons of multilocus recombination distributions. *Proc Natl Acad Sci USA* 75:6332–6336.

Kerem, B., J. A. Buchanan, P. Durie, et al. 1989. DNA Marker haplotype association with pancreatic sufficiency in cystic fibrosis. *Am J Hum Genet* 44:827–834.

Kidd, K. K., and J. Ott. 1984. Power and sample size in linkage studies. *Human Gene Mapping* 7:510–511.

Kong, A., M. Frigge, M. Irwin, et al. 1992. *Importance sampling (I): computing multi-model p-values in linkage analysis.* Technical Report No. 337—University of Chicago Dept. of Statistics.

Kwan, S.-P., J. Terwilliger, R. Parmley, et al. 1990. Identification of a closely linked DNA marker, DXS178, to further refine the X-linked agammaglobulinemia locus. *Genomics* 6:238–242.

Lalouel, J.-M., and S. Yee. 1980. *POINTER: a computer program for complex segregation analysis with pointers.* Technical Report, Population Genetics Laboratory, University of Hawaii, Honolulu.

Lander, E. S., and D. Botstein. 1986. Mapping complex genetic traits in humans: new methods using a complete RFLP linkage map. *Cold Spring Harb Symp Quant Biol* 51:49–62.

Lander, E. S., and D. Botstein. 1987. Homozygosity mapping: a way to map human recessive traits with the DNA of inbred children. *Science* 236:1567–1570.

Lander, E., and P. Green. 1987. Construction of multilocus genetic linkage maps in humans. *Proc Natl Acad Sci USA* 84:2363–2367.

Lander, E. S., P. Green, J. Abrahamson, et al. 1987. MAPMAKER: an interactive computer package for constructing primary genetic linkage maps of experimental and natural populations. *Genomics* 1:174–181.

Lange, K., D. Weeks, and M. Boehnke. 1988. Programs for pedigree analysis: MENDEL, FISHER, and dGENE. *Genet Epidemiol* 5:471–472.

Lathrop, G. M., J. M. Lalouel, C. Julier, et al. 1984. Strategies for multilocus linkage analysis in humans. *Proc Natl Acad Sci USA* 81:3443–3446.

Lathrop, G. M., and J. Ott. 1990. Analysis of complex diseases under oligogenic models and intrafamilial heterogeneity by the LINKAGE programs. *Am J Hum Genet* 47:A188.

Liberman, U., and S. Karlin. 1984. Theoretical models of genetic map functions. *Theor Popul Biol* 25:331–346.

Lindenbaum, S. 1979. *Kuru sorcery.* Palo Alto, Calif.: Mayfield.

MacLean, C. J., L. M. Ploughman, S. R. Diehl, et al. 1992. A new test for linkage in the presence of locus heterogeneity. *Am J Hum Genet* 50:1259–1266.

Malcolm, S., J. Clayton-Smith, H. Nichols, et al. 1990. Uniparental paternal disomy in Angelman's syndrome. *Lancet* 337:694–697.

McKusick, V. A. 1990. *Mendelian inheritance of man,* 9th ed. Baltimore: Johns Hopkins University Press.

Merette, C., M. C. King, and J. Ott. 1992. Heterogeneity analysis of breast cancer families by using age at onset as a covariate. *Am J Hum Genet* 50:515–519.

Mills, K. A., K. H. Buetow, Y. Xu, et al. 1992. Genetic and physical maps of human chromosome 4 based on dinucleotide repeats. *Genomics* 14:209–219.

Morton, N. E. 1955. Sequential tests for the detection of linkage. *Am J Hum Genet* 7:277–318.

Morton, N. E., and V. Andrews. 1989. MAP, an expert system for multiple pairwise linkage analysis. *Ann Hum Genet* 53:263–269.

Morton, N. E., and C. J. MacLean. 1974. Analysis of family resemblance. III. Complex segregation of quantitative traits. *Am J Hum Genet* 26:489–503.

Ott, J. 1974. Estimation of the recombination fraction in human pedigrees: efficient computation of the likelihood for human linkage studies. *Am J Hum Genet* 26:588–597.

Ott, J. 1976. A computer program for linkage analysis of general human pedigrees. *Am J Hum Genet* 28:528–529.

Ott, J. 1985. *Analysis of Human Genetic Linkage*, 1st ed. Baltimore: Johns Hopkins University Press.

Ott, J. 1989. Computer-simulation methods in human linkage analysis. *Proc Natl Acad Sci USA* 86:4175–4178.

Ott, J. 1991. *Analysis of Human Genetic Linkage*, 2nd ed. Baltimore, Johns Hopkins University Press.

Ott, J. 1992. Strategies for characterizing highly polymorphic markers in human gene mapping. *Am J Hum Genet* 51:283–290.

Ott, J. 1993a. Molecular and statistical approaches to the detection and correction of errors in genotype databases. *Am J Hum Genet* (in press).

Ott, J. 1993b. Choice of genetic models for linkage analysis of psychiatric traits. In: *Genetic approaches to mental disorders*, American Psychiatric Press (in press).

Ott, J., and J. D. Terwilliger. 1992. Assessing the evidence for linkage in psychiatric genetics. In: *Genetic research in psychiatry*, edited by J. Mendlewicz and H. Hippius. Berlin: Springer-Verlag, pp. 245–249.

Ott, J., J. D. Terwilliger, and X. Xie. 1992. Determining the informativeness of untyped individuals in a pedigree analysis. *Am J Hum Genet* 51:A197.

Ott, J., J. D. Terwilliger, and G. M. Lathrop. 1994. Testing for chiasma interference in human genetic maps (Submitted for Publication).

Petrukhin, K. E., M. C. Speer, E. Cayanis, et al. 1993. A microsatellite genetic linkage map of human chromosome 13. *Genomics* 15:76–85.

Risch, N. 1988. A new statistical test for linkage heterogeneity. *Am J Hum Genet* 42:353–364.

Risch, N. 1990a. Linkage strategies for genetically complex traits. I. Multilocus models. *Am J Hum Genet* 46:222–228.

Risch, N. 1990b. Linkage strategies for genetically complex traits. II. The power of affected relative pairs. *Am J Hum Genet* 46:229–241.

Round, A. P. 1990. Computerized pedigree drawing in the SCHESIS risk calculation and linkage package. *Am J Hum Genet* 46:A75.

Rubinstein, P., M. Walker, C. Carpenter, et al. 1981. Genetics of HLA disease associations. The use of the haplotype relative risk (HRR) and the "haplo-delta" (Dh) estimates in juvenile diabetes from three racial groups. *Hum Immunol* 3:384 (abstr.).

Sandkuyl, L. A. 1989. Analysis of affected sib-pairs using information from extended families. In: *Multipoint Mapping and Linkage Based Upon Affected Pedigree Members: Genetic Analysis Workshop 6*, edited by R. C. Elston, M. A. Spence, S. E. Hodge, et al. New York: Alan R. Liss.

Sarfarazi, M. 1990. A database management system for linkage analysis. Proceedings of the European Society of Human Genetics Meeting, Corfu.

Schork, N. J., M. Boehnke, J. D. Terwilliger, et al. 1993. Two trait locus linkage analysis: a powerful strategy for mapping complex genetic traits. *Am J Hum Genet* 53:1127–1136.

Seuchter, S. A., and M. H. Skolnick. 1988. HGDBMS: a human genetics database management system. *Comput Biomed Res* 21:478–487.

Sherrington, R., J. Brynjolfsson, H. Petursson, et al. 1988. Localization of a susceptibility locus for schizophrenia on chromosome 5. *Nature* 336:164–167.

Shugart, Y. Y., and J. Ott. 1992. Significance tests relating to heterozygosity. *Am J Hum Genet* 51:A159.

Smith, C. A. B. 1953. The detection of linkage in human genetics. *J R Statist Soc* 15B:153–184.

Smith, C. A. B. 1963. Testing for heterogeneity of recombination fraction values in human genetics. *Ann Hum Genet* 27:175–182.

Speer, M., J. D. Terwilliger, and J. Ott. 1992. A chromosome-based method for rapid computer simulation. *Am J Hum Genet* 51:A202.

Spence, M. A., D. T. Bishop, M. Boehnke, et al. 1993. Methodological issues in linkage analyses for psychiatric disorders: secular trends, assortative mating, bilineal pedigrees. Report of the MacArthur Foundation Network I Task Force on Methodological Issue. *Hum Hered* 43:166–172.

Spielman, R. S., R. E. McGinnis, and W. J. Ewens. 1993. Transmission test for linkage disequilibrium: the insulin gene region and insulin-dependent diabetes mellitus (IDDM). *Am J Hum Genet* 52:506–516.

Sturt, E. 1976. A mapping function for human chromosomes. *Ann Hum Genet* 40:147–163.

Suarez, B. K., and P. Van Eerdewegh. 1984. A comparison of three affected-sib-pair scoring methods to detect HLA-linked disease susceptibility genes. *Am J Med Genet* 18:135–146.

te Meerman, G. J. 1991. *A logic programming approach to pedigree analysis.* Amsterdam: Thesis Publishers.

Terwilliger, J. D., Y. Ding, and J. Ott. 1992. On the relative importance of heterozygosity and intermarker distance in gene mapping. *Genomics* 13:951–956.

Terwilliger, J. D., G. M. Lathrop, and J. Ott. 1993a. Multipoint analysis to detect and quantify interference on CEPH chromosome 10 consortium data. (In preparation).

Terwilliger, J. D., T. Lehner, and J. Ott. 1991. *Differential sex dependent penetrances of autosomal dominant diseases mimic linkage to the boundary of the pseudoautosomal region.* Abstract to International Congress of Human Genetics.

Terwilliger, J. D., and J. Ott. 1990. Laboratory errors in the reading of marker alleles cause massive reductions in lod score and lead to gross overestimation of the recombination fraction. *Am J Hum Genet* 47:A201.

Terwilliger, J. D., and J. Ott. 1992a. A multi-sample bootstrap approach to the estimation of maximized-over-models lod score distributions. *Cytogenet Cell Genet* 59:142–144.

Terwilliger, J. D., and J. Ott. 1992b. A haplotype-based haplotype relative risk statistic. *Hum Hered* 42:337–346.

Terwilliger, J. D., and J. Ott. 1992c. A novel approach to combining data from multiple linked loci into a maximally heterozygous "super-locus" yields greatly increased power in 2-point linkage and sib-pair analysis. *Am J Hum Genet* 51:A202.

Terwilliger, J. D., and J. Ott. 1993. A novel polylocus method for linkage analysis using the lod score or affected sib-pair methods. *Genet Epidemiol* (in press).

Terwilliger, J. D., M. C. Speer, and J. Ott. 1993b. A chromosome-based method for rapid computer simulation in human genetic linkage analysis. *Genet Epidemiol* 10:217–224.

Thompson, M. W., R. R. McInnes, and H. F. Willard. 1991. *Thompson and Thompson: Genetics in Medicine,* 5th ed. Philadelphia: W. B. Saunders Company.

Tienari, P. J., J. Wikstrum, A. Sajantila, et al. 1992. Genetic susceptibility to multiple sclerosis linked to myelin basic protein gene. *Lancet* 340:987–991.

Trofatter, J. A., J. L. Haines, and P. M. Conneally. 1986. LIPIN: an interactive data entry and management program for LIPED. *Am J Hum Genet* 39:147–148.

Vogel, F., and A. G. Motulsky. 1986. *Human genetics.* New York: Springer.

Weeks, D. E. 1991. Human linkage analysis: strategies for locus ordering. In: *Advanced techniques in chromosome research,* edited by K. W. Adolph, New York: Marcel Dekker, pp. 297–330.

Weeks, D. E., and K. Lange. 1988. The affected-pedigree-member method of linkage analysis. *Am J Hum Genet* 42:315–326.

Weeks, D. E., T. Lehner, E. Squires-Wheeler, et al. 1990a. Measuring the inflation of the lod score due to its maximization over model parameter values in human linkage analysis. *Genet Epidemiol* 7:237–243.

Weeks, D. E., J. Ott, and G. M. Lathrop. 1990b. SLINK: a general simulation program for linkage analysis. *Am J Hum Genet* 47:A204.

Weeks, D. E., J. Ott, and G. M. Lathrop. 1991. Multipoint mapping under different models of interference using the LINKAGE programs. *Am J Hum Genet* 49:372.

Weir, B. S. 1990. *Genetic data analysis.* Sunderland, Mass.: Sinauer Associates, Inc.

Weissenbach, J., G. Gyapay, C. Dib, et al. 1992. A second-generation linkage map of the human genome. *Nature* 359:794–801.

White, R. L., J. -M. Lalouel, Y. Nakamura, et al. 1990. The CEPH consortium primary linkage map of human chromosome 10. *Genomics* 6:393–412.

Wolak, G. R., and M. Sarfarazi. 1987. Plot 2000: a Universal Pedigree plotting program. *J Med Genet* 24:246–247.

Wright, S. 1968. *The genetics of human populations: a treatise in four volumes.* Paperback edition 1984. Chicago: University of Chicago Press.

Xie, X., and J. Ott. 1990. Determining the effect of a change in the affection status on the lod score. *Am J Hum Genet* 47:A205.

Xie, X., and J. Ott. 1992. Finding all loops in a pedigree. *Am J Hum Genet* 51:A206.

Zonta, L. A., S. D. Jayakar, M. Bosisio, et al. 1987. Genetic analysis of human obesity in an Italian sample. *Hum Hered* 37:129–139.

Index

COMPUTER PROGRAMS

About the Authors

Joseph D. Terwilliger received a Ph.D. in Genetics and Development in 1993 from Columbia University. He is currently a post-doctoral fellow at the Institute of Molecular Medicine and the Nuffield Department of Clinical Medicine, University of Oxford, U.K. He has taught courses in linkage analysis in the United States and Europe for the last four years.

Jurg Ott received a Ph.D. in zoology from the University of Zurich in 1967 and an M.S. in biomathematics from the University of Washington in 1972. He is Professor of Genetics and Development in the Department of Genetics and Development and the Department of Psychiatry at Columbia University, and a research scientist at the New York State Psychiatric Institute. He serves on various editorial boards, is editor-in-chief of *Human Heredity,* and is a member of HUGO. He wrote the first generally available computer program on linkage analysis (LIPED).